U0235290

连续层次局部解剖
彩色图谱

Colour Atlas of Regional Anatomy of Continuous Layer

主　编　段坤昌　王振宇

主　审　方秀斌

副主编　潘　峰　段维轶　富长海　邵　博

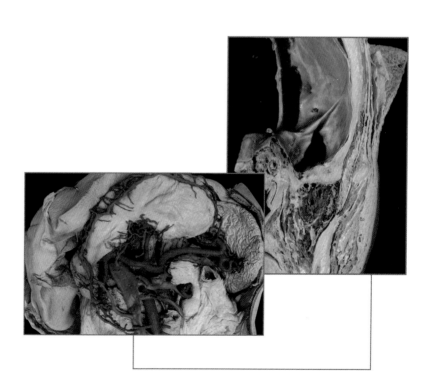

人民卫生出版社

图书在版编目（CIP）数据

连续层次局部解剖彩色图谱 / 段坤昌，王振宇主编 . —北京：
人民卫生出版社，2016
　ISBN 978-7-117-23853-3

　Ⅰ . ①连…　Ⅱ . ①段…②王…　Ⅲ . ①局部解剖学 - 图谱
Ⅳ . ①R323–64

　中国版本图书馆 CIP 数据核字（2016）第 310766 号

人卫智网	www.ipmph.com	医学教育、学术、考试、健康，购书智慧智能综合服务平台
人卫官网	www.pmph.com	人卫官方资讯发布平台

连续层次局部解剖彩色图谱

主　　编：段坤昌　王振宇
出版发行：人民卫生出版社（中继线 010-59780011）
地　　址：北京市朝阳区潘家园南里 19 号
邮　　编：100021
E - mail：pmph @ pmph.com
购书热线：010-59787592　010-59787584　010-65264830
印　　刷：三河市宏达印刷有限公司（胜利）
经　　销：新华书店
开　　本：889×1194　1/16　印张：20
字　　数：634 千字
版　　次：2017 年 8 月第 1 版　2017 年 8 月第 1 版第 1 次印刷
标准书号：ISBN 978-7-117-23853-3/R · 23854
定　　价：169.00 元

打击盗版举报电话：010-59787491　E-mail：WQ @ pmph.com
（凡属印装质量问题请与本社市场营销中心联系退换）

编委

前　言

　　局部解剖学是临床医学的重要基础学科，是解剖学重要分支，通过由浅入深的剖析正常人体各局部器官和结构的位置、形态、层次和毗邻关系，阐述人体的构造。人体的器官、结构形态各异，分布走行错综复杂，个体差异多而复杂，如要做到熟识人体每一局部的解剖结构，能在较小的视野中辨清微小结构之间的毗邻和相互位置关系，理清头绪，自我驾驭，是成为一名优秀的临床医师的必修课。为此，我们按着局部解剖学教材各章节内容的编排顺序，采用栩栩如生的实物标本彩色图像，编著了局部解剖学教材的辅助配套教材《连续层次局部解剖彩色图谱》。

　　本图谱是已出版的《系统解剖学彩色图谱》的姐妹篇。该图谱以临床医学专业五年制和八年制国家级规划教材《局部解剖学》架构为导向，按人体的局部划分章节，全书内容分为8章，即：头部、颈部、胸部、腹部、盆部与会阴、脊柱、上肢和下肢等。采集了540幅精心设计、细心解剖制作的实物标本图像，扩展了局部解剖学知识内容。因此，本图谱不仅可作为医学院校学习局部解剖学和指导学生尸体解剖实习的辅助教材，而且可供临床医师，特别是外科医师和医学康复科医师学习参考。

　　本图谱具有局部解剖结构层次分明、毗邻关系清楚、内容翔实、一目了然的特点。重点的局部内容，采取由浅入深的连续层次解剖的方法，逐层解剖局部的结构，其实物图像选用不同的方位、多角度，充分展示各器官、结构的相互关系。连续图像叠加利于读者整合、建立局部立体观的感性认识。其目的是力求能为医学本科生、研究生和临床医师熟识和掌握解剖学知识，而提供一本有价值的工具书。

　　图谱初稿完成后，编委会进行了认真的审校和修改。书中的名词以全国自然科学名词审定委员会《人体解剖学名词》为准，并进行中英文双语标注，便于学生对主要英语词汇的掌握和记忆。

　　最后我们期望该图谱能够符合全国医学院校教改的要求，适合教学实际的需要，为提高局部解剖学教学质量起到推动作用。由于我们的水平有限，错误疏漏之处在所难免，敬请解剖界同仁、医务工作者和医学生提出宝贵意见，以便日后修订，日臻完善。

段坤昌

2016 年 11 月 28 日

目　录

第四章　腹部 Chapter4　Abdomen ·················· 113

第五章　盆部和会阴 Chapter5　Pelvis and perineum ············· 165

第六章　脊柱区 Chapter6　Vertebral region ················· 197

第八章　下肢 Chapter8　Lower limb ···259

绪　　论

Introduction

　　学习局部解剖学，进行尸体解剖操作和认知，首先必须了解和掌握人体体表的骨性标志（图1）、人体解剖常用皮肤切口（图2）和常用的解剖器械的准备及使用。

　　常用的解剖器械包括解剖刀、解剖镊（无齿镊和有齿镊）、解剖剪、止血钳、拉钩、肋骨剪、咬骨钳、骨凿、板锯、弓形锯和椎管锯（图3）。

常用解剖器械的持执方法： 首先要掌握持刀、持镊、持剪和止血钳的持钳方法（见图4）。

解剖刀持刀法：（1）执笔法：用拇指、示指、中指捏持刀柄前端。
　　　　　　　　（2）执弓法：用拇指与中指、环指和小指夹持刀柄、示指按于刀柄背部。

解剖镊持镊法： 用拇指、示指、中指、捏持解剖镊的中部。一般为左手持解剖镊钳夹结构，右手持刀、剪或止血钳进行切、剪或剥离。

解剖剪持剪法： 用拇指和无名指各伸入解剖剪的一个环内，中指放在无名指环的前方，示指按压在剪刀运动轴处。

解剖止血钳持钳法： 如同持剪法。在开合时，拇指向内稍施推力，中指和无名指向外轻轻施一拉力，钳口方可张开。

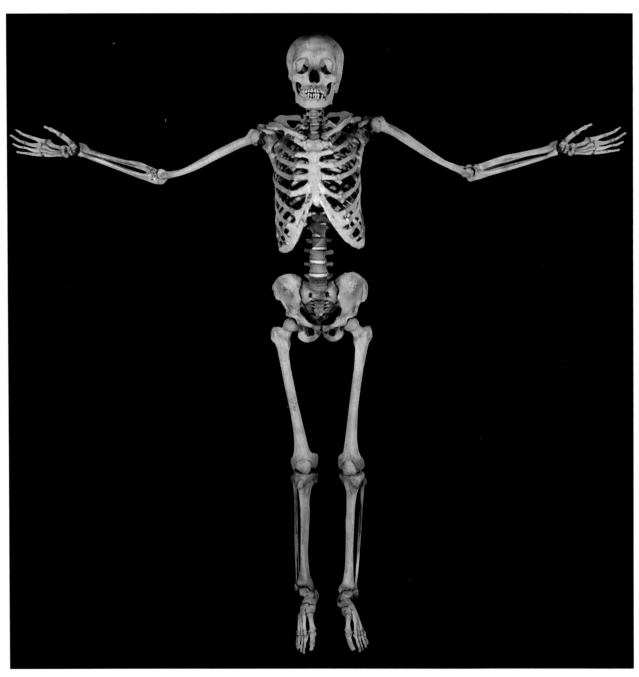

▲ 图1 全身骨骼
Skeleton

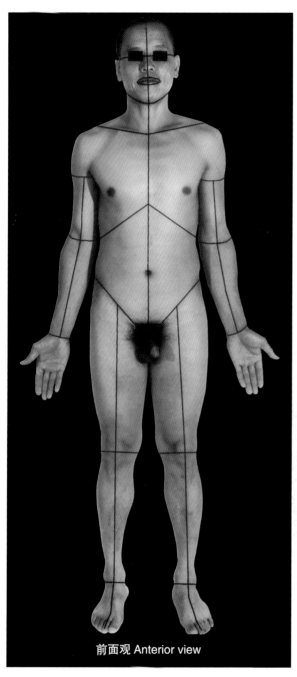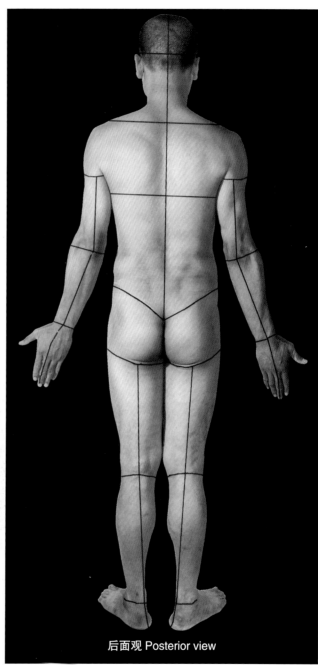

前面观 Anterior view　　后面观 Posterior view

▲ 图 2　人体解剖常用皮肤切口
Common skin incision for body dissection

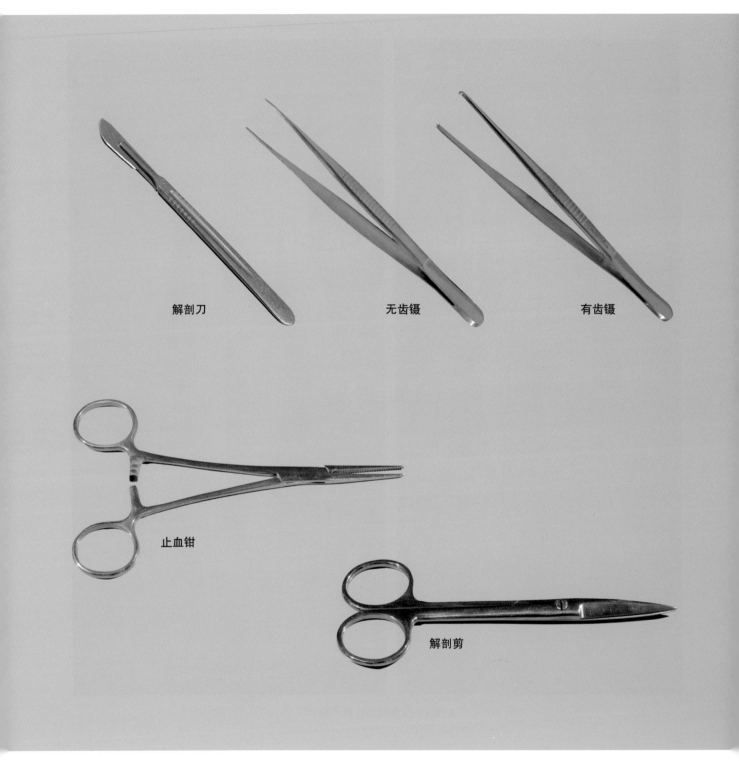

解剖刀　　　无齿镊　　　有齿镊

止血钳

解剖剪

▲ 图 3　常用解剖器械
Commoly used dissecting instruments

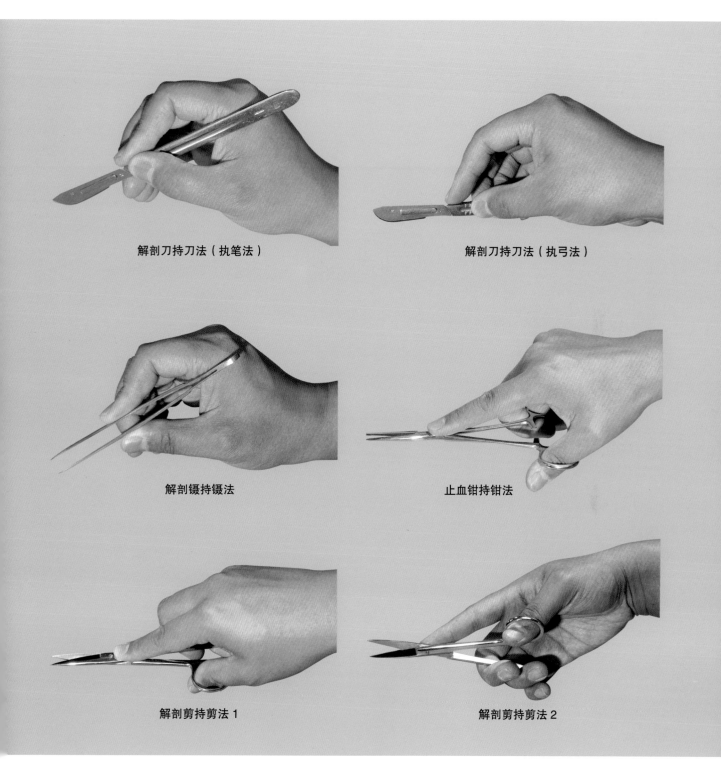

解剖刀持刀法（执笔法）　　　　　解剖刀持刀法（执弓法）

解剖镊持镊法　　　　　止血钳持钳法

解剖剪持剪法 1　　　　　解剖剪持剪法 2

▲ 图 4　常用解剖器械持执法
Common holding methods of dissecting instrument

连续层次局部解剖

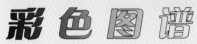

彩色图谱

第一章

头 部

Chapter 1 Head

　　头部由颅和面两部分组成。两者借眶上缘、颧弓上缘、外耳门上缘和乳突的连线为界，分为前下方的面部和后上方的颅部。头部又借下颌骨下缘、下颌角、乳突尖端、上项线和枕外隆凸之间的连线与颈部分界。

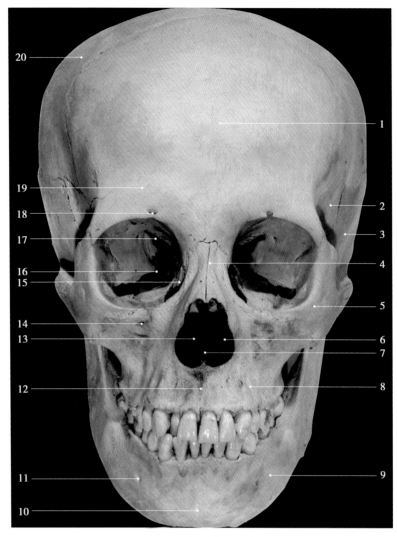

▲ 图 5 颅（前面观）
Skull.Anterior view

1. 额骨 frontal bone
2. 蝶骨大翼 greater wing of sphenoid bone
3. 颞骨 temporal bone
4. 鼻骨 nasal bone
5. 颧骨 zygomatic bone
6. 下鼻甲 inferior nasal concha
7. 鼻中隔 nasal septum
8. 上颌骨 maxilla
9. 下颌骨 mandible
10. 颏隆凸 mental protuberance

11. 颏孔 mental foramen
12. 上颌间缝 intermaxillary suture
13. 鼻腔 nasal cavity
14. 眶下孔 infraorbital foramen
15. 泪骨 lacrimal bone
16. 眶下裂 inferior orbital fissure
17. 眶上裂 superior orbital fissure
18. 眶上孔 supraorbital foramen
19. 眉弓 superciliary arch
20. 顶骨 parietal bone

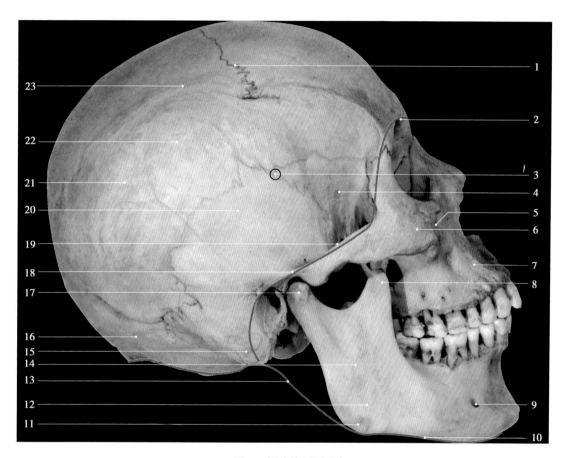

▲ 图 6 颅（外侧面观）
Skull.Lateral view

1. 冠状缝 coronal suture
2. 眶上缘 supraorbital margin
3. 翼点 pterion
4. 蝶骨大翼 greater wing of sphenoid bone
5. 眶下孔 infraorbital foramen
6. 颧骨 zygomatic bone
7. 上颌骨 maxilla
8. 冠突 coronoid process
9. 颏孔 mental foramen
10. 下颌骨下缘 inferior border of mandible
11. 下颌角 angle of mandible
12. 咬肌粗隆 masseteric tuberosity
13. 颈部上界 upper bound of neck
14. 下颌支 ramus of mandible
15. 乳突 mastoid process
16. 枕骨 occipital bone
17. 下颌头 head of mandible
18. 面部与颅界线 border of face and skull
19. 颧弓上缘 superior border of zygomatic arch
20. 颞骨 temporal bone
21. 顶骨 parietal bone
22. 下颞线 inferior temporal line
23. 上颞线 superior temporal line

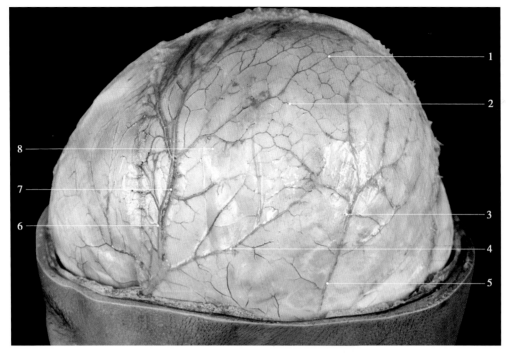

▲ 图 7 硬脑膜的血管
Blood vessels of cerebral dura mater

1. 硬脑膜动脉网 arterial rete of cerebral dura mater
2. 吻合支 anastomotic branch
3. 脑膜中静脉后支 posterior branch of middle meningeal v.
4. 脑膜中动脉顶孔支 parietal foramen branch of middle meningeal a.
5. 脑膜中动脉后支 posterior branch of middle meningea a.
6. 脑膜中动脉前支 anterior branch of middle meningeal a.
7. 脑膜中静脉前支 anterior branch of middle meningeal v.
8. 硬脑膜 cerebral dura mater

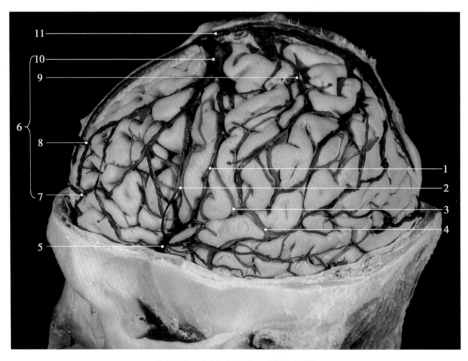

▲ 图 8 大脑主要沟、回的血管
Blood vessels of main sulcus and gyrus

1. 上吻合静脉 superior anastomotic v.
2. 中央前沟动脉 artery of precentral sulcus
3. 中央沟动脉 arlery of central sulcus
4. 颞中动脉 middle temporal a.
5. 大脑中浅静脉 superficial middle cerebral v.
6. 大脑上静脉 superior cerebral v.
7. 额前静脉 prefrontal v.
8. 额静脉 frontal v.
9. 顶静脉 parietal v.
10. 中央沟静脉 vein of central sulcus
11. 上矢状窦 superior sagittal sinus

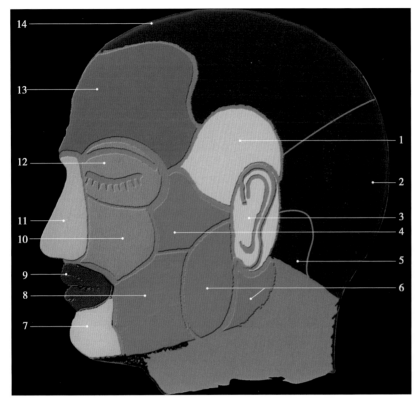

◀ 图 9 头面部的分区
Regions of head and face

1. 颞区 temporal region
2. 枕区 occipital region
3. 耳区 auricular region
4. 颧区 zygomatic region
5. 乳突区 mastoid region
6. 腮腺咬肌区 parotideomasseteric region
7. 颏区 mental region
8. 颊区 buccal region
9. 口区 oral region
10. 眶下区 infraorbital region
11. 鼻区 nasal region
12. 眶区 orbital region
13. 额区 frontal region
14. 顶区 parietal region

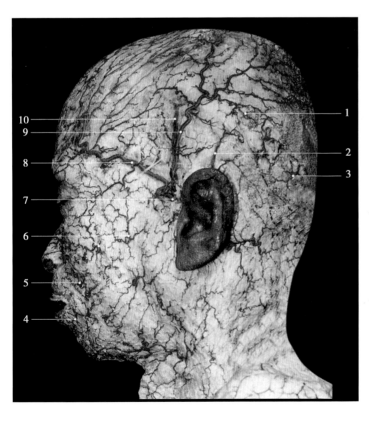

◀ 图 10 头面部的皮动脉（侧面观）
Cutaneous arteries of head and face.Lateral view

1. 吻合支 anastomotic branch
2. 耳后动脉 posterior auricular a.
3. 枕区动脉网 arterial rete of occipital region
4. 下唇动脉皮支 cutaneous branch of inferior labial a.
5. 上唇动脉皮支 cutaneous branch of superior labial a.
6. 面横动脉皮支 cutaneous branch of transverse facial a.
7. 颞浅动脉 superficial temporal a.
8. 颞浅动脉额支 frontal branch of superficial temporal a.
9. 颞浅动脉顶支 parietal branch of superficial temporal a.
10. 颞浅静脉顶支 parietal branch of superficial temporal v.

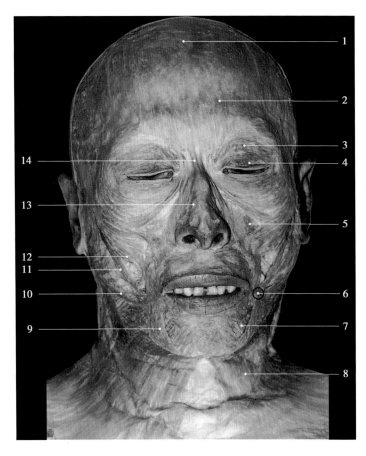

◀图 11　面部表情肌（1）
Facial muscles（1）

1. 帽状腱膜 galea aponeurotica
2. 枕额肌额腹 frontal belly of occipitofrontalis
3. 眼轮匝肌眶部 orbital part of orbicularis oculi
4. 眼轮匝肌睑部 palpebral part of orbicularis oculi
5. 提上唇肌 levator labii superioris
6. 口轴 modiolus
7. 降下唇肌 depressor labii inferioris
8. 颈阔肌 platysma
9. 降口角肌 depressor anguli oris
10. 笑肌 risorius
11. 颧大肌 zygomaticus major
12. 颧小肌 zygomaticus minor
13. 鼻肌 nasalis
14. 降眉间肌 procerus

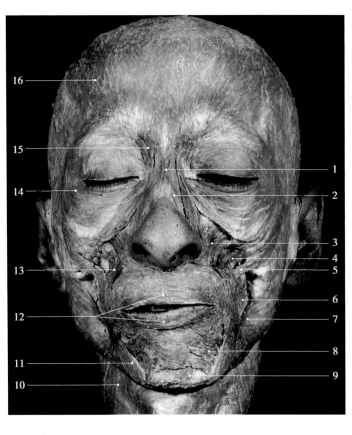

◀图 12　面部表情肌（2）
Facial muscles（2）

1. 降眉间肌 procerus
2. 鼻肌 nasalis
3. 提上唇肌 levator labii superioris
4. 颧小肌 zygomaticus minor
5. 颧大肌 zygomaticus major
6. 颊肌 buccinator
7. 笑肌 risorius
8. 降下唇肌 depressor labii inferioris
9. 颏肌 mentalis
10. 颈阔肌 platysma
11. 降口角肌 depressor anguli oris
12. 口轮匝肌 orbicularis oris
13. 提口角肌 levator anguli oris
14. 眼轮匝肌 orbicularis oculi
15. 皱眉肌 corrugator supercilii
16. 枕额肌额腹 frontal belly of occipitofrontalis

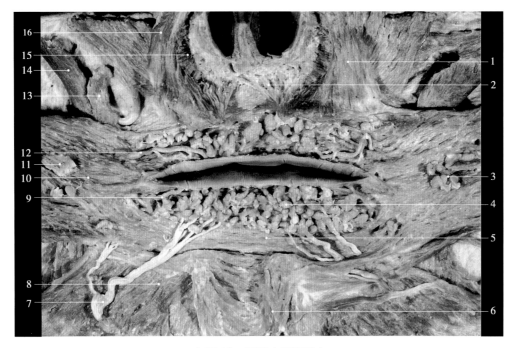

▲ 图 13　唇腺（后面观）
Labial glands.Posterior view

1. 提上唇肌 levator labii superioris
2. 降鼻中隔肌 depressor septi
3. 颊腺 buccal glands
4. 唇腺 labial glands
5. 口轮匝肌 orbicularis oris
6. 颏肌 mentalis
7. 颏神经 mental n.
8. 降下唇肌 depressor labii inferioris
9. 下唇动脉 inferior labial a.
10. 颊肌 buccinator
11. 腮腺管 parotid duct
12. 上唇动脉 superior labial a.
13. 颧小肌 zygomaticus minor
14. 颧大肌 zygomaticus major
15. 鼻肌翼部 alar part of nasalis
16. 提上唇鼻翼肌 levator labii superioris alaeque nasi

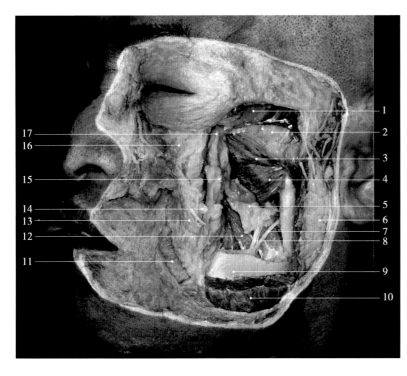

◀ 图 14　颊脂肪垫
Buccal fat pad

1. 颞深脂肪垫 deep temporal fat pad
2. 颞骨 temporal bone
3. 翼外肌上头 superior head of lateral pterygoid
4. 翼外肌下头 inferior head of lateral pterygoid
5. 颊脂肪垫翼突 pterygoid process of buccal fat pad
6. 腮腺 parotid gland
7. 下牙槽动脉 inferior alveolar a.
8. 下牙槽神经 inferior alveolar n.
9. 下颌骨 mandible
10. 咬肌 masseter
11. 颊肌 buccinator
12. 翼内肌 medial pterygoid
13. 颊脂肪垫颊突 buccal process of buccal fat pad
14. 腮腺管 parotid duct
15. 颊脂肪垫体部 body part of buccal fat pad
16. 颊脂肪垫眶下突 infraorbital process of buccal fat pad
17. 颊脂肪垫颞突 temporal process of buccal fat pad

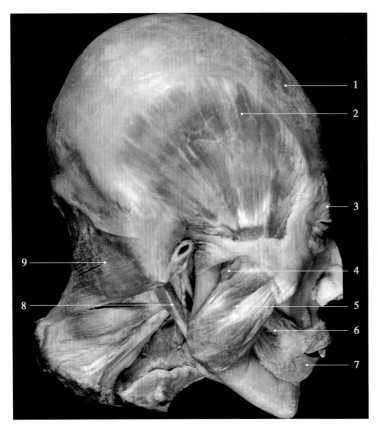

◀图 15　咀嚼肌（1）
Masticatory muscles（1）

1. 额骨 frontal bone
2. 颞肌 temporalis
3. 眶隔 orbital septum
4. 咬肌深部 deep part of masseter
5. 咬肌浅部 superficial part of masseter
6. 颊肌 buccinator
7. 口轮匝肌 orbicularis oris
8. 二腹肌后腹 posterior belly of digastric
9. 头夹肌 splenius capitis

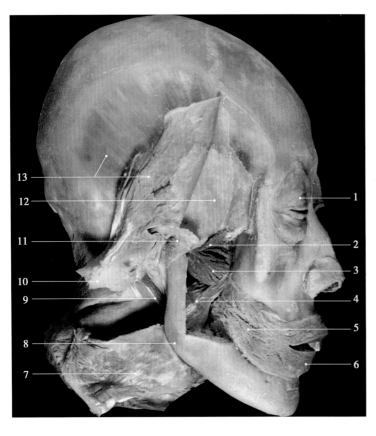

◀图 16　咀嚼肌（2）
Masticatory muscles（2）

1. 眶隔 orbital septum
2. 翼外肌上头 superior head of lateral pterygoid
3. 翼外肌下头 inferior head of lateral pterygoid
4. 翼内肌 medial pterygoid
5. 颊肌 buccinator
6. 口轮匝肌 orbicularis oris
7. 咬肌 masseter
8. 下颌角 angle of mandible
9. 二腹肌后腹 posterior belly of digastric
10. 冠突 coronoid process
11. 颞下颌关节 temporomandibular joint
12. 颞窝 temporal fossa
13. 颞肌 temporalis

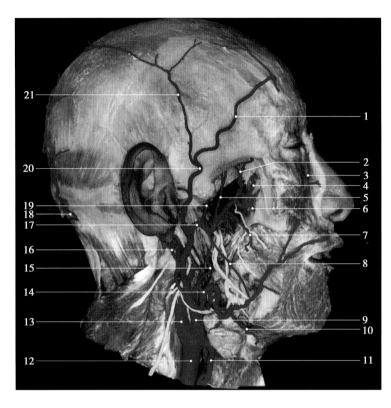

◀ 图 17 头面部动脉（1）
Arteries of head and face（1）

1. 颞浅动脉额支 frontal branch of superficial temporal a.
2. 颞深前动脉 anterior deep temporal a.
3. 内眦动脉 angular a.
4. 蝶腭动脉 sphenopalatine a.
5. 颞深后动脉 posterior deep temporal a.
6. 上牙槽后动脉 posterior superior alveolar a.
7. 颊动脉 buccal a.
8. 下牙槽动脉 inferior alveolar a.
9. 颈外动脉 external carotid a.
10. 颏下动脉 submental a.
11. 甲状腺上动脉 superior thyroid a.
12. 颈总动脉 common carotid a.
13. 颈内动脉 internal carotid a.
14. 面动脉 facial a.
15. 腭升动脉 ascending palatine a.
16. 耳后动脉 posterior auricular a.
17. 上颌动脉 maxillary a.
18. 枕动脉 occipital a.
19. 脑膜中动脉 middle meningeal a.
20. 颞浅动脉 superficial temporal a.
21. 颞浅动脉顶支 parietal branch of superficial temporal a.

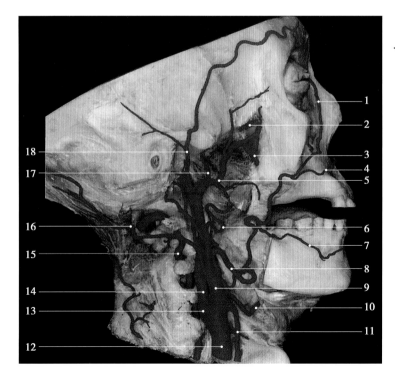

◀ 图 18 头面部动脉（2）
Arteries of head and face（2）

1. 内眦动脉 angular a.
2. 蝶腭动脉 sphenopalatine a.
3. 上牙槽后动脉 posterior superior alveolar a.
4. 上唇动脉 superior labial a.
5. 上颌动脉 maxillary a.
6. 腭升动脉 ascending palatine a.
7. 下唇动脉 inferior labial a.
8. 面动脉 facial a.
9. 颈外动脉 external carotid a.
10. 舌动脉 lingual a.
11. 甲状腺上动脉 superior thyroid a.
12. 颈总动脉 common carotid a.
13. 颈动脉窦 carotid sinus
14. 颈内动脉 internal carotid a.
15. 椎动脉 vertebral a.
16. 枕动脉 occipital a.
17. 脑膜中动脉 middle meningeal a.
18. 颞浅动脉 superficial temporal a.

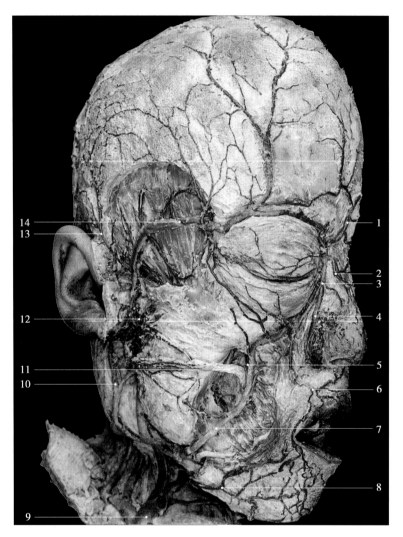

▲ 图 19 头面部静脉（1）
Veins of head and face（1）

1. 滑车上静脉 supratrochlear v.
2. 鼻背静脉 dorsal nasal v.
3. 内眦静脉 angular v.
4. 鼻外侧静脉 lateral nasal v.
5. 面深静脉 deep facial v.
6. 上唇静脉 superior labial v.
7. 面静脉 facial v.
8. 下唇静脉 inferior labial v.
9. 颈外静脉 external jugular v.
10. 耳后静脉 posterior auricular v.
11. 腮腺管 parotid duct
12. 上颌静脉 maxillary v.
13. 颞浅静脉 superficial temporal v.
14. 颞中静脉 middle temporal v.

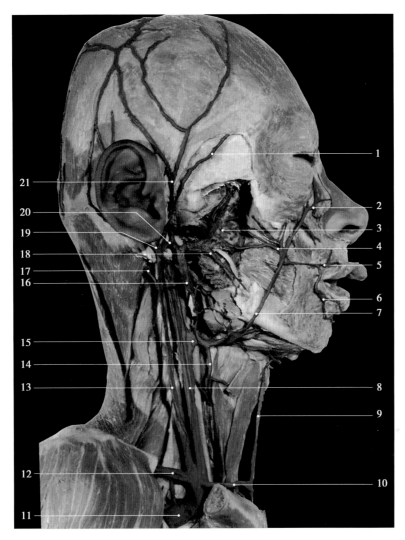

▲ 图 20　头面部静脉（2）
Veins of head and face（2）

1.　颞中静脉 middle temporal v.
2.　内眦静脉 angular v.
3.　翼静脉丛 pterygoid venous plexus
4.　面深静脉 deep facial v.
5.　上唇静脉 superior labial v.
6.　下唇静脉 inferior labial v.
7.　面静脉 facial v.
8.　颈内静脉 internal jugular v.
9.　颈前静脉 anterior jugular v.
10.　颈静脉弓 jugular venous arch
11.　锁骨下静脉 subclavian v.

12.　肩胛上静脉 suprascapular v.
13.　颈外静脉 external jugular v.
14.　甲状腺上静脉 superior thyroid v.
15.　面总静脉 common facial v.
16.　下颌后静脉 retromandibular v.
17.　枕静脉 occipital v.
18.　下牙槽静脉 inferior alveolar v.
19.　耳后静脉 posterior auricular v.
20.　上颌静脉 maxillary v.
21.　颞浅静脉 superficial temporal v.

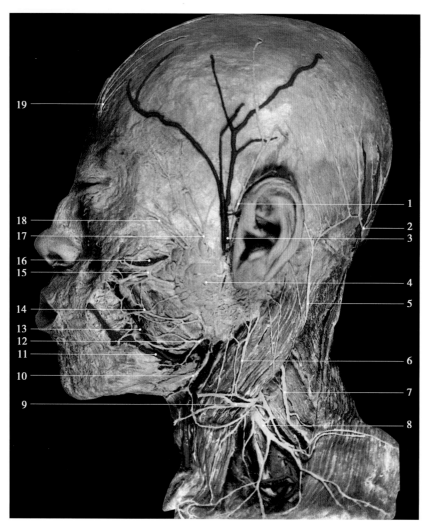

▲ 图 21　面神经（1）
Facial nerve（1）

1. 耳颞神经 auriculotemporal n.
2. 枕大神经 greater occipital n.
3. 颞浅动脉 superficial temporal a.
4. 腮腺 parotid gland
5. 枕小神经 lesser occipital n.
6. 耳大神经 great auricular n.
7. 副神经 accessory n.
8. 锁骨上神经 supraclavicular n.
9. 颈横神经 transverse nerve of neck
10. 颈支 cervical branch
11. 面动脉 facial a.
12. 下颌缘支 marginal mandibular branch
13. 面静脉 facial v.
14. 下颊支 inferior buccal branches
15. 上颊支 superior buccal branches
16. 面横动脉 transverse facial a.
17. 颞支 temporal branches
18. 颧支 zygomatic branches
19. 眶上神经 supraorbital n.

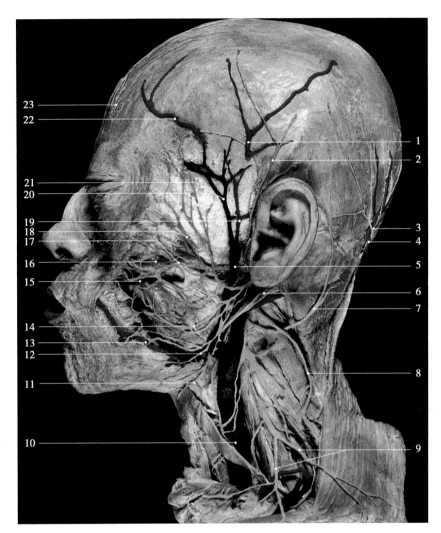

▲ 图 22 面神经（2）
Facial nerve（2）

1. 颞浅动脉顶支 parietal branch of superficial temporal a.
2. 耳颞神经 auriculotemporal n.
3. 枕大神经 greater occipital n.
4. 枕动脉 occipital a.
5. 颞浅静脉 superficial temporal v.
6. 二腹肌后腹 posterior belly of digastric
7. 枕小神经 lesser occipital n.
8. 副神经 accessory n.
9. 锁骨上神经 supraclavicular n.
10. 颈内静脉 internal jugular v.
11. 颈支 cervical branch
12. 下颌缘支 marginal mandibular branch
13. 面动脉 facial a.
14. 下颊支 inferior buccal branches
15. 腮腺管 parotid duct
16. 面横动脉 transverse facial a.
17. 上颊支 superior buccal branches
18. 颧支 zygomatic branches
19. 颞中动脉 middle temporal a.
20. 颞支 temporal branches
21. 颞中静脉 middle temporal v.
22. 颞浅动脉额支 frontal branch of superficial temporal a.
23. 眶上神经 supraorbital n.

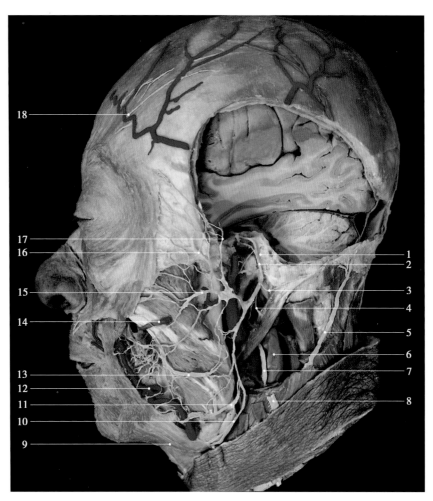

▲ 图 23　面神经（3）
Facial nerve（3）

1. 茎乳孔 stylomastoid foramen
2. 面神经 facial n.
3. 面神经后支 posterior branch of facial n.
4. 二腹肌后腹肌支 muscular branch of posterior belly of digastric
5. 枕小神经 lesser occipital n.
6. 颈内静脉 internal jugular v.
7. 舌下神经 hypoglossal n.
8. 耳大神经 great auricular n.
9. 颈阔肌 platysma
10. 颈支 cervical branch
11. 下颌缘支 marginal mandibular branch
12. 面动脉 facial a.
13. 下颊支 inferior buccal branches
14. 腮腺管 parotid duct
15. 上颊支 superior buccal branches
16. 颧支 zygomatic branches
17. 颞支 temporal branches
18. 眶上神经 supraorbital n.

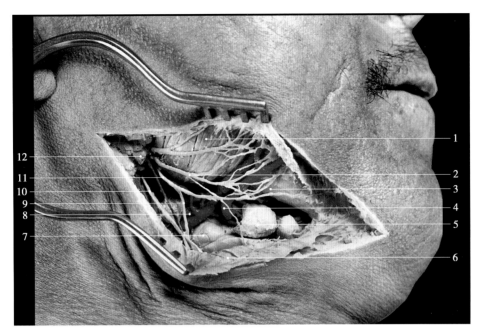

▲ 图 24 面神经的下颌缘支
Marginal mandibular branch of facial nerve

1. 咬肌 masseter
2. 下颌缘支上支 superior branch of marginal mandibular branch
3. 下颌骨下缘 inferior margin of mandible
4. 面动脉 facial a.
5. 下颌下淋巴结 submandibular lymph nodes
6. 颈阔肌 platysma
7. 下颌下腺 submandibular gland
8. 面静脉 facial v.
9. 颈支交通支 communicating branch with cervical branch
10. 面神经颈支 cervical branch of facial n.
11. 下颌缘支下支 inferior branch of marginal mandibular branch
12. 腮腺下缘 inferior border of parotid gland

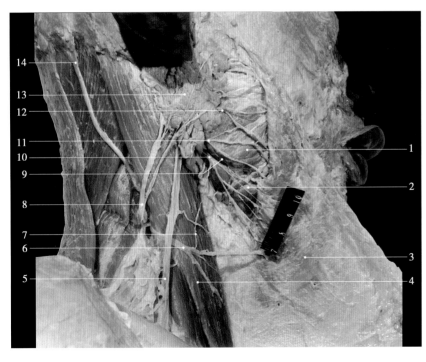

◀ 图 25 面神经的颈支
Cervical branch of facial nerve

1. 咬肌 masseter
2. 下颌下腺 submandibular gland
3. 颈阔肌 platysma
4. 胸锁乳突肌 sternocleidomastoid
5. 颈外静脉 external jugular v.
6. 颈横神经 transverse nerve of neck
7. 颈横神经交通支 communicating branch with transverse nerve of neck
8. 耳大神经 great auricular n.
9. 下颌角 angle of mandible
10. 面神经颈支 cervical branch of facial n.
11. 下颌缘支 marginal mandibular branch
12. 下颊支 inferior buccal branches
13. 腮腺 parotid gland
14. 枕小神经 lesser occipital n.

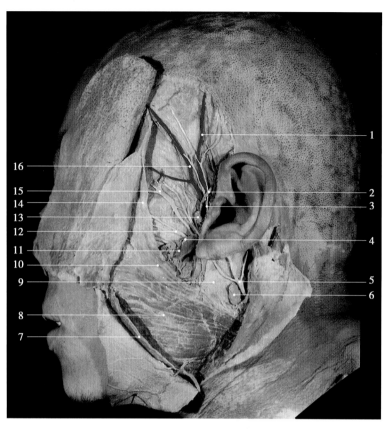

◀ 图 26　腮腺浅部的结构（1）
Superficial structures of parotid gland（1）

1. 颞浅动脉顶支
　parietal branch of superficial temporal a.
2. 颞浅静脉 superficial temporal v.
3. 耳颞神经 auriculotemporal n.
4. 腮腺上缘 superior border of parotid gland
5. 耳大神经 great auricular n.
6. 耳下淋巴结 infraauricular lymph nodes
7. 浅筋膜 superficial fascia
8. 颈阔肌 platysma
9. 腮腺筋膜 parotid gland fascia
10. SMAS-肌 SMAS-muscle
11. 腮腺 parotid gland
12. 颧支 zygomatic branches
13. 耳前淋巴结 preauricular lymph nodes
14. SMAS-筋膜 SMAS-fascia
15. 颞支 temporal branches
16. 颞浅动脉额支
　frontal branch of superficial temporal a.

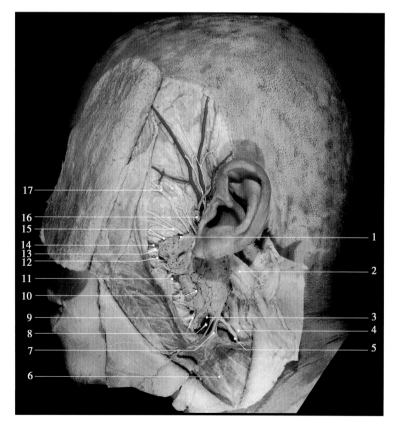

◀ 图 27　腮腺浅部的结构（2）
Superficial structures of parotid gland（2）

1. 腮腺上缘 superior border of parotid gland
2. 腮腺筋膜 parotid gland fascia
3. 腮腺下缘 inferior border of parotid gland
4. 颈外静脉 external jugular v.
5. 颈支 cervical branch
6. 颈阔肌 platysma
7. 腮腺 – 颈阔肌韧带
　parotid gland–platysma muscle lig.
8. 下颌缘支 marginal mandibular branch
9. 下颊支 inferior buccal branches
10. 腮腺 parotid gland
11. 腮腺前缘 anterior border of parotid gland
12. 腮腺管 parotid duct
13. 上颊支 superior buccal branches
14. 面横动脉 transverse facial a.
15. 颧支 zygomatic branches
16. 耳前淋巴结 preauricular lymph nodes
17. 颞支 temporal branches

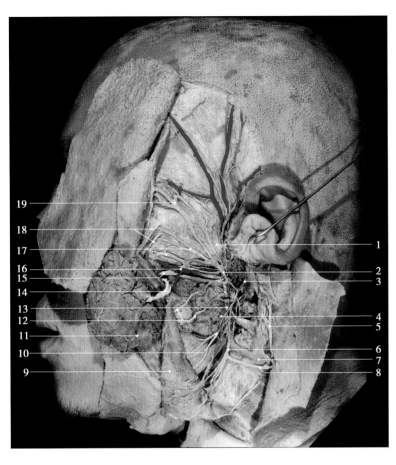

◀ 图 28 腮腺深部的结构（1）
Deep structures of parotid gland（1）

1. 颞中静脉 middle temporal v.
2. 面神经腮腺段（染绿色部）
   facial nerve in parotid gland
3. 面神经 facial n.
4. 腮腺深部 deep part of parotid gland
5. 耳大神经 great auricular n.
6. 颈支 cervical branch
7. 颈外静脉 external jugular v.
8. 颈横神经交通支 communicating branch with
   transverse nerve of neck
9. SMAS- 肌 SMAS-muscle
10. 下颌缘支 marginal mandibular branch
11. 腮腺浅部 superficial part of parotid gland
12. 下颊支 inferior buccal branches
13. 颞浅静脉 superficial temporal v.
14. 腮腺管 parotid duct
15. 上颊支 superior buccal branches
16. 面横动脉 transverse facial a.
17. 颧支 zygomatic branches
18. 颧韧带 zygomatic lig.
19. 颞支 temporal branches

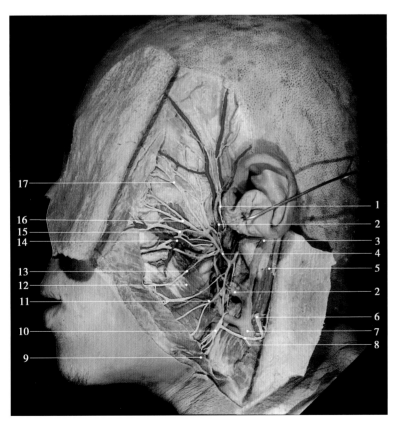

◀ 图 29 腮腺深部的结构（2）
Deep structures of parotid gland（2）

1. 耳颞神经 auriculotemporal n.
2. 颞浅静脉 superficial temporal v.
3. 耳后静脉 posterior auricular v.
4. 面神经腮腺段 facial nerve in parotid gland
5. 胸锁乳突肌 sternocleidomastoid
6. 耳大神经 great auricular n.
7. 颈外静脉 external jugular v.
8. 交通支 communicating branches
9. 颈阔肌 platysma
10. 颈支 cervical branch
11. 下颌缘支 marginal mandibular branch
12. 咬肌 masseter
13. 下颊支 inferior buccal branches
14. 面横动脉 transverse facial a.
15. 上颊支 superior buccal branches
16. 颧支 zygomatic branches
17. 颞支 temporal branches

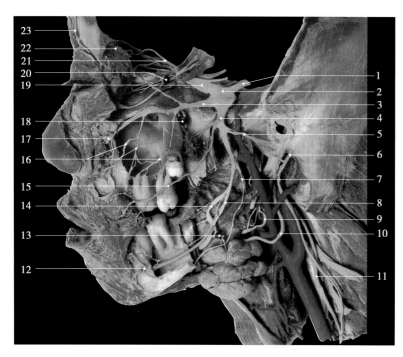

◀ 图 30　三叉神经（外侧面观）
Trigeminal nerve.Lateral view

1. 三叉神经 trigeminal n.
2. 三叉神经节 trigeminal ganglion
3. 上颌神经 maxillary n.
4. 下颌神经 mandibular n.
5. 耳颞神经 auriculotemporal n.
6. 面神经 facial n.
7. 下颌舌骨肌神经 mylohyoid n.
8. 下牙槽神经 inferior alveolar n.
9. 舌咽神经 glossopharyngeal n.
10. 舌下神经 hypoglossal n.
11. 迷走神经 vagus n.
12. 颏神经 mental n.
13. 下颌下神经节 submandibular ganglion
14. 舌神经 lingual n.
15. 颊神经 buccal n.
16. 上牙槽神经 superior alveolar n.
17. 眶下神经 infraorbital n.
18. 翼腭神经节 pterygopalatine ganglion
19. 眼神经 ophthalmic n.
20. 睫状神经节 ciliary ganglion
21. 泪腺神经 lacrimal n.
22. 泪腺 lacrimal gland
23. 眶上神经 supraorbital n.

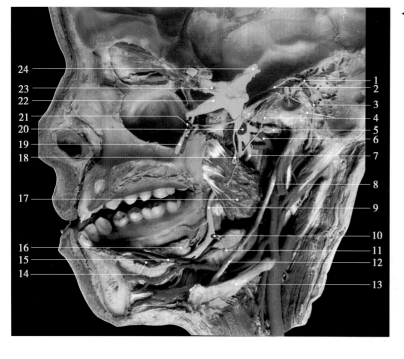

◀ 图 31　三叉神经（内侧面观）
Trigeminal nerve.Medial view

1. 膝神经节 geniculate ganglion
2. 岩大神经 greater petrosal n.
3. 面神经 facial n.
4. 鼓索 chorda tympani
5. 耳颞神经 auriculotemporal n.
6. 脑膜中动脉 middle meningeal a.
7. 下牙槽神经 inferior alveolar n.
8. 茎突 styloid process
9. 舌神经 lingual n.
10. 下颌下神经节 submandibular ganglion
11. 下颌下腺 submandibular gland
12. 茎突舌骨韧带 stylohyoid lig.
13. 舌骨 hyoid bone
14. 舌下腺大管 major sublingual duct
15. 下颌下腺管 submandibular duct
16. 舌下腺 sublingual gland
17. 翼内肌 medial pterygoid
18. 翼内肌神经 medial pterygoid n.
19. 腭大神经 greater palatine n.
20. 耳神经节 otic ganglion
21. 翼腭神经节 pterygopalatine ganglion
22. 上颌神经 maxillary n.
23. 眼神经 ophthalmic n.
24. 三叉神经 trigeminal n.

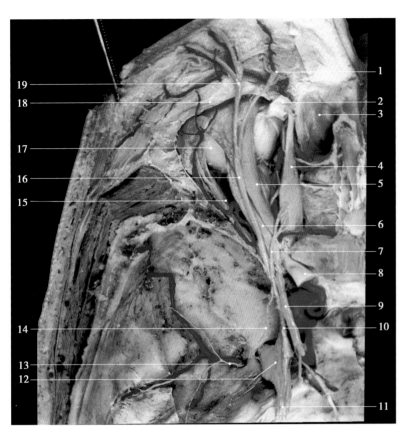

◀ 图 32 眼神经
Ophthalmic nerve

1. 滑车上神经 supratrochlear n.
2. 滑车 trochlea
3. 额窦 frontal sinus
4. 上斜肌 superior obliquus
5. 上睑提肌 levator palpebrae superioris
6. 上直肌 superior rectus
7. 滑车神经 trochlear n.
8. 视神经 optic n.
9. 动眼神经 oculomotor n.
10. 眼神经 ophthalmic n.
11. 三叉神经 trigeminal n.
12. 三叉神经节 trigeminal ganglion
13. 脑膜支 meningeal branch
14. 小脑幕支 tentorial branch
15. 外直肌 lateral rectus
16. 额神经 frontal n.
17. 眼球 eyeball
18. 眶隔 orbital septum
19. 眶上神经 supraorbital n.

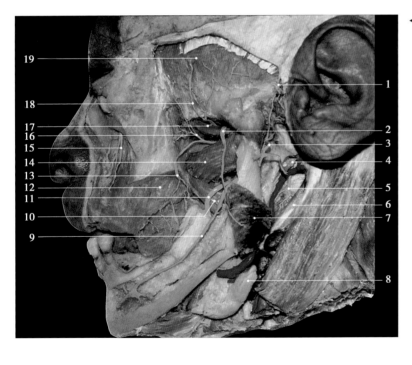

◀ 图 33 下颌神经
Mandibular nerve

1. 耳颞神经 auriculotemporal n.
2. 咬肌神经 masseteric n.
3. 面神经交通支 communicating branch with facial n.
4. 面神经 facial n.
5. 二腹肌后腹肌支
   muscular branch of posterior belly of digastric
6. 二腹肌 digastric
7. 咬肌 masseter
8. 下颌下腺 submandibular gland
9. 下牙槽神经 inferior alveolar n.
10. 翼内肌 medial pterygoid
11. 舌神经 lingual n.
12. 颊肌 buccinator
13. 颊神经 buccal n.
14. 翼外肌下头 inferior head of lateral pterygoid
15. 眶下神经 infraorbital n.
16. 颞深前神经 deep anterior temporal n.
17. 翼外肌上头 superior head of lateral pterygoid
18. 颞深后神经 deep posterior temporal n.
19. 颞肌 temporalis

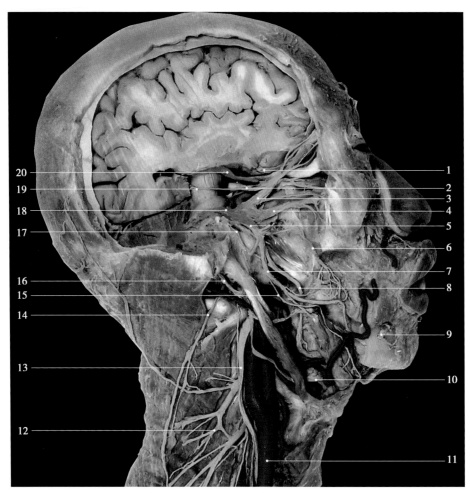

▲ 图 34 脑神经（外侧面观）
Cranial nerves.lateral view

1. 嗅束 olfactory tract
2. 动眼神经 oculomotor n.
3. 眼神经 ophthalmic n.
4. 上颌神经 maxillary n.
5. 下颌神经 mandibular n.
6. 颊神经 buccal n.
7. 下牙槽神经 inferior alveolar n.
8. 舌神经 lingual n.
9. 颏神经 mental n.
10. 舌下神经 hypoglossal n.
11. 颈总动脉 common carotid a.
12. 颈丛 cervical plexus
13. 迷走神经 vagus n.
14. 副神经 accessory n.
15. 下颌舌骨肌神经 mylohyoid n.
16. 面神经 facial n.
17. 鼓索 chorda tympani
18. 三叉神经 trigeminal n.
19. 滑车神经 trochlear n.
20. 视束 optic tract

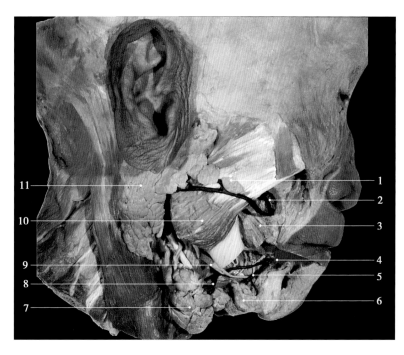

◀ 图 35 口腔腺
Glands of oral cavity

1. 副腮腺 accessory parotid gland
2. 腮腺管 parotid duct
3. 颊肌 buccinator
4. 舌下阜 sublingual caruncle
5. 舌下腺大管 major sublingual duct
6. 舌下腺 sublingual gland
7. 下颌下腺 submandibular gland
8. 下颌下腺管 submandibular duct
9. 舌神经 lingual n.
10. 咬肌 masseter
11. 腮腺 parotid gland

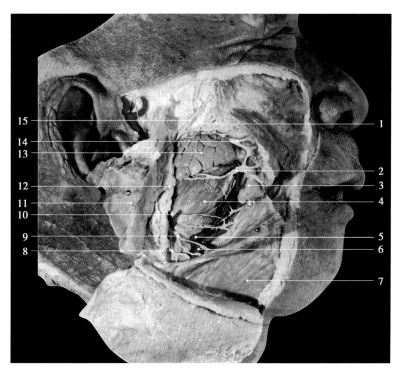

◀ 图 36 腮腺咬肌区的结构（1）
Structures of parotideomassetertic region（1）

1. 颧弓 zygomatic arch
2. 上颊支 superior buccal branches
3. 颊脂肪垫 buccal fat pad
4. 咬肌 masseter
5. 面动脉 facial a.
6. 面静脉 facial v.
7. 颈阔肌 platysma
8. 颈支 cervical branch
9. 下颌缘支 marginal mandibular branch
10. 下颊支 inferior buccal branches
11. 腮腺筋膜 parotid fascia
12. 腮腺 parotid gland
13. 副腮腺 accessory parotid gland
14. 颧支 zygomatic branches
15. 颞支 temporal branches

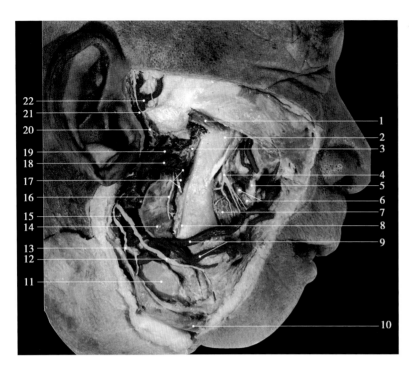

◀ 图 37　腮腺咬肌区的结构（2）
Structures of parotideomassetertic region（2）

1. 颞肌 tempralis
2. 冠突 coronoid process
3. 翼静脉丛 pterygoid venous plexus
4. 颊神经 buccal n.
5. 腮腺管 parotid duct
6. 颊腺 buccal glands
7. 颊肌 buccinator
8. 下颌支 ramus of mandible
9. 面动、静脉 facial a.and v.
10. 颈阔肌 platysma
11. 下颌下腺 submandibular gland
12. 下颌缘支 marginal mandibular branch
13. 颈支 cervical branch
14. 翼内肌 medial pterygoid
15. 下颌静脉 retromandibular v.
16. 下颌舌骨肌神经 mylohyoid n.
17. 下牙槽动、静脉、神经 inferior alveolar a., v.and n.
18. 上颌静脉 maxillary v.
19. 上颌动脉 maxillary a.
20. 耳颞神经 auriculotemporal n.
21. 颞浅静脉 superficial temporal v.
22. 颞浅动脉 superficial temporal a.

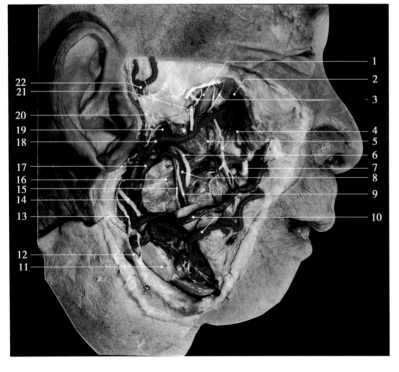

◀ 图 38　腮腺咬肌区的结构（3）
Structures of parotideomassetertic region（3）

1. 颞深动脉 deep temporal a.
2. 蝶腭动脉 sphenopalatine a.
3. 颞深神经 deep temporal n.
4. 上牙槽动脉 superior alveolar a.
5. 颊动脉、颊神经 buccal a. and n.
6. 舌神经 lingual n.
7. 腮腺管 parotid duct
8. 下牙槽动脉 inferior alveolar a.
9. 下牙槽神经 inferior alveolar n.
10. 面动、静脉 facial a.and v.
11. 下颌下腺 submandibular gland
12. 颈阔肌 platysma
13. 颈支 cervical branch
14. 下颌缘支 marginal mandibular branch
15. 下颌舌骨肌神经 mylohyoid n.
16. 翼内肌 medial pterygoid
17. 上颌静脉 maxillary v.
18. 上颌动脉 maxillary a.
19. 脑膜中动脉 middle meningeal a.
20. 耳颞神经 auriculotemporal n.
21. 咬肌神经 masseteric n.
22. 颞浅动脉 superficial temporal a.

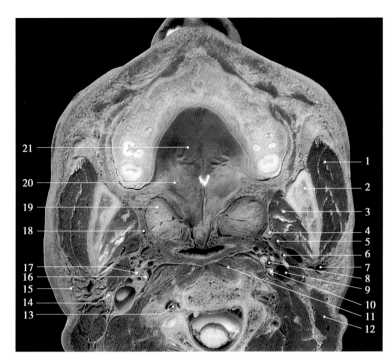

◀图 39 腮腺和面侧区的水平切面
Horizontal plane through parotid gland and lateral region of face

1. 咬肌 masseter
2. 下颌支 ramus of mandible
3. 翼内肌 medial pterygoid
4. 咽旁间隙 parapharyngeal space
5. 茎突及其周围肌 styloid process and its around muscle
6. 颈外动脉 external carotid a.
7. 下颌后静脉 retromandibular v.
8. 颈内动脉 internal corotid a.
9. 颈内静脉 internal jugular v.
10. 迷走神经 vagus n.
11. 椎前肌 anterior vertebral muscles
12. 胸锁乳突肌 sternocleidomastoid
13. 椎动脉 vertebral a.
14. 副神经 accessory n.
15. 腮腺 parotid gland
16. 交感干 sympathetic trunk
17. 舌下神经 hypoglossal n.
18. 颊咽筋膜 buccopharyngeal fascia
19. 腭扁桃体 palatine tonsil
20. 软腭 soft palate
21. 硬腭 hand palate

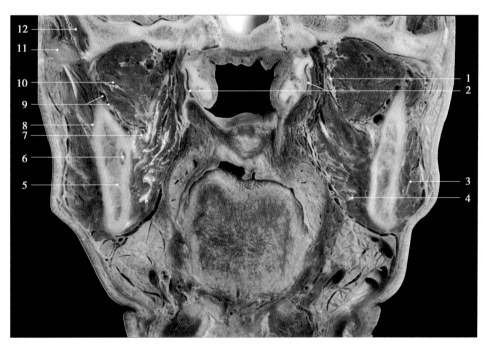

▲图 40 面部间隙（冠状切面）
Facial gap.Coronal section

1. 下颌神经 maxillary n.
2. 咽鼓管 auditory tube
3. 咬肌 masseter
4. 翼内肌 medial pterygoid
5. 下颌支 ramus of mandible
6. 下牙槽神经、动脉 inferior alveolar n.and a.
7. 翼下颌间隙 pterygomandibular space
8. 咬肌间隙 masseter space
9. 上颌动、静脉 maxillary a.and v.
10. 翼外肌 lateral pterygoid
11. 颧弓 zygomatic arch
12. 颞肌 temporalis

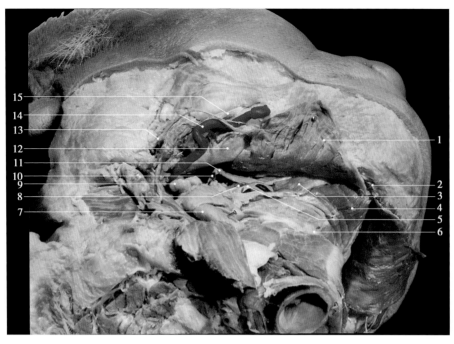

▲ 图 41　舌下间隙（1）
Sublingual space（1）

1. 下颌舌骨肌 mylohyoid
2. 二腹肌前腹 anterior belly of digastric
3. 下颌下腺深部 deep part of submandibular gland
4. 颏舌骨肌 geniohyoid
5. 舌下神经 hypoglossal n.
6. 舌骨 hyoid bone

7. 下颌下腺浅部 superficial part of
   submandibular gland
8. 下颌下腺管 submandibular duct
9. 下颌下淋巴结 submandibular lymph nodes
10. 下颌下神经节 submandibular ganglion

11. 舌神经 lingual n.
12. 下颌骨下缘 inferior border of mandible
13. 下颌缘支 marginal mandibular branch
14. 面动脉 facial a.
15. 面静脉 facial v.

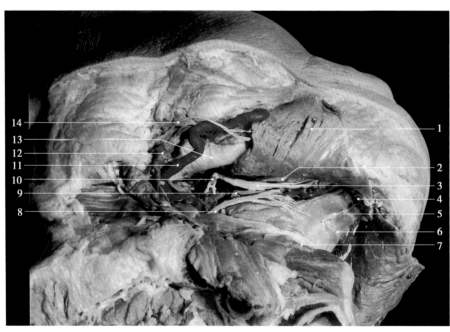

▲ 图 42　舌下间隙（2）
Sublingual space（2）

1. 下颌舌骨肌 mylohyoid
2. 舌下腺 sublingual gland
3. 舌神经 lingual n.
4. 颏舌骨肌 geniohyoid
5. 舌中隔 septum of tongue

6. 颏舌肌 genioglossus
7. 舌骨 hyoid bone
8. 舌下神经 hypoglossal n.
9. 下颌下腺管 submandibular duct
10. 下颌下神经节 submandibular ganglion

11. 面动脉 facial a.
12. 面静脉 facial v.
13. 下颌骨下缘 inferior border of mandible
14. 下颌缘支 marginal mandibular branch

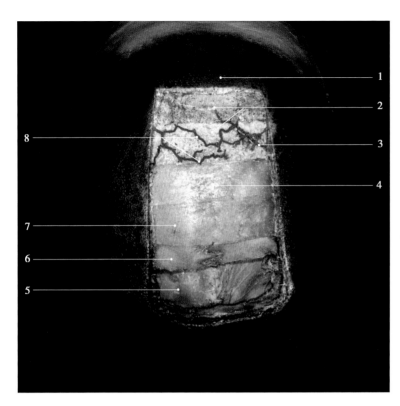

◀ 图 43 颅顶层次
Different layers of top of head

1. 皮肤 skin
2. 浅筋膜 superficial fascia
3. 头皮静脉 scalp v.
4. 帽状腱膜 galea aponeurotica
5. 硬脑膜 cerebral dura mater
6. 颅骨 cranial bone
7. 颅骨膜 pericranium
8. 头皮动脉网 arterial rete of scalp

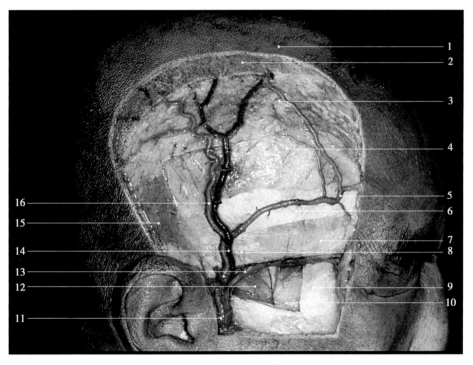

▲ 图 44 颞筋膜
Temporal fascia

1. 皮肤 skin
2. 浅筋膜 superficial fascia
3. 颞浅筋膜 superficial temporal fascia
4. 颞中筋膜 middle temporal fascia
5. 额支 frontal branch
6. 颞深筋膜 deep temporal fascia
7. 颞浅脂肪垫 superficial temporal fat pad
8. 颞深筋膜浅层 superficial layer of deep temporal fascia
9. 颞深筋膜深层 deep layer of deep temporal fascia
10. 颞深脂肪垫 deep temporal fat pad
11. 颞浅动脉 superficial temporal a.
12. 颞肌 temporalis
13. 颞中静脉 middle temporal v.
14. 颞浅静脉 superficial temporal v.
15. 耳上肌 auricularis superior
16. 顶支 parietal branch

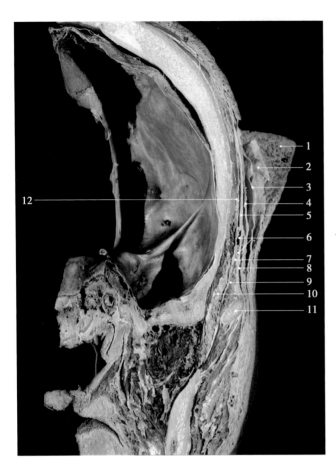

◀ 图 45　颞筋膜（冠状切面）
Temporal fascia.Coronal section

1. 皮肤 skin
2. 浅筋膜 superficial fascia
3. 颞浅筋膜 superficial temporal fascia
4. 颞中筋膜 middle temporal fascia
5. 颞深筋膜 deep temporal fascia
6. 颞中动、静脉 middle temporal a.and v.
7. 颞深筋膜深层 deep layer of deep temporal fascia
8. 颞深筋膜浅层 superficial layer of deep temporal fascia
9. 颞浅脂肪垫 superficial temporal fat pad
10. 颞深脂肪垫 deep temporal fat pad
11. 颧弓 zygomatic arch
12. 颞肌 temporalis

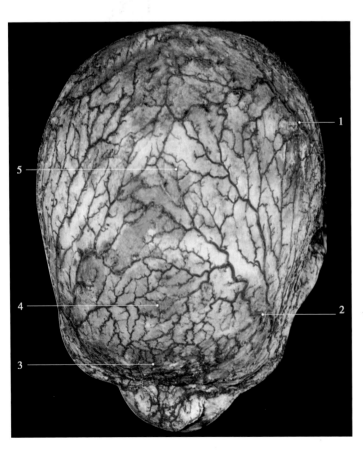

◀ 图 46　颅顶浅筋膜及皮动脉
Superficial fascia and cutaneous arteries of top of head

1. 顶支 parietal branch
2. 额支 frontal branch
3. 眶上动脉 supraorbital a.
4. 额区动脉网 arterial rete of frontal region
5. 顶区动脉网 arterial rete of parietal region

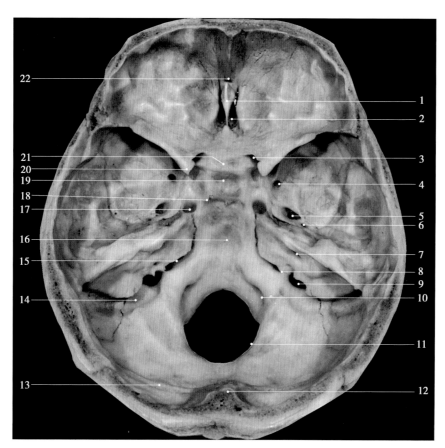

▲ 图 47　颅底（内面观）
Base of skull.Internal view

1. 鸡冠 crista galli
2. 筛板 cribriform plate
3. 视神经管 optic canal
4. 圆孔 foramen rotundum
5. 卵圆孔 foramen ovale
6. 棘孔 foramen spinosum
7. 内耳门 internal acoustic pore
8. 岩枕裂 petrooccipital fissure
9. 颈静脉孔 jugular foramen
10. 舌下神经管 hypoglossal canal
11. 枕骨大孔 foramen magnum of occipital bone

12. 枕内隆凸 internal occipital protuberance
13. 横窦沟 sulcus for transverse sinus
14. 乙状窦沟 sulcus for sigmoid sinus
15. 岩下窦沟 sulcus for inferior petrosal sinus
16. 斜坡 clivus
17. 破裂孔 foramen lacerum
18. 后床突 posterior clinoid process
19. 垂体窝 hypophysial fossa
20. 前床突 anterior clinoid process
21. 鞍结节 tuberculum sellae
22. 盲孔 foramen cecum

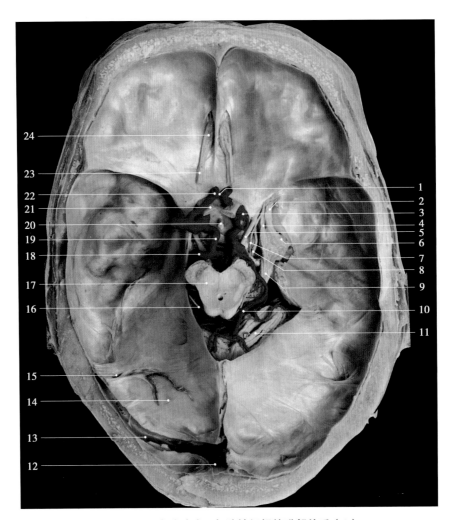

▲ 图 48　大脑动脉环与脑神经根的毗邻关系（1）
Adjacent relationship of cranial nervous roots and cerebral arterial circle（1）

1. 前交通动脉 anterior communicating a.
2. 上颌神经 maxillary n.
3. 颈内动脉 internal carotid a.
4. 眼神经 ophthalmic n.
5. 动眼神经 oculomotor n.
6. 下颌神经 mandibular n.
7. 滑车神经 trochlear n.
8. 展神经 abducent n.
9. 三叉神经 trigeminal n.
10. 小脑上动脉 superior cerebellar a.
11. 小脑 cerebellum
12. 窦汇 confluence of sinuses
13. 横窦 transverse sinus
14. 小脑幕 tentorium of cerebellum
15. 大脑下静脉 inferior cerebral v.
16. 滑车神经 trochlear n.
17. 中脑 midbrain
18. 大脑后动脉 posterior cerebral a.
19. 后交通动脉 posterior communicating a.
20. 漏斗 infundibulum
21. 视神经 optic n.
22. 大脑前动脉 anterior cerebral a.
23. 嗅束 olfactory tract
24. 嗅球 olfactory bulb

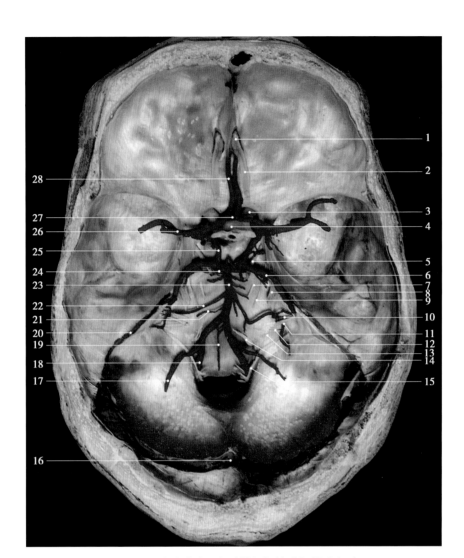

▲ 图 49 大脑动脉环与脑神经根的毗邻关系（2）
Adjacent relationship of cranial nervous roots and cerebral arterial circle（2）

1. 嗅球 olfactory bulb
2. 嗅束 olfactory tract
3. 视神经 optic n.
4. 视交叉 optic chiasma
5. 动眼神经 oculomotor n.
6. 大脑后动脉 posterior cerebral a.
7. 展神经 abducent n.
8. 三叉神经 trigeminal n.
9. 滑车神经 trochlear n.
10. 前庭蜗神经 vestibulocochlear n.
11. 面神经 facial n.
12. 舌咽神经 glossopharyngeal n.
13. 迷走神经 vagus n.
14. 舌下神经 hypoglossal n.
15. 副神经 accessory n.
16. 窦汇 confluence of sinuses
17. 小脑下后动脉 posterior inferior cerebellar a.
18. 椎动脉 vertebral a.
19. 脊髓前动脉 anterior spinal a.
20. 岩上窦 superior petrosal sinus
21. 迷路动脉 labyrinthine a.
22. 小脑下前动脉 anterior inferior cerebellar a.
23. 基底动脉 basilar a.
24. 小脑上动脉 superior cerebellar a.
25. 后交通动脉 posterior communicating a.
26. 大脑中动脉 middle cerebral a.
27. 前交通动脉 anterior communicating a.
28. 大脑前动脉 anterior cerebral a.

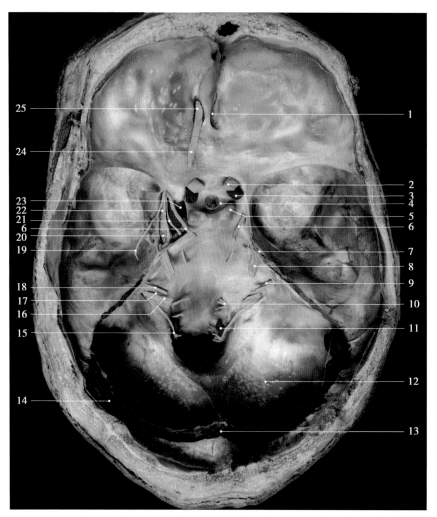

▲ 图 50　颅底内面脑神经出口
Passage for cranial nerves on internal surface of base of skull

1. 筛板 cribriform plate
2. 视神经 optic n.
3. 颈内动脉 internal carotid a.
4. 鞍膈 diaphragma sellae
5. 后床突 posterior clinoid process
6. 动眼神经 oculomotor n.
7. 岩上窦 superior petrosal sinus
8. 三叉神经 trigeminal n.
9. 面神经 facial n.
10. 舌下神经 hypoglossal n.
11. 椎动脉 vertebral a.
12. 颅后窝 posterior cranial fossa
13. 窦汇 confluence of sinuses
14. 横窦 transverse sinus
15. 副神经脊髓根 spinal root of accessory n.
16. 迷走神经 vagus n.
17. 舌咽神经 glossopharyngeal n.
18. 前庭蜗神经 vestibulocochlear n.
19. 滑车神经 trochlear n.
20. 三叉神经节 trigeminal ganglion
21. 展神经 abducent n.
22. 眼神经 ophthalmic n.
23. 颈内动脉海绵窦段 cavernous part of
    internal carotid a.
24. 嗅束 olfactory tract
25. 嗅球 olfactory bulb

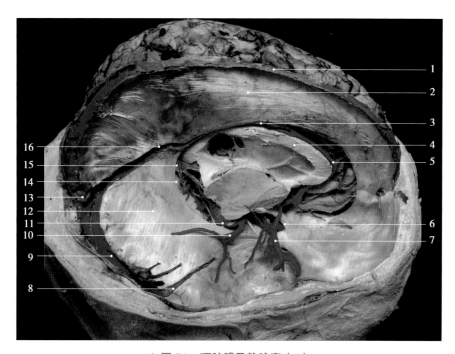

▲ 图 51 硬脑膜及静脉窦（1）
Cerebral dura mater and venous sinuses（1）

1. 上矢状窦 superior sagittal sinus
2. 大脑镰 cerebral falx
3. 下矢状窦 inferior sagittal sinus
4. 胼胝体 corpus callosum
5. 大脑前动脉 anterior cerebral a.
6. 视神经 optic n.
7. 大脑中动脉 middle cerebral a.
8. 岩上窦 superior petrosal sinus
9. 横窦 transverse sinus
10. 大脑后动脉 posterior cerebral a.
11. 小脑上动脉 superior cerebellar a.
12. 小脑幕 tentorium of cerebellum
13. 窦汇 confluence of sinuses
14. 幕切迹 tentorial incisure
15. 大脑大静脉 great cerebral v.
16. 直窦 straight sinus

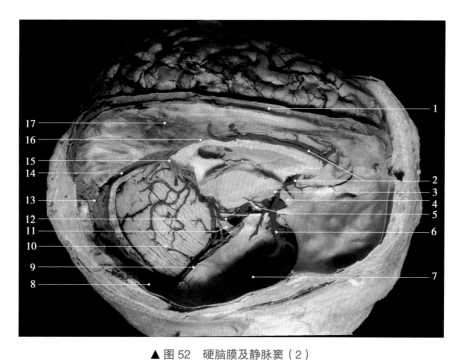

▲ 图 52 硬脑膜及静脉窦（2）
Cerebral dura mater and venous sinuses（2）

1. 上矢状窦 superior sagittal sinus
2. 大脑前动脉 anterior cerebral a.
3. 视交叉 optic chiasma
4. 视神经 optic n.
5. 动眼神经 oculomotor n.
6. 大脑中动脉 middle cerebral a.
7. 颅中窝 middle cranial fossa
8. 横窦 transverse sinus
9. 岩上窦 superior petrosal sinus
10. 小脑 cerebellum
11. 三叉神经 trigeminal n.
12. 小脑上动脉 superior cerebellar a.
13. 窦汇 confluence of sinuses
14. 直窦 straight sinus
15. 大脑大静脉 great cerebral v.
16. 下矢状窦 inferior sagittal sinus
17. 大脑镰 cerebral falx

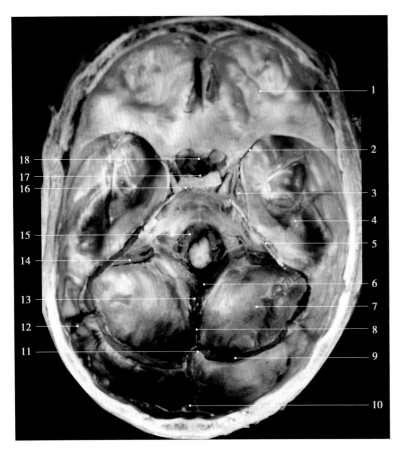

◀ 图 53　硬脑膜及静脉窦（3）
Cerebral dura mater and venous sinuses（3）

1. 颅前窝 anterior cranial fossa
2. 蝶顶窦 sphenopariatal sinus
3. 海绵窦 cavernous sinus
4. 颅中窝 middle cranial fossa
5. 岩上窦 superior petrosal sinus
6. 边缘窦 marginal sinus
7. 颅后窝 posterior cranial fossa
8. 枕窦 occipital sinus
9. 横窦 transverse sinus
10. 上矢状窦 superior sagittal sinus
11. 窦汇 confluence of sinuses
12. 大脑下静脉 inferior cerebral v.
13. 脑膜后动脉 posterior meningeal a.
14. 乙状窦 sigmoid sinus
15. 椎动脉 vertebral a.
16. 基底静脉丛 basilar venous plexus
17. 海绵间后窦 posterior intercavernous sinus
18. 海绵间前窦 anterior intercavernous sinus

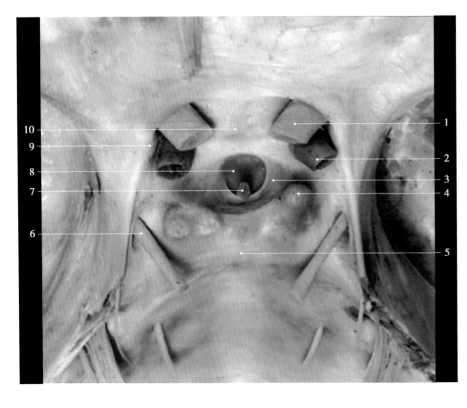

◀ 图 54　鞍膈
Diaphragma sellae

1. 视神经 optic n.
2. 颈内动脉 internal carotid a.
3. 鞍膈 diaphragma sellae
4. 后床突 posterior clinoid process
5. 斜坡 clivus
6. 动眼神经 oculomotor n.
7. 漏斗 infundibulum
8. 垂体 hypophysis
9. 前床突 anterior clinoid process
10. 交叉前沟 sulcus prechiasmaticus

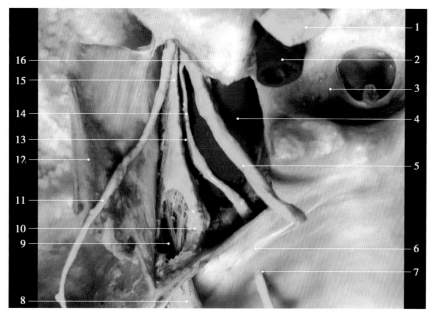

▲ 图 55 海绵窦腔内的结构（1）
Structures inside cavernous sinus（1）

1. 视神经 optic n.
2. 颈内动脉 internal carotid a.
3. 鞍膈 diaphragma sellae
4. 颈内动脉海绵窦部 cavernous part of internal carotid a.
5. 动眼神经 oculomotor n.
6. 上蝶岩韧带 superior sphenopetrosal lig.
7. Dorollo 管 Dorollo canal
8. 三叉神经 trigeminal n.
9. 三叉神经腔（Meckerl's 腔）trigeminal cavity
10. 三叉神经节 trigeminal ganglion
11. 滑车神经 trochlear n.
12. 硬脑膜 cerebral dura mater
13. 海绵窦 cavernous sinus
14. 展神经 abducent n.
15. 眼神经 ophthalmic n.
16. 前床突 anterior clinoid process

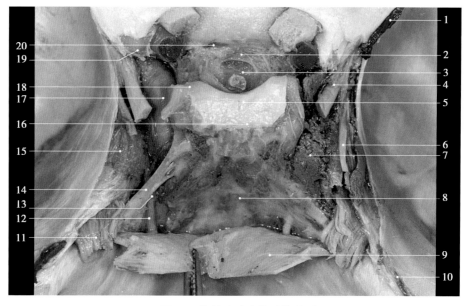

▲ 图 56 海绵窦腔内的结构（2）
Structures inside cavernous sinus（2）

1. 蝶顶窦 sphenoparietal sinus
2. 鞍膈 diaphragma sellae
3. 垂体 hypophysis
4. 动眼神经 oculomotor n.
5. 鞍背 dorsum sellae
6. 滑车神经 trochlear n.
7. 海绵窦 cavernous sinus
8. 基底静脉丛 basilar venous plexus
9. 硬脑膜 cerebral dura mater
10. 岩上窦 superior petrosal sinus
11. 三叉神经 trigeminal n.
12. 展神经 abducent n.
13. Dorollo 管 Dorollo canal
14. 上蝶岩韧带 superior sphenopetrosal lig.
15. 三叉神经节 trigeminal ganglion
16. 斜坡 clivus
17. 颈内动脉海绵窦部
cavernous part of internal carotid a.
18. 后床突 posterior clinoid process
19. 前床突 anterior clinoid process
20. 海绵间前窦 anterior intercavernous sinus

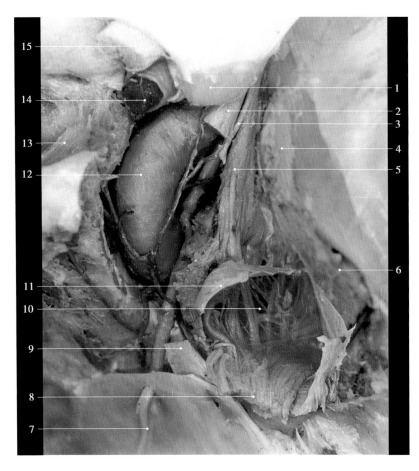

◀ 图 57　三叉神经腔
Trigeminal cavity

1. 前床突 anterior clinoid process
2. 动眼神经 oculomotor n.
3. 滑车神经 trochlear n.
4. 上颌神经 maxillary n.
5. 眼神经 ophthalmic n.
6. 下颌神经 mandibular n.
7. 展神经 abducent n.
8. 三叉神经 trigeminal n.
9. 上蝶岩韧带 superior sphenopetrosal lig.
10. 三叉神经腔（Meckerl's 腔）trigeminal cavity
11. 蛛网膜囊 arachnoid bursa
12. 颈内动脉海绵窦部 cavernous part of internal carotid a.
13. 鞍膈 diaphragma sellae
14. 颈内动脉 internal carotid a.
15. 视神经 optic n.

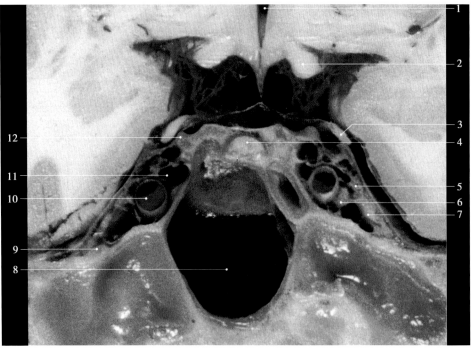

▲ 图 58　海绵窦（冠状切面）
Cavernous sinus.Coronal section

1. 第三脑室 the 3rd ventricle
2. 视束 optic tract
3. 动眼神经 oculomotor n.
4. 垂体 hypophysis
5. 滑车神经 trochlear n.
6. 展神经 abducent n.
7. 眼神经 ophthalmic n.
8. 蝶窦 sphenoidal sinus
9. 上颌神经 maxillary n.
10. 颈内动脉海绵窦部 cavernous part of internal carotid a.
11. 海绵窦 cavernous sinus
12. 后床突 posterior clinoid process

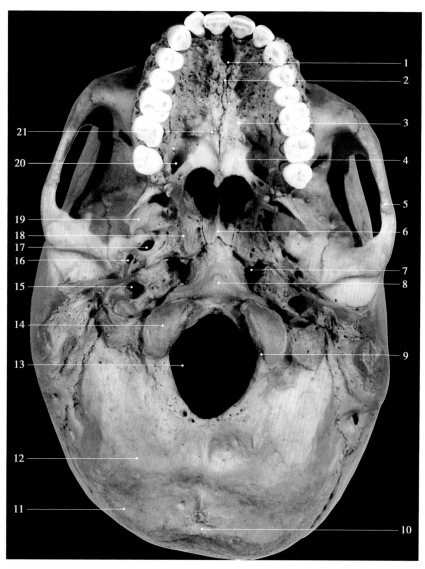

▲ 图 59 颅底（外面观 1）
Base of skull.External view（1）

1. 切牙孔 incisive foramina
2. 腭正中缝 median palatine suture
3. 上颌骨腭突 palatine process of maxilla
4. 腭骨水平板 horizontal plate of palatine bone
5. 颧弓 zygomatic arch
6. 犁骨 vomer
7. 破裂孔 foramen lacerum
8. 咽结节 pharyngeal tubercle
9. 髁管 condylar canal
10. 枕外隆凸 external occipital protuberance
11. 上项线 superior nuchal line
12. 下项线 inferior nuchal line
13. 枕骨大孔 foramen magnum of occipital bone
14. 枕髁 occipital condyle
15. 颈动脉管 carotid canal
16. 棘孔 foramen spinosum
17. 卵圆孔 foramen ovale
18. 翼突内侧板 medial pterygoid plate
19. 翼突外侧板 lateral pterygoid plate
20. 腭大孔 greater palatine foramen
21. 腭横缝 transverse palatine suture

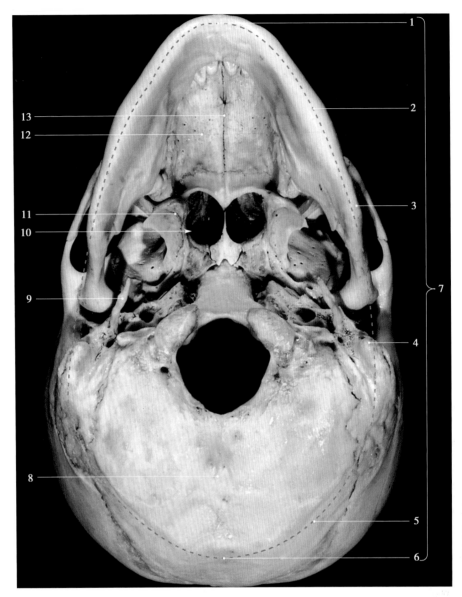

▲ 图 60　颅底（外面观 2）
Base of skull.External view（2）

1. 颏下点 menton
2. 下颌骨下缘 inferior border of mandible
3. 下颌角 angle of mandible
4. 乳突 mastoid process
5. 上项线 superior nuchal line
6. 枕外隆凸 external occipital protuberance
7. 头与颈的界线 terminal line of head and neck
8. 枕外嵴 external occipital crest
9. 茎突 styloid process
10. 鼻后孔 posterior nasal apertures
11. 翼窝 pterygoid fossa
12. 上颌骨腭突 palatine process of maxilla
13. 腭正中缝 median palatine suture

第二章

颈   部

Chapter 2   Neck

颈部上界以下颌骨下缘、下颌角、乳突尖、上项线和枕外隆凸的连线与头部分界。下界以胸骨颈静脉切迹、胸锁关节、锁骨上缘和肩峰至第 7 颈椎棘突的连线，分别与胸部及上肢为界。

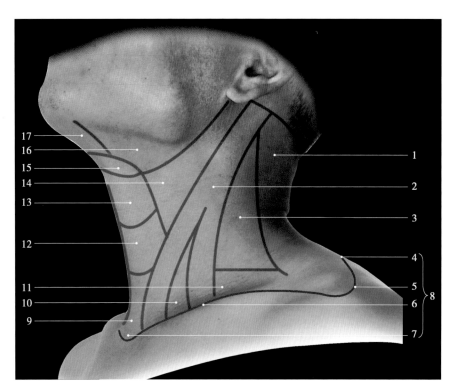

◀ 图 61　颈部的分区（侧面观）
Regions of neck.Lateral view

1. 颈后区 posterior region of neck
2. 胸锁乳突肌区 sternocleidomastoid region
3. 枕三角 occipital triangle
4. 第 7 颈椎棘突 spinous process of the 7th cervical vertebra
5. 肩峰 acromion
6. 锁骨上缘 superior border of clavicle
7. 颈静脉切迹 jugular notch
8. 颈部下界 lower bound of neck
9. 胸骨上窝 suprasternal fossa
10. 锁骨上小窝 lesser supraclavicular fossa
11. 锁骨上大窝 greater supraclavicular fossa
12. 甲状腺区 thyroid region
13. 喉区 laryngeal region
14. 颈动脉三角 carotid triangle
15. 舌骨区 hyoid region
16. 下颌下三角 submandibular triangle
17. 颏下三角 submental triangle

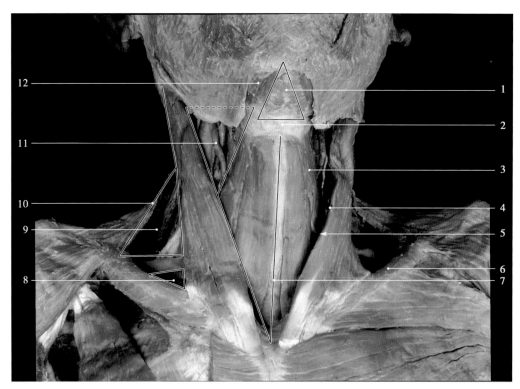

▲ 图 62　颈部三角（前面观）
Triangles of neck.Anterior view

1. 颏下三角 submental triangle
2. 舌骨 hyoid bone
3. 肩胛舌骨肌上腹 superior belly of omohyoid
4. 胸锁乳突肌前缘 anterior border of sternocleidomastoid
5. 肌三角 muscular triangle
6. 锁骨上缘 superior border of clavicle
7. 颈前正中线 anterior median line of neck
8. 锁骨上大窝 greater supraclavicular fossa
9. 枕三角 occipital triangle
10. 斜方肌前缘 anterior border of trapezius
11. 颈动脉三角 carotid triangle
12. 二腹肌前腹 anterior belly of digastric

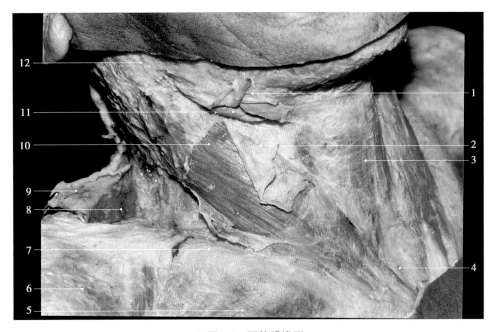

▲ 图 63　颈筋膜浅层
Superficial cervical fascia

1. 下颌下腺筋膜鞘 fascial sheath of submandibular gland
2. 胸锁乳突肌筋膜鞘 fascial sheath of sternocleidomastoid
3. 颈筋膜浅层 superficial layer of cervical fascia
4. 胸骨上窝 suprasternal fossa
5. 胸肌筋膜 pectoral fascia
6. 三角肌筋膜 deltoid fascia
7. 锁骨 clavicle
8. 斜方肌 trapezius
9. 斜方肌筋膜鞘 fascial sheath of trapezius
10. 胸锁乳突肌 sternocleidomastoid
11. 下颌下腺 submandibular gland
12. 腮腺筋膜 parotid fascia

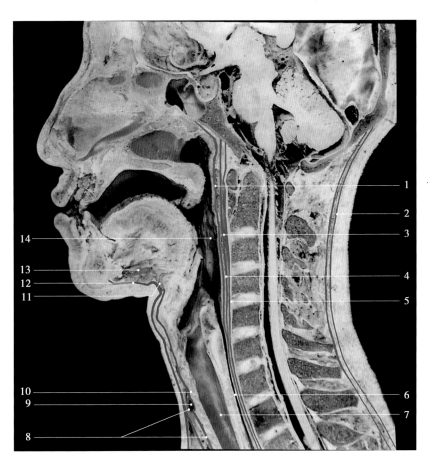

◀ 图 64　颈筋膜（正中矢状切面）
Cervical fascia.Median sagittal section

1. 颊咽筋膜 buccopharyngeal fascia
2. 颈筋膜浅层 superficial layer of cervical fascia
3. 翼状筋膜 alar fascia
4. 咽后间隙 retropharyngeal space
5. 椎前筋膜 prevertebral fascia
6. 食管 esophagus
7. 气管 trachea
8. 气管前筋膜 anterior fascia of trachea
9. 甲状腺 thyroid gland
10. 气管前间隙 pretracheal space
11. 舌骨 hyoid bone
12. 颏舌骨筋膜 geniohyoid fascia
13. 颏舌骨肌 geniohyoid
14. 咽 pharynx

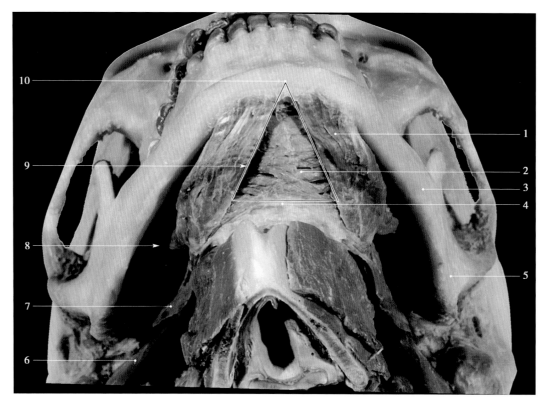

▲ 图 65　下颌下三角和颏下三角
Submandibular triangle and submental triangle

1. 二腹肌前腹 anterior belly of digastric
2. 下颌舌骨肌 mylohyoid
3. 下颌骨下缘 inferior border of mandible
4. 舌骨 hyoid bone
5. 下颌角 angle of mandible
6. 二腹肌后腹 posterior belly of digastric
7. 茎突舌骨肌 stylohyoid
8. 下颌下三角 submandibular triangle
9. 颏下三角 submental triangle
10. 颏下点 menton

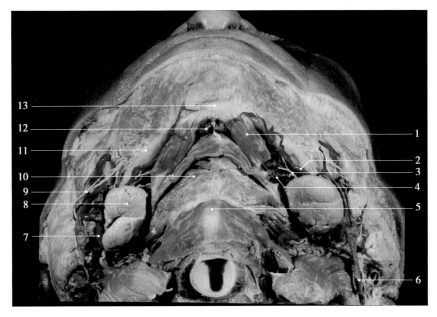

▲ 图 66　舌骨上区（前面观 1）
Suprahyoid region.Anterior view（1）

1. 二腹肌前腹 anterior belly of digastric
2. 颏下动脉 submental a.
3. 下颌舌骨肌神经 mylohyoid n.
4. 下颌下淋巴结 submandibular lymph nodes
5. 喉结 laryngeal prominence
6. 面静脉 facial v.
7. 面动脉 facial a.
8. 下颌下腺浅部 superficial part of submandibular gland
9. 下颌缘支 marginal mandibular branch
10. 下颌舌骨肌 mylohyoid
11. 下颌骨下缘 inferior border of mandible
12. 颏下淋巴结 submental lymph node
13. 颏下点 menton

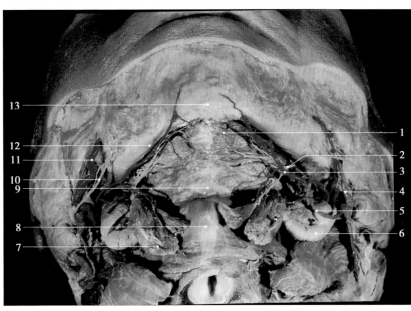

▲ 图 67　舌骨上区（前面观 2）
Suprahyoid region.Anterior view（2）

1. 下颌舌骨肌 mylohyoid
2. 下颌舌骨肌神经 mylohyoid n.
3. 颏下动脉 submental a.
4. 面静脉 facial v.
5. 颏下静脉 submental v.
6. 下颌下腺浅部 superficial part of submandibular gland
7. 二腹肌前腹 anterior belly of digastric
8. 喉结 laryngeal prominence
9. 舌骨体 body of hyoid bone
10. 面神经下颌缘支 marginal mandibular branch of facial n.
11. 面动脉 facial a.
12. 下颌骨下缘 inferior border of mandible
13. 颏下点 menton

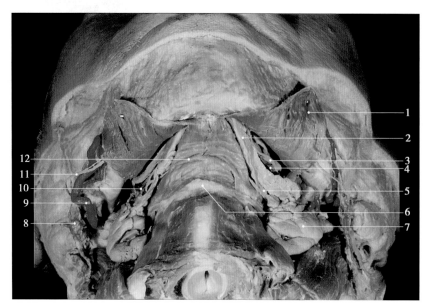

▲ 图 68　舌骨上区（前面观 3）
Suprahyoid region.Anterior view（3）

1. 下颌舌骨肌 mylohyoid
2. 下颌下腺深部 deep part of submandibular gland
3. 舌神经 lingual n.
4. 下颌下腺管 submandibular duct
5. 舌下神经 hypoglossal n.
6. 舌骨体 body of hyoid bone
7. 下颌下腺浅部 superficial part of submandibular gland
8. 面静脉 facial v.
9. 面动脉 facial a.
10. 下颌下神经节 submandibular ganglion
11. 下颌缘支 marginal mandibular branch
12. 颏舌骨肌 geniohyoid

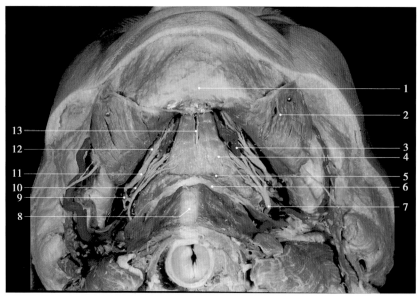

▲ 图 69　舌骨上区（前面观 4）
Suprahyoid region.Anterior view（4）

1. 颏下点 menton
2. 下颌舌骨肌 mylohyoid
3. 舌下动脉 sublingual a.
4. 颏舌肌 genioglossus
5. 颏舌骨肌 geniohyoid
6. 舌骨体 body of hyoid bone
7. 舌下神经 hypoglossal n.
8. 喉结 laryngeal prominence
9. 下颌下神经节 submandibular ganglion
10. 下颌下腺管 submandibular duct
11. 舌神经 lingual n.
12. 舌下腺 sublingual gland
13. 舌中隔 septum of tongue

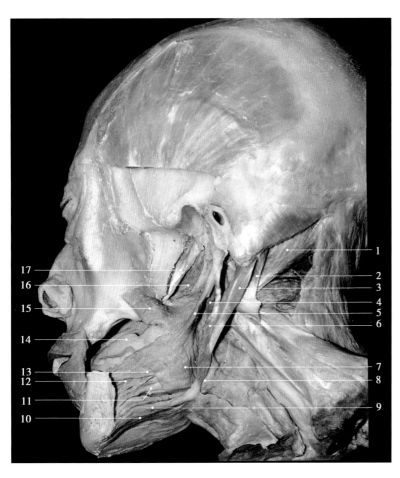

◀ 图 70　舌骨上区（侧面观 1）
Suprahyoid region.Lateral view（1）

1. 头上斜肌 obliquus capitis superior
2. 头外侧直肌 rectus capitis lateralis
3. 二腹肌后腹 posterior belly of digastric
4. 茎突咽肌 stylopharyngeus
5. 茎突舌肌 styloglossus
6. 茎突舌骨肌 stylohyoid
7. 舌骨舌肌 hyoglossus
8. 舌骨大角 greater horn of hyoid bone
9. 下颌舌骨肌 mylohyoid
10. 二腹肌前腹 anterior belly of digastric
11. 颏舌骨肌 geniohyoid
12. 颏舌肌 genioglossus
13. 下纵肌 inferior longitudinal m.
14. 舌 tongue
15. 颊肌 buccinator
16. 腭帆提肌 levator veli palatini
17. 腭帆张肌 tensor veli palatini

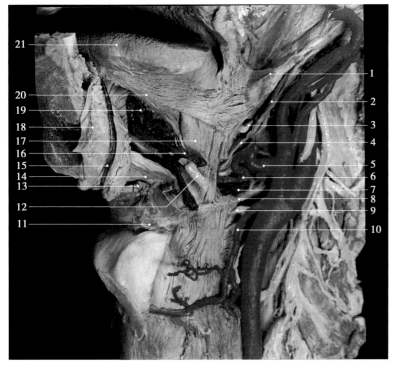

◀ 图 71　舌骨上区（侧面观 2）
Suprahyoid region.Lateral view（2）

1. 茎突舌肌 styloglossus
2. 茎突咽肌 stylopharyngeus
3. 舌咽神经 glossopharyngeal n.
4. 茎突舌骨韧带 stylohyoid lig.
5. 舌面干 linguofacial trunk
6. 舌动脉 lingual a.
7. 舌静脉 lingual v.
8. 舌骨大角 greater horn of hyoid bone
9. 喉上神经内支 internal branch of superior laryngeal n.
10. 甲状腺上动脉 superior thyroid a.
11. 舌骨体 body of hyoid bone
12. 舌下神经 hypoglossal n.
13. 下颌舌骨肌 mylohyoid
14. 颏舌骨肌 geniohyoid
15. 下颌下腺管 submandibular duct
16. 舌下神经伴行静脉 accompanying vein of hypoglossal n.
17. 舌骨舌肌 hyoglossus
18. 舌下腺 sublingual gland
19. 舌深动脉 deep lingual a.
20. 下纵肌 inferior longitudinal m.
21. 舌 tongue

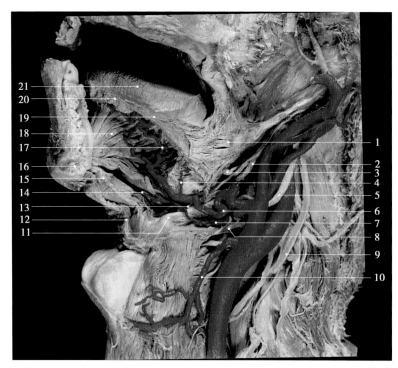

◀ 图 72 舌骨上区（侧面观 3）
Suprahyoid region.Lateral view（3）

1. 茎突舌肌 styloglossus
2. 茎突咽肌 stylopharyngeus
3. 舌咽神经 glossopharyngeal n.
4. 舌背支 dorsal lingual branches
5. 舌下神经 hypoglossal n.
6. 舌动脉 lingual a.
7. 舌静脉 lingual v.
8. 舌骨大角 greater horn of hyoid bone
9. 迷走神经 vagus n.
10. 甲状腺上动脉 superior thyroid a.
11. 舌骨小角 lesser horn of hyoid bone
12. 下颌舌骨肌 mylohyoid
13. 舌骨上支 suprahyoid branch
14. 舌下动脉 hypoglossal a.
15. 颏舌骨肌 geniohyoid
16. 下颌骨 mandible
17. 舌深动脉 deep lingual a.
18. 颏舌肌 genioglossus
19. 下纵肌 inferior longitudinal m.
20. 舌腺 lingual glands
21. 舌 tongue

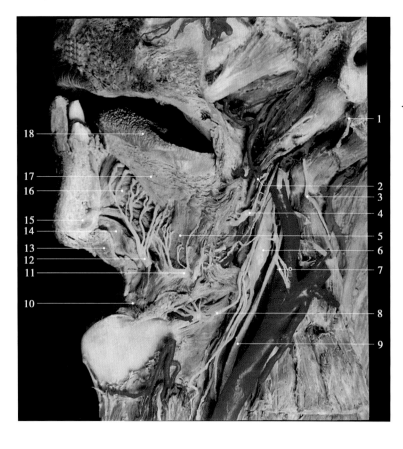

◀ 图 73 舌骨上区（侧面观 4）
Suprahyoid region.Lateral view（4）

1. 面神经 facial n.
2. 腭升动脉 ascending palatine a.
3. 副神经 accessory n.
4. 舌咽神经 glossopharyngeal n.
5. 舌骨舌肌 hyoglossus
6. 颈上神经节 superior cervical ganglion
7. 颈动脉窦支 carotid sinus branch
8. 喉上神经内支 internal branch of superior laryngeal n.
9. 迷走神经 vagus n.
10. 舌骨体 body of hyoid bone
11. 舌下神经 hypoglossal n.
12. 舌神经 lingual n.
13. 下颌舌骨肌 mylohyoid
14. 颏舌骨肌 geniohyoid
15. 下颌骨 mandible
16. 颏舌肌 genioglossus
17. 下纵肌 inferior longitudinal m.
18. 舌 tongue

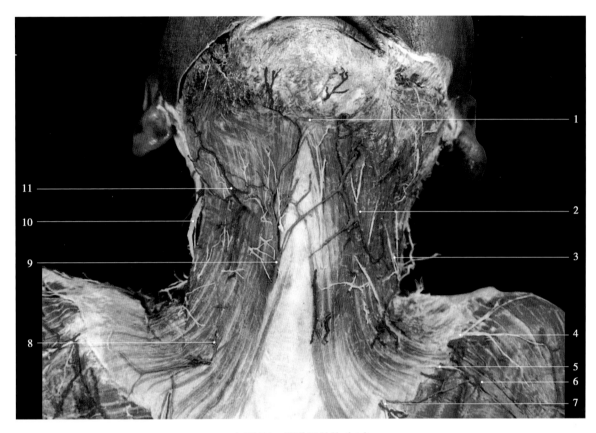

▲ 图 74 颈前区结构（1）
Structures of anterior region of neck（1）

1. 颏横肌 transverses menti
2. 颈阔肌 platysma
3. 颈横神经 transverse nerve of neck
4. 锁骨上外侧神经 lateral supraclavicular n.
5. 锁骨上中间神经 intermediate supraclavicular n.
6. 头静脉 cephalic v.
7. 锁骨上内侧神经 medial supraclavicular n.
8. 颈静脉弓皮支 cutaneous branch of jugular venous arch
9. 颈前静脉皮支 cutaneous branch of anterior jugular v.
10. 耳大神经 great auricular n.
11. 甲状腺上动脉皮支 cutaneous branch of superior thyroid a.

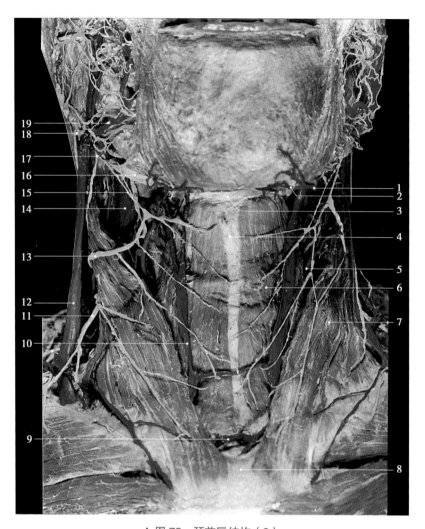

▲ 图 75　颈前区结构（2）
Structures of anterior region of neck（2）

1. 颏下动脉 submental a.
2. 颏下静脉 submental v.
3. 舌骨 hyoid bone
4. 喉结 laryngeal prominence
5. 甲状腺上动脉 superior thyroid a.
6. 胸骨舌骨肌 sternohyoid
7. 胸锁乳突肌 sternocleidomastoid
8. 颈静脉切迹 jugular notch
9. 颈静脉弓 jugular venous arch
10. 颈前静脉 anterior jugular v.
11. 锁骨上神经 supraclavicular n.
12. 颈外静脉 external jugular v.
13. 颈横神经 transverse nerve of neck
14. 颈内静脉 internal jugular v.
15. 面神经交通支 communicating branch with facial n.
16. 下颌下腺 submandibular gland
17. 面神经颈支 cervical branch of facial n.
18. 面神经下颌缘支 marginal mandibular branch of facial n.
19. 面动脉 facial a.

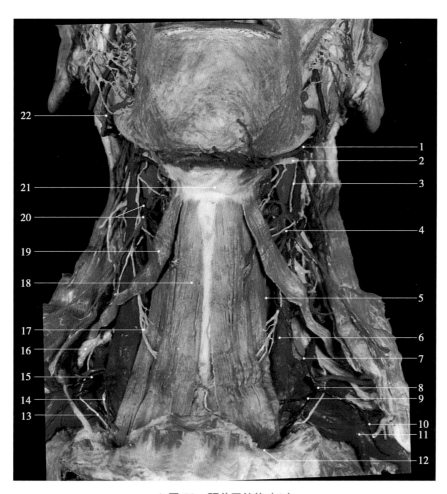

▲ 图 76 颈前区结构（3）
Structures of anterior region of neck（3）

1. 颏下动脉 submental a.
2. 舌下神经 hypoglossal n.
3. 上根 superior root
4. 肩胛舌骨肌支 omohyoid branch
5. 颈总动脉 common carotid a.
6. 颈内静脉 internal jugular v.
7. 左颈干 left jugular trunk
8. 胸导管 thoracic duct
9. 左支气管纵隔干 left bronchomediastinal trunk
10. 左锁骨下干 left subclavian trunk
11. 左锁骨下静脉 left subclavian v.
12. 锁切迹 clavicular notch
13. 副膈神经 accessory phrenic n.
14. 膈神经 phrenic n.
15. 右淋巴导管 right lymphatic duct
16. 臂丛 brachial plexus
17. 胸骨舌骨肌支 sternohyoid branch
18. 胸骨舌骨肌 sternohyoid
19. 肩胛舌骨肌上腹 superior belly of omohyoid
20. 甲状腺上动、静脉 superior thyroid a.and v.
21. 舌骨 hyoid bone
22. 面动脉 facial a.

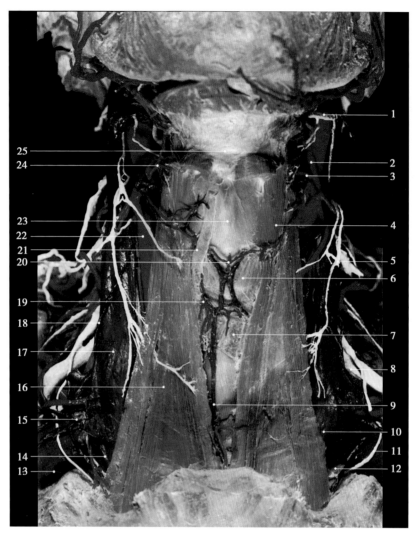

▲ 图 77　颈前区结构（4）
Structures of anterior region of neck（4）

1. 舌下神经 hypoglossal n.
2. 甲状腺上动脉 superior thyroid a.
3. 喉上动脉 superior laryngeal a.
4. 甲状舌骨肌 thyrohyoid
5. 颈襻 ansa cervicalis
6. 环甲肌 cricothyroid
7. 甲状腺 thyroid gland
8. 臂丛 brachial plexus
9. 甲状腺下静脉 inferior thyroid v.
10. 左头臂静脉 left brachiocephalic v.
11. 膈神经 phrenic n.
12. 胸膜顶 cupula of pleura
13. 右锁骨下静脉 right subclavian v.
14. 右头臂静脉 right brachiocephalic v.
15. 右淋巴导管 right lymphatic duct
16. 胸骨甲状肌 sternothyroid
17. 右颈内静脉 right internal jugular v.
18. 右颈干 right jugular trunk
19. 前腺支 anterior glandular branch
20. 甲状腺上动脉吻合支 anastomotic branch with superior thyroid a.
21. 甲状腺锥状叶 pyramidal lobe of thyroid gland
22. 颈总动脉 common carotid a.
23. 喉结 laryngeal prominence
24. 舌骨下支 infrahyoid branch
25. 舌骨 hyoid bone

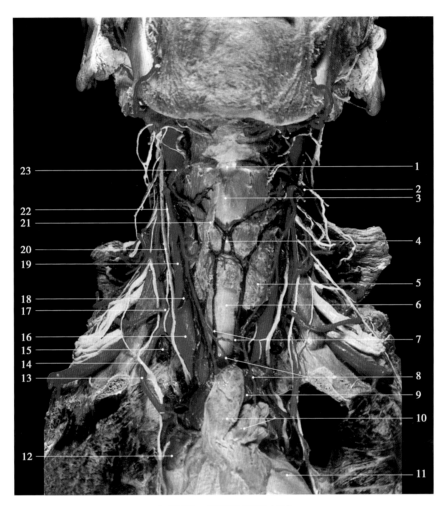

▲ 图 78　颈前区结构（5）
Structures of anterior region of neck（5）

1. 甲状舌骨膜 thyrohyoid membrane
2. 甲状腺上静脉 superior thyroid v.
3. 喉结 laryngeal prominence
4. 环状软骨 cricoid cartilage
5. 甲状腺左叶 left lobe of thyroid gland
6. 气管 trachea
7. 甲状腺下静脉 inferior thyroid v.
8. 胸腺支 thymic branch
9. 左头臂静脉 left brachiocephalic v.
10. 胸腺 thymus
11. 心包 pericardium
12. 上腔静脉 superior vena cava
13. 胸廓内动脉 internal thoracic a.
14. 膈神经 phrenic n.
15. 颈深静脉 deep cervical v.
16. 头臂干 brachiocephalic trunk
17. 甲状颈干 thyrocervical trunk
18. 甲状腺中静脉 middle thyroid v.
19. 颈总动脉 common carotid a.
20. 迷走神经 vagus n.
21. 锥状叶 pyramidal lobe
22. 颈交感干 cervical sympathetic trunk
23. 甲状腺上动脉 superior thyroid a.

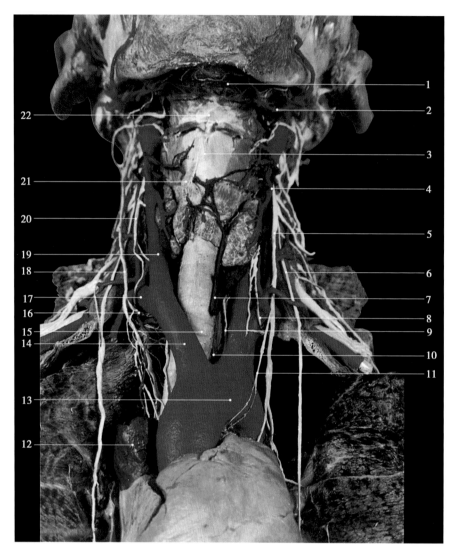

▲ 图 79　颈前区结构（6）
Structures of anterior region of neck（6）

1. 下颌舌骨肌 mylohyoideus
2. 颏下动脉 submental a.
3. 喉结 laryngeal prominence
4. 甲状腺上动脉 superior thyroid a.
5. 左迷走神经 left vagus n.
6. 左膈神经 left phrenic n.
7. 甲状腺下静脉 inferior thyroid v.
8. 锁骨下襻 ansa subclavia
9. 左喉返神经 left recurrent laryngeal n.
10. 食管 esophagus
11. 迷走神经心上支 superior cardiac branches of vagus n.
12. 上腔静脉 superior vena cava
13. 主动脉弓 aortic arch
14. 头臂干 brachiocephalic trunk
15. 气管 trachea
16. 右喉返神经 right recurrent laryngeal n.
17. 右锁骨下动脉 right subclavian a.
18. 右迷走神经 right vagus n.
19. 右颈总动脉 right common carotid a.
20. 右颈交感干 right cervical sympathetic trunk
21. 锥状叶 pyramidal lobe
22. 舌骨 hyoid bone

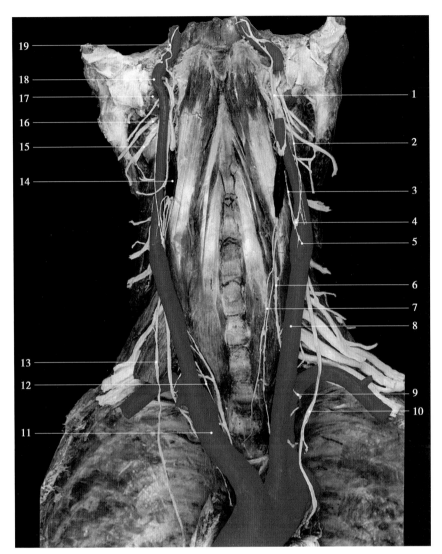

▲ 图 80 颈前区结构（7）
Structures of anterior region of neck（7）

1. 颈内动脉神经 internal carotid n.
2. 颈动脉窦支 carotid sinus branch
3. 颈动脉体支 branch of carotid body
4. 颈动脉小球 carotid glomus
5. 颈动脉窦 carotid sinus
6. 交感干 sympathetic trunk
7. 颈上心神经 superior cervical cardiac n.
8. 颈总动脉 common carotid a.
9. 锁骨下襻 ansa subclavia
10. 迷走神经 vagus n.
11. 头臂干 brachiocephalic trunk
12. 颈中心神经 middle cervical cardiac n.
13. 膈神经 phrenic n.
14. 颈上神经节 superior cervical ganglion
15. 舌下神经 hypoglossal n.
16. 副神经 accessory n.
17. 颈内静脉 internal jugular v.
18. 颈内动脉 internal carotid a.
19. 颈内动脉丛 internal carotid plexus

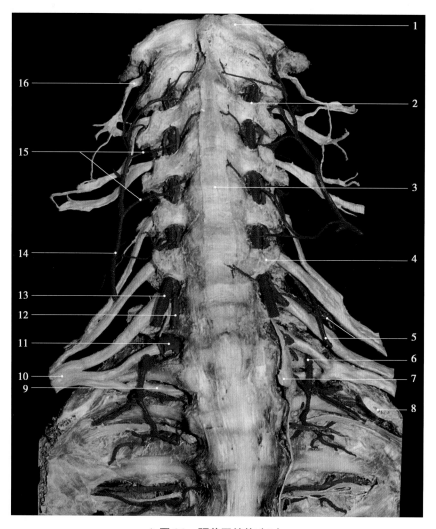

▲ 图 81　颈前区结构（8）
Structures of anterior region of neck（8）

1. 寰椎 atlas
2. 横突孔 transverse foramen
3. 前纵韧带 anterior longitudinal lig.
4. 第 6 颈椎横突 transverse process of the 6th cervical vertebra
5. 颈深动、静脉 deep cervical a. and v.
6. 肋间最上动脉 supreme intercostal a.
7. 颈胸神经节 cervicothoracic ganglion
8. 第 1 肋 the 1st rib
9. 第 1 胸神经前支 anterior branch of the 1st thoracic n.
10. 臂丛 brachial plexus
11. 肋间最上静脉 highest intercostal v.
12. 椎静脉 vertebral v.
13. 椎动脉 vertebral a.
14. 颈升动脉 ascending cervical a.
15. 脊支 spinal branches
16. 第 2 颈神经 the 2nd cervical n.

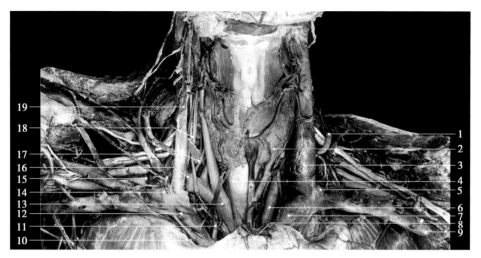

▲ 图 82 颈根部（1）
Root of neck（1）

1. 颈横动脉 transverse cervical a.
2. 甲状腺 thyroid gland
3. 左颈内静脉 left internal jugular v.
4. 气管 trachea
5. 静脉角 venous angle
6. 左颈总动脉 left common carotid a.
7. 左头臂静脉 left brachiocephalic v.

8. 颈静脉切迹 jugular notch
9. 左锁骨下静脉 left subclavian v.
10. 锁切迹 clavicular notch
11. 甲状腺下静脉 inferior thyroid v.
12. 右头臂静脉 right brachiocephalic v.
13. 头臂干 brachiocephalic trunk
14. 右锁骨下静脉 right subclavian v.

15. 右锁骨下动脉 right subclavian a.
16. 右甲状颈干 right thyrocervical trunk
17. 甲状腺下动脉 inferior thyroid a.
18. 迷走神经 vagus n.
19. 右颈内静脉 right internal jugular v.

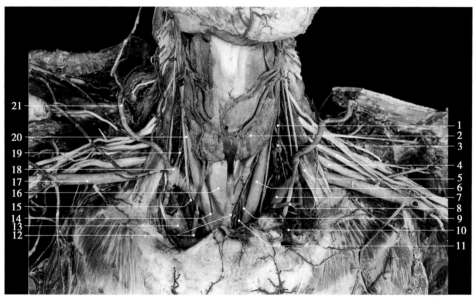

▲ 图 83 颈根部（2）
Root of neck（2）

1. 颈交感干 cervical sympathetic trunk
2. 甲状腺 thyroid gland
3. 颈中神经节 middle cervical ganglion
4. 臂丛 brachial plexus
5. 前斜角肌 scalenus anterior
6. 颈总动脉 common carotid a.
7. 锁骨下动脉 subclavian a.

8. 胸导管 thoracic duct
9. 食管 esophagus
10. 左静脉角 left venous angle
11. 左喉返神经 left recurrent laryngeal n.
12. 甲状腺下静脉 inferior thyroid v.
13. 右头臂静脉 right brachiocephalic v.
14. 头臂干 brachiocephalic trunk

15. 膈神经 phrenic n.
16. 气管 trachea
17. 右锁骨下动脉 right subclavian a.
18. 甲状颈干 thyrocervical trunk
19. 甲状腺下动脉 inferior thyroid a.
20. 颈总动脉 common carotid a.
21. 颈横动脉 transverse cervical a.

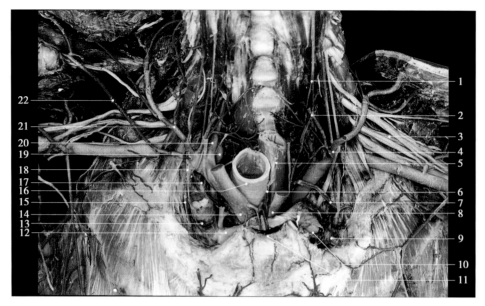

▲ 图 84　颈根部（3）
Root of neck（3）

1. 颈交感干 cervical sympathetic trunk
2. 颈中神经节 middle cervical ganglion
3. 臂丛 brachial plexus
4. 甲状颈干 thyrocervical trunk
5. 食管 esophagus
6. 左喉返神经 left recurrent laryngeal n.
7. 胸导管 thoracic duct
8. 左颈总动脉 left common carotid a.

9. 左静脉角 left venous angle
10. 左颈内静脉 left internal jugular v.
11. 颈静脉切迹 jugular notch
12. 左头臂静脉 left brachiocephalic v.
13. 右头臂静脉 right brachiocephalic v.
14. 头臂干 brachiocephalic trunk
15. 胸廓内动脉 internal thoracic a.
16. 气管 trachea

17. 胸膜顶 cupula of pleura
18. 膈神经 phrenic n.
19. 颈深静脉 deep cervical v.
20. 椎动脉 vertebral a.
21. 颈横动脉 transverse cervical a.
22. 肩胛上动脉 suprascapular a.

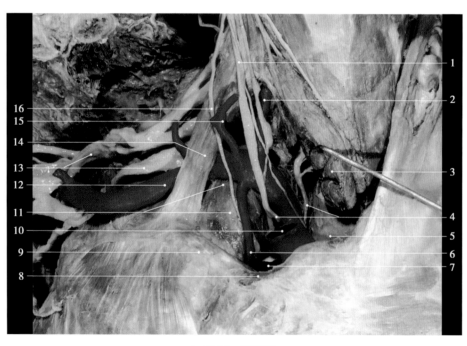

▲ 图 85　胸膜顶
Cupula of pleura

1. 迷走神经 vagus n.
2. 椎动脉 vertebral a.
3. 甲状腺 thyroid gland
4. 喉返神经 recurrent laryngeal n.
5. 气管 trachea
6. 胸廓内动脉 internal thoracic a.

7. 右头臂静脉 right brachiocephalic v.
8. 锁切迹 clavicular notch
9. 第 1 肋 the 1st rib
10. 颈总动脉 common carotid a.
11. 胸膜顶 cupula of pleura
12. 锁骨下动脉 subclavian a.

13. 臂丛 brachial plexus
14. 前斜角肌 anterior scalenus
15. 甲状颈干 thyrocervical trunk
16. 膈神经 phrenic n.

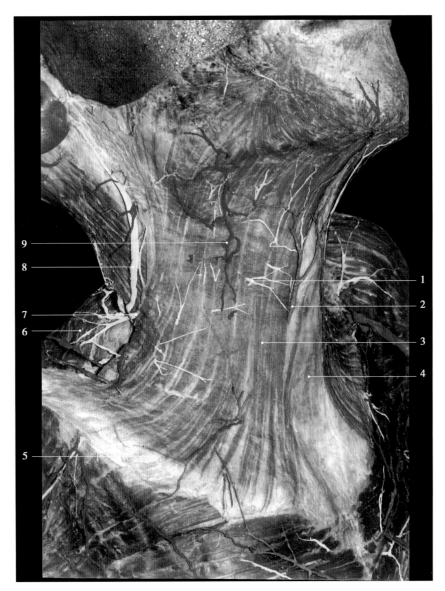

▲ 图 86　颈部的血管、神经（侧面观 1）
Blood vessels and nerves of neck.Lateral view（1）

1. 皮神经 cutaneous n.
2. 颈前静脉皮支 cutaneous branch of anterior jugular v.
3. 颈阔肌 platysma
4. 颈筋膜 cervical fascia
5. 锁骨 clavicle
6. 斜方肌 trapezius
7. 锁骨上外侧神经 lateral supraclavicular n.
8. 耳大神经 great auricular n.
9. 甲状腺上动脉皮支 cutaneous branch of superior thyroid a.

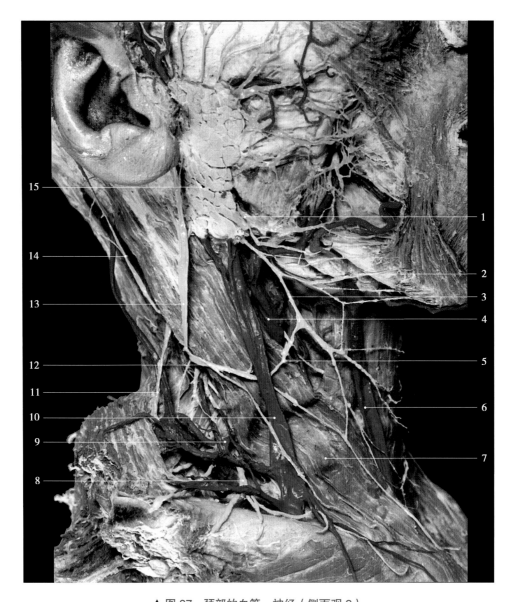

▲ 图 87　颈部的血管、神经（侧面观 2）
Blood vessels and nerves of neck.Lateral view（2）

1. 面神经下颌缘支 marginal mandibular branch of facial n.
2. 下颌下腺 submandibular gland
3. 面神经颈支 cervical branch of facial n.
4. 颈内静脉 internal jugular v.
5. 面神经交通支 communicating branch with facial n.
6. 颈前静脉 anterior jugular v.
7. 胸锁乳突肌 sternocleidomastoid
8. 锁骨上神经 supraclavicular n.
9. 颈横动脉 transverse cervical a.
10. 颈外静脉 external jugular v.
11. 副神经 accessory n.
12. 颈横神经 transverse nerve of neck
13. 耳大神经 great auricular n.
14. 枕小神经 lesser occipital n.
15. 腮腺 parotid gland

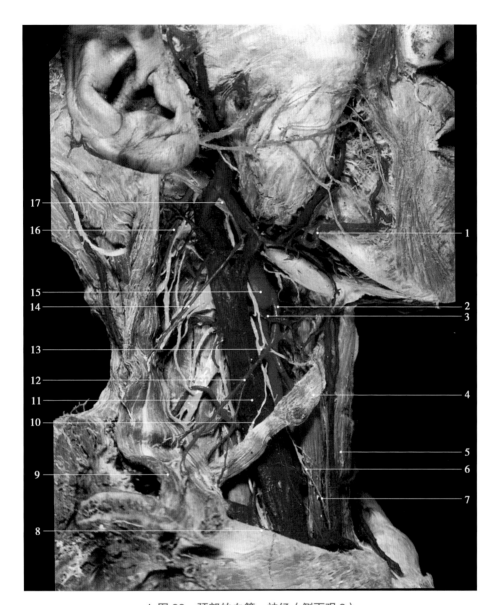

▲ 图 88　颈部的血管、神经（侧面观 3）
Blood vessels and nerves of neck.Lateral view（3）

1. 面动脉 facial a.
2. 甲状腺上动脉 superior thyroid a.
3. 甲状腺上静脉 superior thyroid v.
4. 肩胛舌骨肌 omohyoid
5. 胸骨舌骨肌 sternohyoid
6. 胸骨甲状肌支 sternothyroid branch
7. 胸骨舌骨肌支 sternohyoid branch
8. 锁骨 clavicle.
9. 胸锁乳突肌 sternocleidomastoid
10. 肩胛舌骨肌支 omohyoid branch
11. 颈内静脉 internal jugular v.
12. 胸锁乳突肌支（甲状腺上动脉）
    sternocleidomastoid branch of superior thyroid a.
13. 颈襻 ansa cervicalis
14. 胸锁乳突肌支（颈外动脉）
    sternocleidomastoid branch of external carotid a.
15. 颈外动脉 external carotid a.
16. 胸锁乳突肌支（枕动脉）
    sternocleidomastoid branch of occipital a.
17. 二腹肌后腹 posterior belly of digastric

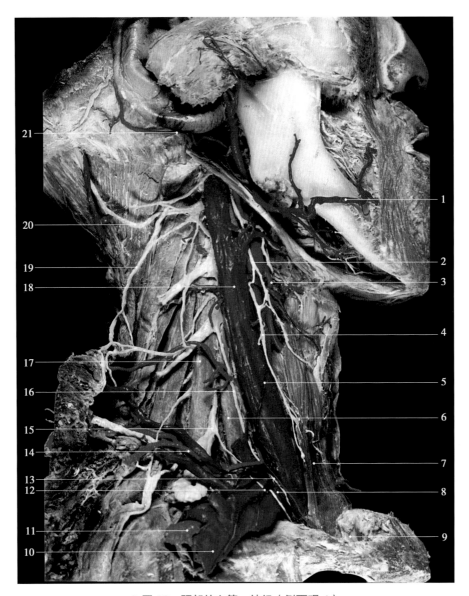

▲ 图 89　颈部的血管、神经（侧面观 4）
Blood vessels and nerves of neck.Lateral view（4）

1. 面动脉 facial a.
2. 上根（舌下神经）superior root
3. 甲状腺上动脉 superior thyroid a.
4. 胸骨甲状肌支 sternothyroid branch
5. 右颈干 right jugular trunk
6. 前斜角肌 scalenus anterior
7. 胸骨甲状肌 sternothyroid
8. 右支气管纵隔干 right bronchomediastinal trunk
9. 锁切迹 clavicular notch
10. 锁骨下静脉 subclavian v.
11. 锁骨下动脉 subclavian a.
12. 右锁骨下干 right subclavian trunk
13. 右淋巴导管 right lymphatic duct
14. 颈横动脉 transverse cervical a.
15. 臂丛 brachial plexus
16. 膈神经 phrenic n.
17. 中斜角肌 scalenus middle
18. 颈内静脉 internal jugular v.
19. 副神经 accessory n.
20. 枕小神经 lesser occipital n.
21. 耳后动脉 posterior auricular a.

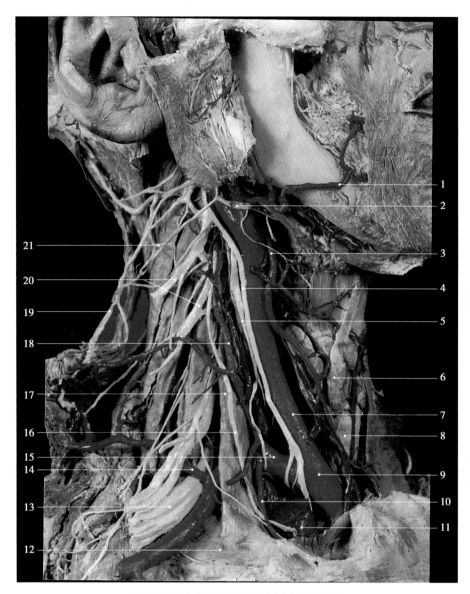

▲ 图 90 颈部的血管、神经（侧面观 5）
Blood vessels and nerves of neck.Lateral view（5）

1. 面动脉 facial a.
2. 舌下神经 hypoglossal n.
3. 甲状腺上动脉 superior thyroid a.
4. 迷走神经 vagus n.
5. 颈交感干 cervical sympathetic trunk
6. 甲状腺 thyroid gland
7. 右颈总动脉 right common carotid a.
8. 气管 trachea
9. 头臂干 brachiocephalic trunk
10. 胸廓内动脉 internal thoracic a.
11. 右头臂静脉 right brachiocephalic v.

12. 第 1 肋 the1st rib
13. 臂丛 brachial plexus
14. 颈横动脉 transverse cervical a.
15. 锁骨下动脉 subclavian a.
16. 膈神经 phrenic n.
17. 前斜角肌 scalenus anterior
18. 颈升动脉 ascending cervical a.
19. 副神经 accessory n.
20. 颈丛 cervical plexus
21. 颈襻 ansa cervicalis

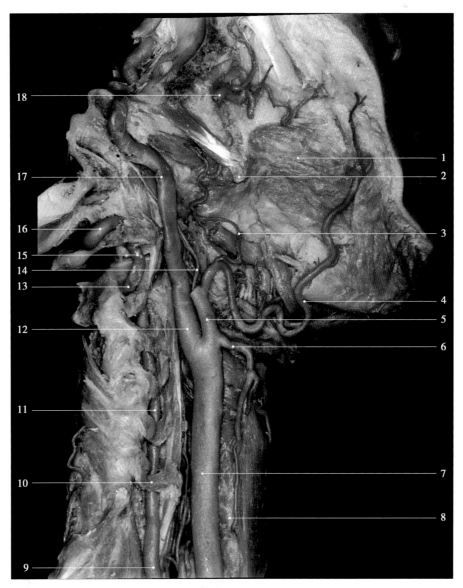

▲ 图 91 颈内动脉及椎动脉（侧面观）
Vertebral artery and internal carotid artery.Lateral view

1. 颊肌 buccinator
2. 翼钩 pterygoid hamulus
3. 腭升动脉 ascending palatine a.
4. 面动脉 facial a.
5. 颈外动脉 external carotid a.
6. 甲状腺上动脉 superior thyroid a.
7. 颈总动脉 common carotid a.
8. 甲状腺 thyroid gland
9. 椎动脉 vertebral a.
10. 第 6 颈椎横突 transverse process of the 6th cervical vertebra
11. 椎动脉 V1 段 V1 portion of vertebral a.
12. 颈动脉窦 carotid sinus
13. 椎动脉 V2 段 V2 portion of vertebral a.
14. 咽升动脉 ascending pharyngeal a.
15. 椎动脉 V3 段 V3 portion of vertebral a.
16. 椎动脉 V4 段 V4 portion of vertebral a.
17. 颈内动脉 internal carotid a.
18. 上颌动脉 maxillary a.

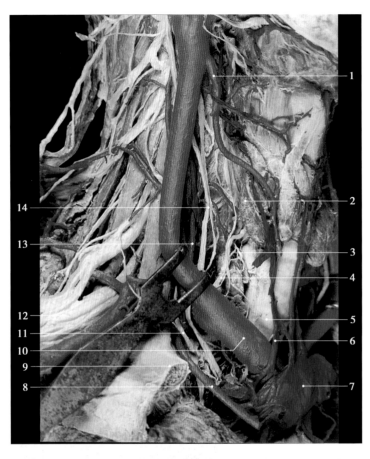

◀ 图 92　右喉返神经（1）
Right recurrent laryngeal nerve（1）

1. 甲状腺上动脉 superior thyroid a.
2. 甲状腺右叶 right lobe of thyroid gland
3. 气管支 tracheal branches
4. 右喉返神经 right recurrent laryngeal n.
5. 气管 trachea
6. 右甲状腺下静脉 right inferior thyroid v.
7. 左头臂静脉 left brachiocephalic v.
8. 胸廓内动脉 iuternal thoracic a.
9. 第一肋骨 the 1st rib
10. 头臂干 brachiocephalic trunk
11. 右膈神经 right phrenic n.
12. 臂丛 brachial plexus
13. 甲状腺下动脉 inferior thyroid a.
14. 右迷走神经 right vagus n.

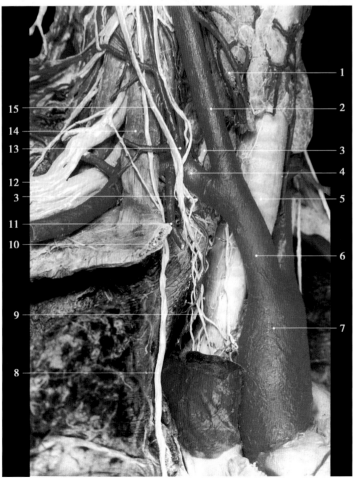

◀ 图 93　右喉返神经（2）
Right recurrent laryngeal nerve（2）

1. 甲状腺右叶 right lobe of thyroid gland
2. 右颈总动脉 right common carotid a.
3. 右喉返神经 right recurrent laryngeal n.
4. 右锁骨下动脉 right subclavian a.
5. 气管 trachea
6. 头臂干 brachiocephalic trunk
7. 主动脉弓 aortic arch
8. 右膈神经 right phrenic n.
9. 迷走神经心丛 cardiac plexus of vagus n.
10. 第 1 肋 the 1st rib
11. 胸廓内动脉 internal thoracic a.
12. 臂丛 brachial plexus
13. 甲状颈干 thyrocervical trunk
14. 前斜角肌 scalenus anterior
15. 迷走神经 vagus n.

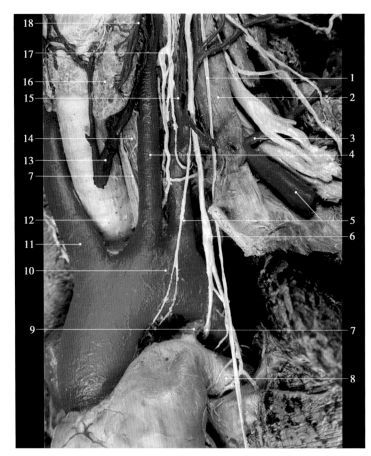

◀ 图 94　左喉返神经
Left recurrent laryngeal nerve

1. 左膈神经 left phrenic n.
2. 前斜角肌 scalenus anterior
3. 颈横动脉 transverse cervical a.
4. 左颈总动脉 left common carotid a.
5. 左锁骨下动脉 left subclavian a.
6. 迷走神经 vagus n.
7. 喉返神经 recurrent laryngeal n.
8. 左肺动脉 left pulminary a.
9. 动脉韧带 arterial lig.
10. 主动脉弓 aortic arch
11. 头臂干 brachiocephalic trunk
12. 气管 trachea
13. 甲状腺下静脉 inferior thyroid v.
14. 食管 esophagus
15. 甲状腺下动脉 inferior thyroid a.
16. 甲状腺左叶 left lobe of thyroid gland
17. 颈交感干 cervical sympathetic trunk
18. 甲状腺上动脉 superior thyroid a.

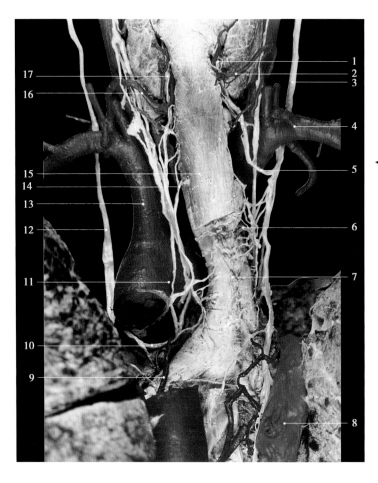

◀ 图 95　喉返神经（后面观）
Recurrent laryngeal nerve.Posterior view

1. 喉下神经 inferior laryngeal n.
2. 右甲状腺下动脉 right inferior thyroid a.
3. 右迷走神经 right vagus n.
4. 右锁骨下动脉 right subclavian a.
5. 右喉返神经 right recurrent laryngeal n.
6. 气管支 tracheal branches
7. 气管 trachea
8. 奇静脉 azygos v.
9. 支气管动脉 branchial a.
10. 左喉返神经 left recurrent laryngeal n.
11. 主动脉弓 aortic arch
12. 左迷走神经 left vagus n.
13. 左锁骨下动脉 left subclavian a.
14. 食管支 esophagus branches
15. 食管 esophagus
16. 左甲状腺下动脉 left inferior thyroid a.
17. 左喉下神经 left inferior laryngeal n.

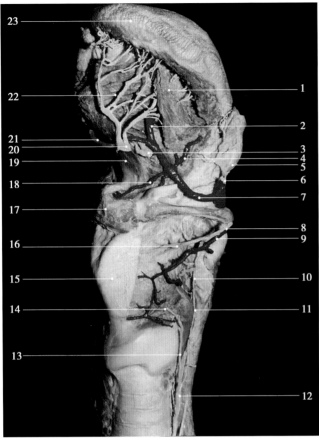

◀ 图 96　喉上神经与喉下神经（侧面观）
Inferior laryngeal nerve and superior laryngeal nerve.
Lateral view

1. 下纵肌 inferior longitudinal m.
2. 舌深动脉 deep lingual a.
3. 舌下神经 hypoglossal n.
4. 舌背支 dorsal lingual branch
5. 腭扁桃体 palatine tonsil
6. 舌咽神经 glossopharyngeal n.
7. 舌动脉 lingual a.
8. 喉上神经内支 internal branch of superior laryngeal n.
9. 喉上动脉 superior laryngeal a.
10. 喉下神经交通支 communicating branch with inferior laryngeal n.
11. 喉下神经后支 posterior branch of inferior laryngeal n.
12. 喉返神经 recurrent laryngeal n.
13. 喉下神经前支 anterior branch of inferior laryngeal n.
14. 甲杓肌支 thyroarytenoid branch
15. 甲状软骨 thyroid cartilage
16. 喉支 larynx branch
17. 舌骨 hyoid bone
18. 舌骨上支 suprahyoid branch
19. 颏舌骨肌 geniohyoid
20. 舌神经 lingual n.
21. 舌下动脉 sublingual a.
22. 颏舌肌 genioglossus
23. 舌 tongue

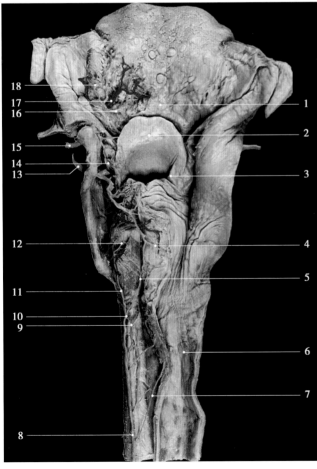

◀ 图 97　喉上神经与喉下神经（后面观）
Inferior laryngeal nerve and superior laryngeal nerve.
Posterior view

1. 舌根 root of tongue
2. 会厌 epiglottis
3. 杓状会厌襞 aryepiglottic fold
4. 喉上神经咽支 pharyngeal branches of superior laryngeal n.
5. 喉下神经交通支 communicating branch with inferior laryngeal n.
6. 食管 esophagus
7. 喉返神经食管支 esophageal branches of recurrent laryngeal n.
8. 喉返神经 recurrent laryngeal n.
9. 喉返神经咽支 pharyngeal branches of recurrent laryngeal n.
10. 喉下神经 inferior laryngeal n.
11. 喉下神经后支 posterior branch of inferior laryngeal n.
12. 杓横肌支 transverse arytenoid branch
13. 喉上神经内支 internal branch of superior laryngeal n.
14. 喉上神经会厌支 epiglottic branch of superior laryngeal n.
15. 舌咽神经 glossopharyngeal n.
16. 舌咽神经舌支 lingual branches of glossopharyngeal n.
17. 扁桃体动脉舌支 lingual branches of tonsilla a.
18. 舌咽神经扁桃体支 tonsillar branches of glossopharyngeal n.

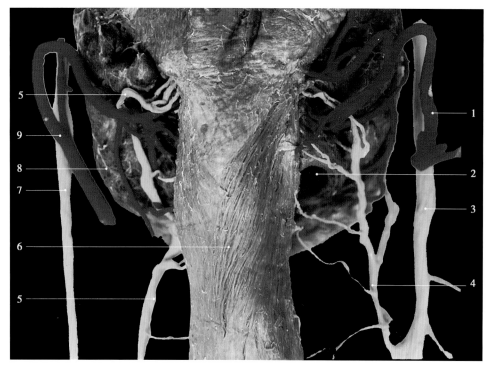

1. 右甲状腺下动脉
   right inferior thyroid a.
2. 气管
   trachea
3. 右迷走神经
   right vagus n.
4. 右喉返神经
   right recurrent laryngeal n.
5. 左喉返神经
   left recurrent laryngeal n.
6. 食管
   esophagus
7. 左迷走神经
   left vagusn
8. 甲状腺左叶
   left lobe of thyroid gland
9. 左甲状腺下动脉
   left inferior thyroid a.

▲ 图 98　甲状腺下动脉与喉返神经的关系（后面观）
Relationship between inferior thyroid artery and recurrent laryngeal nerve.Posterior view

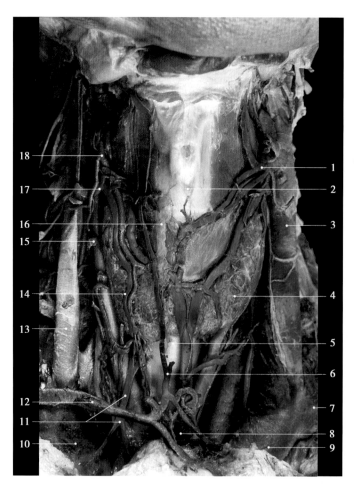

◀图 99　甲状腺静脉
Thyroid veins

1. 左甲状腺上静脉 left superior thyroid v.
2. 喉结 laryngeal prominence
3. 左颈内静脉 left internal jugular v.
4. 甲状腺左叶 left lobe of thyroid gland
5. 气管 trachea
6. 甲状腺下静脉（汇入颈静脉弓）inferior thyroid v.
7. 左锁骨下静脉 left subclavian v.
8. 甲状腺下静脉（汇入左头臂静脉）inferior thyroid v.
9. 左头臂静脉 left brachiocephalic v.
10. 右头臂静脉 right brachiocephalic v.
11. 甲状腺下静脉（汇入右头臂静脉）inferior thyroid v.
12. 颈静脉弓 jugular arch
13. 右颈内静脉 right internal jugular v.
14. 甲状腺右叶 right lobe of thyroid gland
15. 甲状腺中静脉 middle thyroid v.
16. 锥状叶 pyramidal lobe
17. 右甲状腺上静脉 right superior thyroid v.
18. 右甲状腺上动脉 right superior thyroid a.

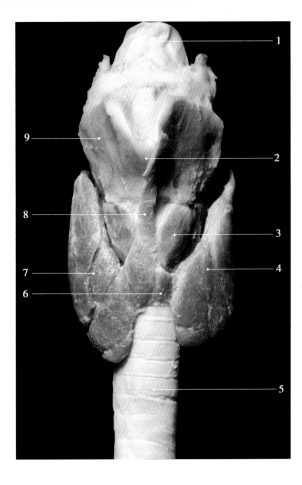

◀ 图 100 甲状腺（前面观）
Thyroid gland.Anterior view

1. 会厌 epiglottis
2. 喉结 laryngeal prominence
3. 环甲肌 cricothyroid
4. 甲状腺左叶 left lobe of thyroid gland
5. 气管 trachea
6. 甲状腺峡 isthmus of thyroid gland
7. 甲状腺右叶 right lobe of thyroid gland
8. 甲状腺锥状叶 pyramidal lobe of thyroid gland
9. 甲状软骨 thyroid cartilage

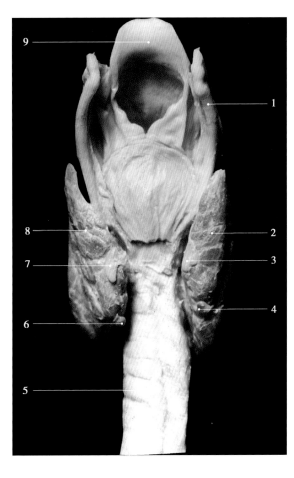

◀ 图 101 甲状旁腺（后面观）
Parathyroid gland.Posterior view

1. 甲状软骨上角 superior cornu of thyroid cartilage
2. 甲状腺右叶 right lobe of thyroid gland
3. 右上甲状旁腺 right superior parathyroid gland
4. 右下甲状旁腺 right inferior parathyroid gland
5. 气管 trachea
6. 左下甲状旁腺 left inferior parathyroid gland
7. 左上甲状旁腺 left superior parathyroid gland
8. 甲状腺左叶 left lobe of thyroid gland
9. 会厌 epiglottis

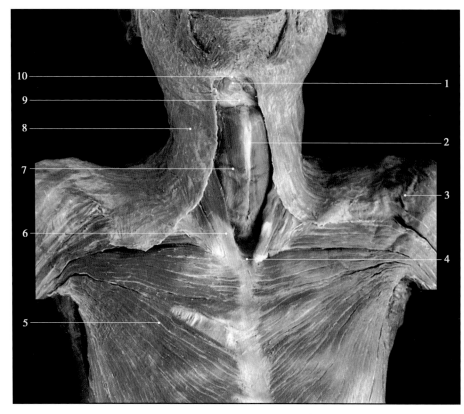

1. 下颌舌骨肌 mylohyoid
2. 喉结 laryngeal prominence
3. 三角肌 deltoid
4. 颈静脉切迹 jugular notch
5. 胸大肌 pectoralis major
6. 胸锁乳突肌胸骨头 sternal head of sternocleidomastoid
7. 胸骨舌骨肌 sternohyoid
8. 颈阔肌 platysma
9. 舌骨 hyoid bone
10. 颏横肌 transversus menti

▲ 图 102 颈部肌（前面观 1）
Muscles of neck.Anterior view（1）

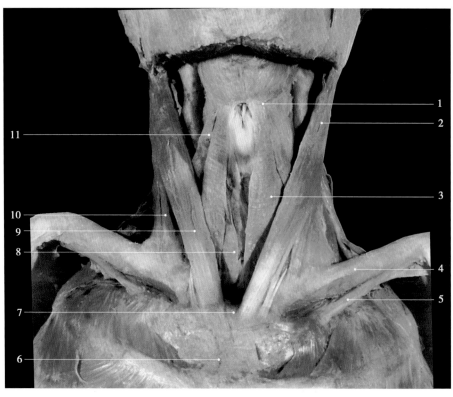

1. 舌骨 hyoid bone
2. 胸锁乳突肌 sternocleidomastoid
3. 胸骨舌骨肌 sternohyoid
4. 锁骨 clavicle
5. 锁骨下肌 subclavius
6. 胸骨柄 manubrium sterni
7. 颈静脉切迹 jugular notch
8. 胸骨甲状肌 sternothyroid
9. 胸锁乳突肌胸骨头 sternal head of sternocleidomastoid
10. 胸锁乳突肌锁骨头 clavicular head of sternocleidomastoid
11. 肩胛舌骨肌 omohyoid

▲ 图 103 颈部肌（前面观 2）
Muscles of neck.Anterior riew（2）

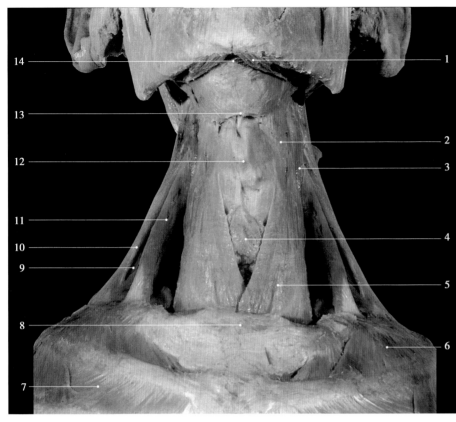

▲ 图 104　颈部肌（前面观 3 ）
Muscles of neck.Anterior view（3）

1. 二腹肌前腹 anterior belly of digastric
2. 甲状舌骨肌 thyrohyoid
3. 头长肌 longus capitis
4. 甲状腺 thyroid gland
5. 胸骨甲状肌 sternothyroid
6. 肋间外肌 intercostales externi
7. 肋间内肌 intercostales interni
8. 胸骨柄 manubrium sterni
9. 斜角肌间隙 scalenus space
10. 中斜角肌 scalenus medius
11. 前斜角肌 scalenus anterior
12. 喉结 laryngeal prominence
13. 舌骨 hyoid bone
14. 下颌舌骨肌 mylohyoid

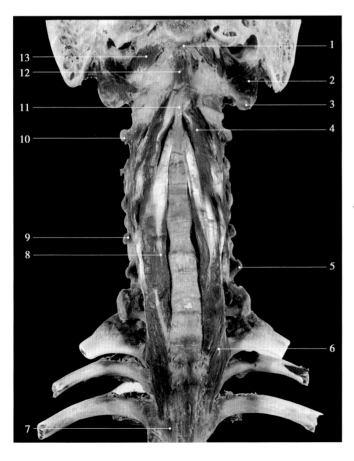

◀ 图 105　颈部肌（前面观 4 ）
Muscles of neck.Anterior view（4）

1. 枕骨基底部 basilar part of occipital bone
2. 头外侧直肌 rectus capitis lateralis
3. 寰椎横突 transverse process of atlas
4. 头长肌 longus capitis
5. 第六颈椎横突 transverse process of the 6th cervical vertebra
6. 颈长肌（下部）longus colli
7. 第三胸椎体 vertebral body of the 3rd thoracic vertebra
8. 颈长肌（中部）longus colli
9. 第五颈椎横突 transverse process of the 5th cervical vertebra
10. 枢椎横突 transverse process of axis
11. 枢椎椎体 vertebral body of axis vertebra
12. 寰椎前结节 anterior tubercle of atlas
13. 头前直肌 rectus capitis anterior

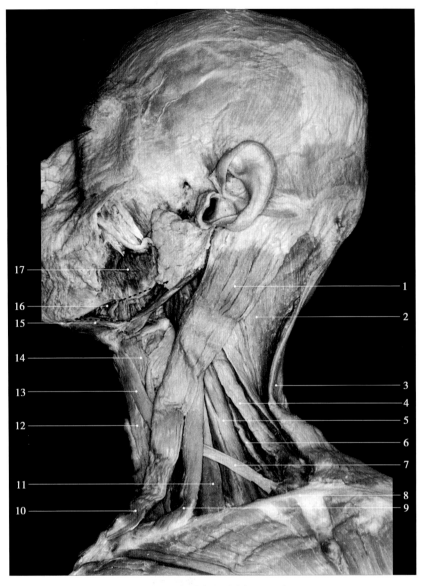

▲ 图 106 颈部肌（侧面观 1）
Muscles of neck.Lateral view（1）

1. 胸锁乳突肌 sternocleidomastoid
2. 头夹肌 splenius capitis
3. 斜方肌 trapezius
4. 肩胛提肌 levator scapulae
5. 中斜角肌 scalenus medius
6. 后斜角肌 scalenus posterior
7. 肩胛舌骨肌下腹 inferior belly of omohyoid
8. 锁骨 clavicle
9. 胸锁乳突肌锁骨头 clavicular head of sternocleidomastoid
10. 胸锁乳突肌胸骨头 sternal head of sternocleidomastoid
11. 前斜角肌 scalenus anterior
12. 胸骨舌骨肌 sternohyoid
13. 肩胛舌骨肌上腹 superior belly of omohyoid
14. 甲状舌骨肌 thyrohyoid
15. 二腹肌前腹 anterior belly of digastric
16. 下颌下三角 submandibular triangle
17. 咬肌 masseter

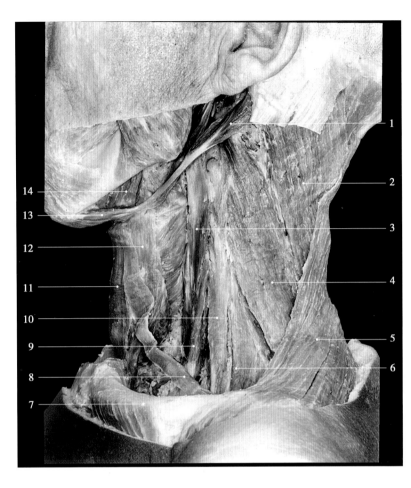

◀图 107　颈部肌（侧面观 2 ）
Muscles of neck.Lateral view (2)

1. 二腹肌后腹 posterior belly of digastric
2. 头夹肌 splenius capitis
3. 头长肌 longus capitis
4. 肩胛提肌 levator scapulae
5. 斜方肌 trapezius
6. 后斜角肌 scalenus posterior
7. 锁骨 clavicle
8. 肩胛舌骨肌 omohyoid
9. 前斜角肌 scalenus anterior
10. 中斜角肌 scalenus medius
11. 胸骨舌骨肌 sternohyoid
12. 甲状舌骨肌 thyrohyoid
13. 二腹肌前腹 anterior belly of digastric
14. 下颌舌骨肌 mylohyoid

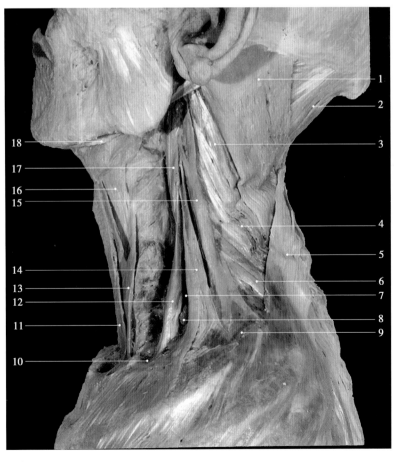

◀图 108　颈部肌（侧面观 3 ）
Muscles of neck.Lateral view (3)

1. 头夹肌 splenius capitis
2. 头半棘肌 semispinalis capitis
3. 颈夹肌 splenius cervicis
4. 颈最长肌 longissimus cervicis
5. 上后锯肌 serratus posterior superior
6. 颈髂肋肌 iliocostalis cervicis
7. 斜角肌间隙 scalenus space
8. 臂丛 brachial plexus
9. 第 2 肋 the 2nd rib
10. 第 1 肋 the 1st rib
11. 胸骨舌骨肌 sternohyoid
12. 前斜角肌 scalenus anterior
13. 胸骨甲状肌 sternothyroid
14. 中斜角肌 scalenus medius
15. 后斜角肌 scalenus posterior
16. 甲状舌骨肌 thyrohyoid
17. 头长肌 longus capitis
18. 二腹肌前腹 anterior belly of digastric

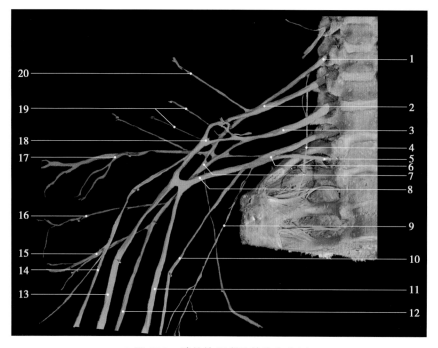

▲ 图 109　臂丛的组成及其分支（1）

Component of brachial plexus and its branches（1）

1. 第 5 颈神经 the 5th cervical n.
2. 上干 superior trunk
3. 中干 middle trunk
4. 膈神经 phrenic n.
5. 第 1 胸神经 the 1st thoracic n.
6. 下干 inferior trunk
7. 后束 posterior cord
8. 内侧束 medial cord
9. 臂内侧皮神经 medial brachial cutaneous n.
10. 前臂内侧皮神经 medial antebrachial cutaneous n.
11. 尺神经 ulnar n.
12. 桡神经 radial n.
13. 正中神经 median n.
14. 肌皮神经 musculocutaneous n.
15. 前臂后神经 posterior antebrachial cutaneous n.
16. 臂下外侧皮神经 inferior lateral brachial cutaneous n.
17. 腋神经 axillary n.
18. 外侧束 lateral cord
19. 肩胛下神经 subscapular n.
20. 肩胛背神经 dorsal scapular n.

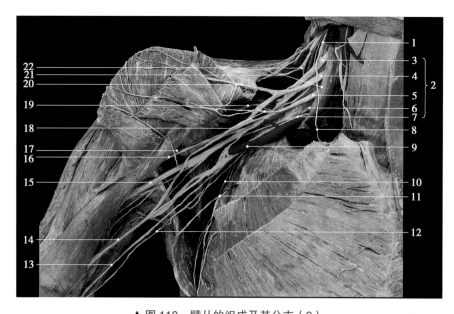

▲ 图 110　臂丛的组成及其分支（2）

Component of brachial plexus and its branches（2）

1. 第 4 颈神经 the 4th cervical n.
2. 臂丛 brachial plexus
3. 第 5 颈神经 the 5th cervical n.
4. 第 6 颈神经 the 6th cervical n.
5. 第 7 颈神经 the 7th cervical n.
6. 第 8 颈神经 the 8th cervical n.
7. 第 1 胸神经 the 1st thoracic n.
8. 膈神经 phrenic n.
9. 腋动脉 axillary a.
10. 胸长神经 long thoracic n.
11. 肋间臂神经 intercostobrachial n.
12. 前臂内侧皮神经 medial antebrachial cutaneous n.
13. 尺神经 ulnar n.
14. 正中神经 median n.
15. 桡神经 radial n.
16. 肌皮神经 musculocutaneous n.
17. 腋神经 axillary n.
18. 胸内侧神经 medial pectoral n.
19. 肩胛上神经 suprascapular n.
20. 胸外侧神经 lateral pectoral n.
21. 前斜角肌 scalenus anterior
22. 肩胛背神经 dorsal scapular n.

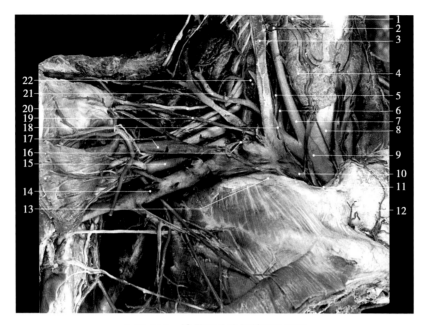

▲ 图 111 锁骨下动脉与锁骨下静脉
Subclavian artery and subclavian vein

1. 甲状腺上动脉 superior thyroid a.
2. 甲状腺上静脉 superior thyroid v.
3. 右颈内静脉 right internal jugular v.
4. 甲状腺 thyroid gland
5. 甲状腺下动脉 inferior thyroid a.
6. 椎动脉 vertebral a.
7. 右颈总动脉 right common carotid a.
8. 气管 trachea
9. 头臂干 brachiocephalic trunk
10. 头臂静脉 brachiocephalic v.
11. 锁切迹 clavicular notch
12. 胸骨柄 manubrium sterni
13. 第 1 肋 the 1st rib
14. 锁骨下静脉 subclavian v.
15. 锁骨下动脉 subclavian a.
16. 右淋巴导管 right lymphatic duct
17. 头静脉 cephalic v.
18. 膈神经 phrenic n.
19. 肩胛上动脉 suprascapular a.
20. 肩胛上神经 suprascapular n.
21. 颈横动脉 transverse cervical a.
22. 前斜角肌 scalenus anterior

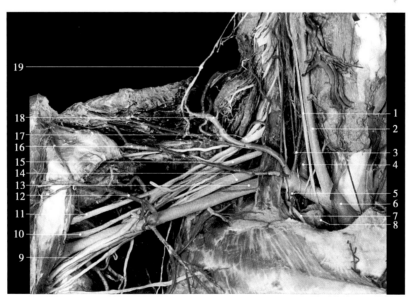

▲ 图 112 锁骨下动脉与臂丛
Subclavian artery and brachial plexus

1. 右迷走神经 right vagus n.
2. 右颈总动脉 right common carotid a.
3. 甲状腺下动脉 inferior thyroid a.
4. 椎动脉 vertebral a.
5. 胸廓内动脉 internal thoracic a.
6. 头臂干 brachiocephalic trunk
7. 膈神经 phrenic n.
8. 右头臂静脉 right brachiocephalic v.
9. 正中神经 median n.
10. 肌皮神经 musculocutaneous n.
11. 腋神经 axillary n.
12. 胸肩峰动脉 thoracoacromial a.
13. 右锁骨下动脉 right subclavian a.
14. 下干 inferior trunk
15. 中干 middle trunk
16. 肩胛上动脉 suprascapular a.
17. 上干 superior trunk
18. 颈横动脉 transverse cervical a.
19. 副神经 accessory n.

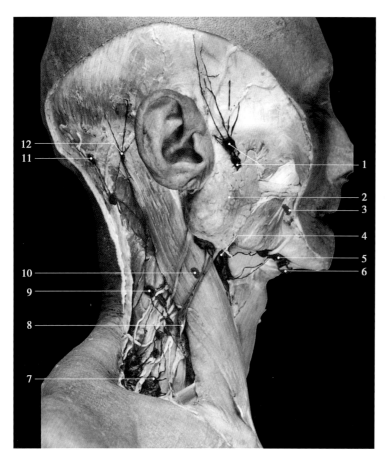

◀ 图 113　颈部的淋巴管和淋巴结（1）
Lymph vessels and nodes of neck（1）

1. 腮腺浅淋巴结 superficial parotid lymph nodes
2. 腮腺 parotid gland
3. 颊肌淋巴结 buccal lymph node
4. 颈内静脉二腹肌淋巴结 jugulodigastric lymph nodes
5. 下颌下淋巴结 submandibular lymph node
6. 颏下淋巴结 submental lymph nodes
7. 锁骨上淋巴结 supraclavicular lymph nodes
8. 颈外静脉 external jugular v.
9. 副神经淋巴结 lymph nodes of accessory n.
10. 颈外侧浅淋巴结 superficial lateral cervical lymph nodes
11. 枕淋巴结 occipital lymph nodes
12. 乳突淋巴结 mastoid lymph nodes

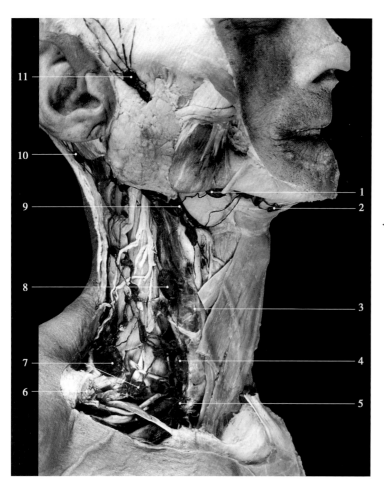

◀ 图 114　颈部的淋巴管和淋巴结（2）
Lymph vessels and nodes of neck（2）

1. 下颌下淋巴结 submandibular lymph nodes
2. 颏下淋巴结 submental lymph nodes
3. 颈内静脉 internal jugular v.
4. 颈外侧下深淋巴结 inferior deep lateral cervical lymph nodes
5. 右淋巴导管 right lymphatic duct
6. 锁骨 clavicle
7. 锁骨上淋巴结 supraclavicular lymph nodes
8. 颈内静脉肩胛舌骨肌淋巴结 juguloomohyoid lymph node
9. 颈内静脉二腹肌淋巴结 jugulodigastric lymph node
10. 乳突淋巴结 mastoid lymph nodes
11. 腮腺浅淋巴结 superficial parotid lymph nodes

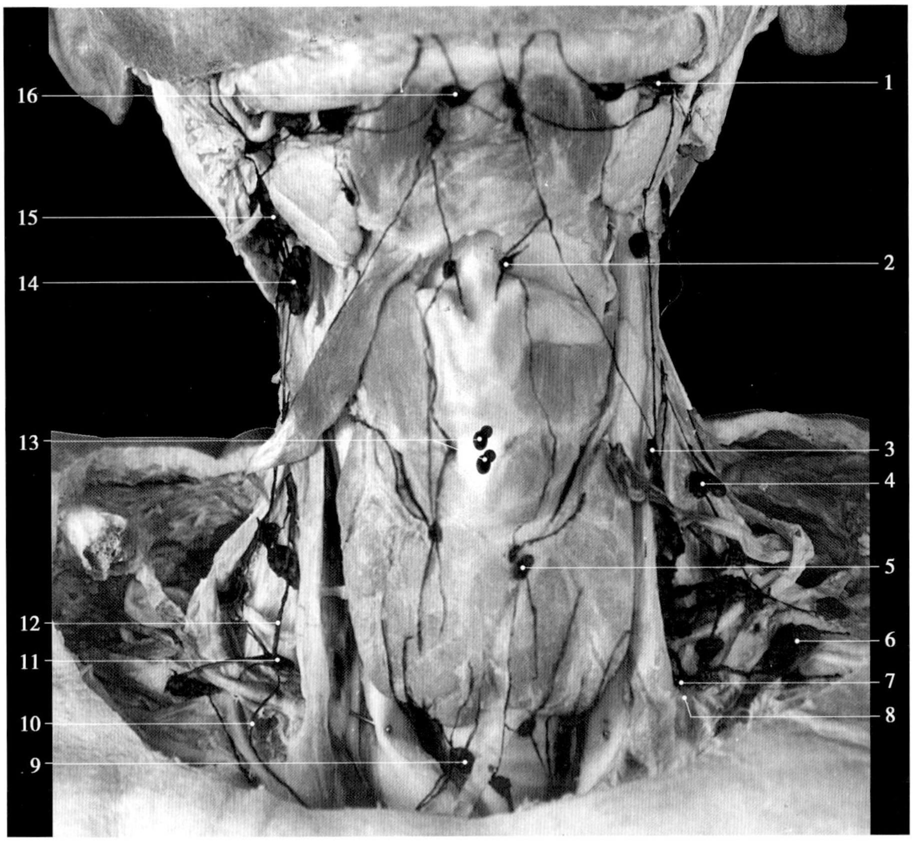

▲ 图 115 颈部的淋巴管和淋巴结（3）
Lymph vessels and nodes of neck（3）

1. 下颌下淋巴结 submandibular lymph nodes
2. 舌骨下淋巴结 infrahyoid lymph nodes
3. 颈内静脉外侧淋巴结 lateral jugular lymph nodes
4. 颈内静脉肩胛舌骨肌淋巴结 juguloomohyoid lymph node
5. 甲状腺淋巴结 thyroid lymph nodes
6. 锁骨上淋巴结 supraclavicular lymph nodes
7. 胸导管 thoracic duct
8. 左静脉角 left venous angle
9. 气管前淋巴结 pretracheal lymph nodes
10. 右支气管纵隔干 right bronchomediastinal trunk
11. 右淋巴导管 right lymphatic duct
12. 右颈干 right jugular trunk
13. 喉前淋巴结 prelaryngeal lymph nodes
14. 颈内静脉前淋巴结 anterior jugular lymph node
15. 颈内静脉二腹肌淋巴结 jugulodigastric lymph nodes
16. 颏下淋巴结 submental lymph nodes

连续层次局部解剖

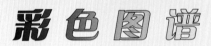

第三章

胸　部

Chapter 3　Thorax

　　胸部上界以颈静脉切迹、胸锁关节、锁骨上缘、肩峰和第 7 颈椎棘突的连线与颈、项部分界。下界自剑胸结合向两侧沿肋弓、第 11 肋前端、第 12 肋下缘至第 12 胸椎棘突与腹部分界。上部两侧以三角肌前、后缘上份和腋前、后襞下缘与胸壁相交处的连线与上肢分界。

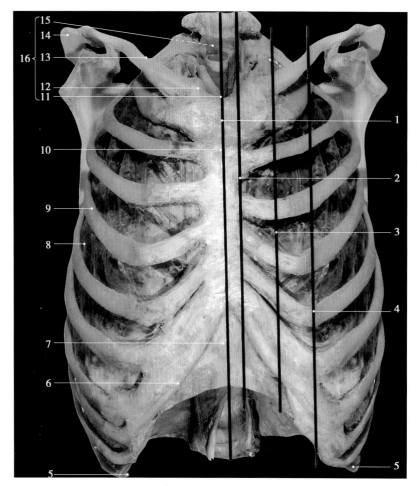

◀ 图 116　胸前壁的标志线
Marking line on anterior thoracic wall

1. 前正中线 anterior median line
2. 胸骨线 sternal line
3. 胸骨旁线 parasternal line
4. 锁骨中线 midclavicular line
5. 第 11 肋前端 anterior extremity of the 11th costal bone
6. 肋弓 costal arch
7. 剑突 xiphoid process
8. 肋间隙 intercostal space
9. 肋骨 costal bone
10. 胸骨角 sternal angle
11. 颈静脉切迹 jugular notch
12. 胸锁关节 sternoclavicular joint
13. 锁骨上缘 superior border of clavicle
14. 肩峰 acromion
15. 第 7 颈椎棘突 spinous process of the 7th cervical vertebra
16. 胸部上界 upper bound of thoracic region

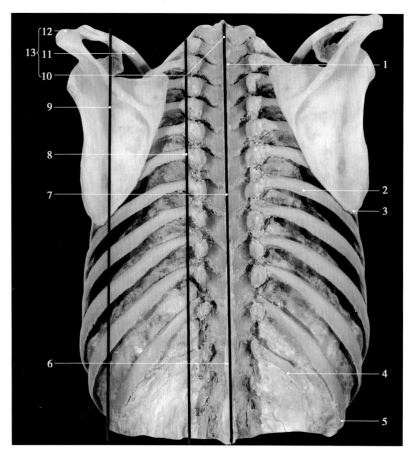

◀ 图 117　胸后壁的标志线
Marking line on posterior thoracic wall

1. 第 1 胸椎棘突 spinous process of the 1st thoracic vertebra
2. 第 7 肋骨 the 7th costal bone
3. 下角 inferior angle
4. 第 12 肋下缘 inferior border of the 12th costal bone
5. 第 11 肋骨 the 11th costal bone
6. 第 12 胸椎棘突 spinous process of the the 12th thoracic vertebra
7. 后正中线 posterior median line
8. 脊柱旁线 paravertebral line
9. 肩胛线 scapular line
10. 第 7 颈椎棘突 spinous process of the 7th cervical vertebra
11. 锁骨上缘 superior border of clavicle
12. 肩峰 acromion
13. 胸部上界 upper bound of thoracic region

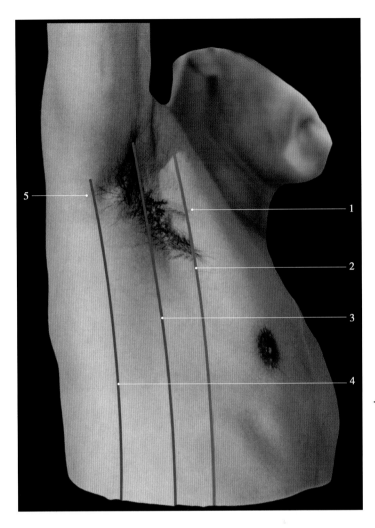

◀图118　胸外侧壁的标志线
Marking line on lateral thoracic wall

1. 腋前襞 plica axillaris anterior
2. 腋前线 anterior axillary line
3. 腋中线 midaxillary line
4. 腋后线 posterior axillary line
5. 腋后襞 plica axillaris posterior

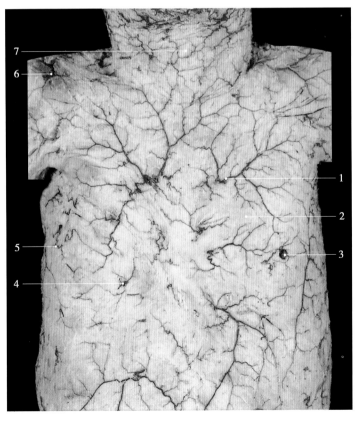

◀图119　胸部浅筋膜及皮动脉
Superficial fascia and cutaneous arteries of thorax

1. 胸廓内动脉第2穿支 the 2nd perforating branch of internal thoracic a.
2. 浅筋膜 superficial fascia
3. 乳头 nipple
4. 胸廓内动脉穿支 perforating branch of internal thoracic a.
5. 肋间后动脉外侧皮支 lateral cutaneous branch of posterior intercostal a.
6. 胸肩峰动脉肩峰支 acromal branch of thoracoacromial a.
7. 颈浅筋膜 superficial cervical fascia

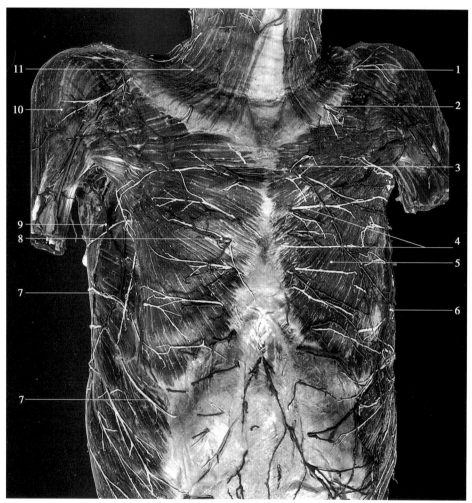

▲ 图 120　胸前外侧壁的浅血管和皮神经
Superficial blood vessels and cutaneous nerves of anterolateral thoracic wall

1. 胸肩峰动脉肩峰支 acromial branch of thoracoacromial a.
2. 锁骨上神经 supraclavicular n.
3. 胸廓内动、静脉穿支 perforating branch of internal thoracic a.and v.
4. 肋间神经前皮支 anterior cutaneous branches of intercostal n.
5. 胸大肌 pectoralis major
6. 胸腹壁静脉 thoracoepigastric v.
7. 肋间神经外侧皮支 lateral culaneous branches of intercostal n.
8. 乳房内侧支（女性）medial marmmary branches
9. 肱胸皮动脉 brachii thoracic cutaneous a.
10. 三角肌 deltoid
11. 颈阔肌 platysma

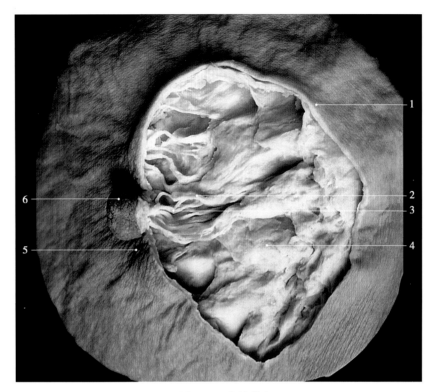

▲ 图 121　女性乳房
Female marmma

1. 皮肤 skin
2. 输乳管 lactiferous duct
3. 输乳管窦 lactiferous sinuses
4. 乳腺小叶 lobule of mammary gland
5. 乳晕 areola of breast
6. 乳头 nipple

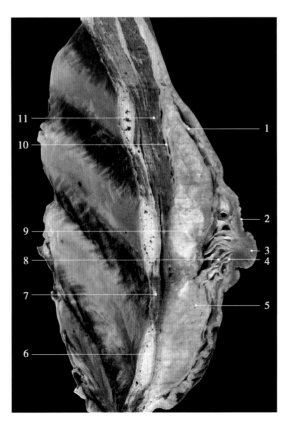

◀ 图 122　女性乳房（矢状切面）
Female mamma.Sagittal section

1. 乳房悬韧带 suspensory ligament of breast
2. 乳晕 areola of breast
3. 乳头 nipple
4. 输乳管窦 lactiferous sinuses
5. 乳房脂肪体 adipose body of mamma
6. 肋骨 costal bone
7. 肋间肌 intercostales
8. 输乳管 lactiferous duct
9. 乳腺小叶 lobules of mammary gland
10. 胸肌筋膜 pectoral fascia
11. 胸大肌 pectoralis major

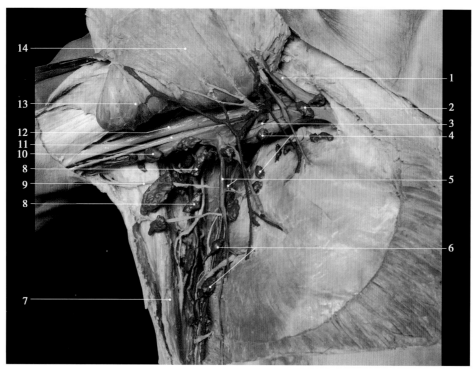

▲ 图 123　腋淋巴结
Axillary lymph nodes

1. 头静脉 cephalic v.
2. 尖淋巴结 apical lymph nodes
3. 腋静脉 axillary v.
4. 中央淋巴结 central lymph nodes
5. 胸外侧动、静脉 lateral thoracica a.and v.
6. 胸肌淋巴结 pectoral lymph nodes
7. 背阔肌 latissimus dorsi

8. 肩胛下淋巴结 subscapular lymph nodes
9. 肋间臂神经 intercostobrachial n.
10. 外侧淋巴结 lateral lymph nodes
11. 尺神经 ulnar n.
12. 正中神经 median n.
13. 胸大肌 pectoralis major
14. 胸小肌 pectoralis minor

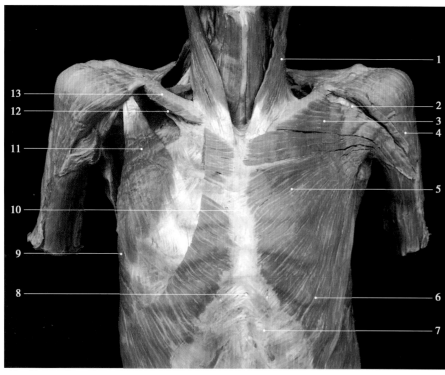

1. 胸锁乳突肌 sternocleidomastoid
2. 三角肌胸肌间沟 deltopectoral groove
3. 胸大肌锁骨部 clavicular part of pectoralis major
4. 三角肌 deltoid
5. 胸大肌胸骨部 sternal part of pectoralis major
6. 胸大肌腹部 abdominal part of pectoralis major
7. 腹直肌鞘前层 anterior layer of sheath of rectus abdominis
8. 剑突 xiphoid process
9. 前锯肌 serratus anterior
10. 胸骨 sternum
11. 胸小肌 pectoralis minor
12. 锁骨下肌 subclavius
13. 锁骨 clavicle

▲ 图 124　胸前外侧壁肌
Muscles of anterolateral thoracic wall

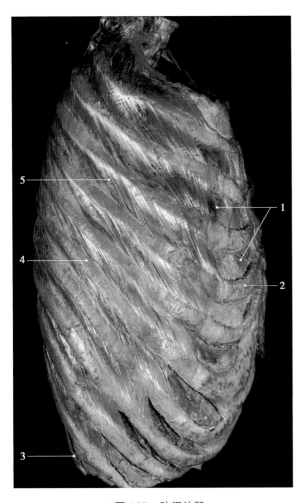

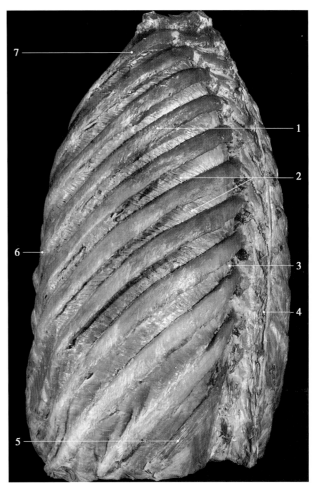

▲ 图 125　肋间外肌
Intercostales externi

1. 壁胸膜 parietal pleura
2. 肋软骨 costal cartilage
3. 第 12 肋 the 12th rib
4. 肋骨 rib
5. 肋间外肌 intercostales externi

▲ 图 126　肋间内肌
Intercostales interni

1. 第 4 肋 the 4th rib
2. 肋间内肌 intercostales interni
3. 壁胸膜 parietal pleura
4. 棘突 spinous process
5. 第 12 肋 the 12th rib
6. 胸骨 sternum
7. 第 1 肋 the 1st rib

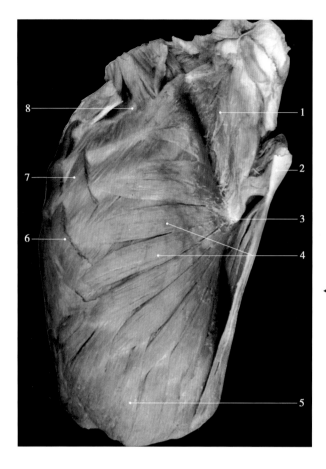

◀ 图 127　前锯肌
Serratus anterior

1. 肩胛下肌 subscapularis
2. 背阔肌 latissimus dorsi
3. 肩胛骨下角 inferior angle of scapula
4. 前锯肌 serratus anterior
5. 腹外斜肌 obliquus externus abdominis
6. 胸大肌（切断）pectoralis major
7. 胸小肌（切断）pectoralis minor
8. 第 1 肋 the 1st rib

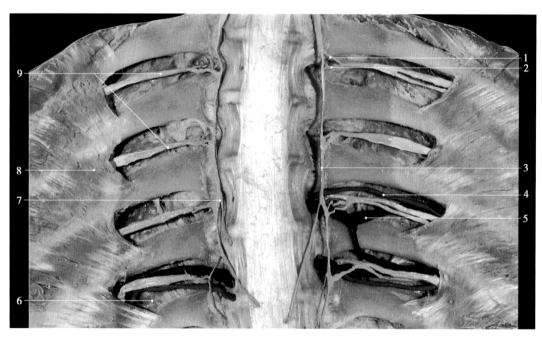

▲ 图 128　肋间神经与肋间后动、静脉
Intercostal nerves and posterior intercostal arteries，veins

1. 灰交通支 gray communicating branch
2. 白交通支 white communicating branch
3. 交感干 sympathetic trunk
4. 肋间后动脉 posterior intercostal a.
5. 肋间后静脉 posterior intercostal v.
6. 肋间外肌 intercostales externi
7. 交感干神经节 ganglia of sympathetic trunk
8. 肋间内肌 intercostales interni
9. 肋间神经 intercostal n.

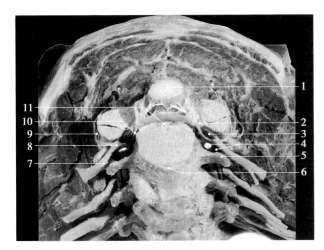

◀图 129 脊神经前、后支（上面观）
Posterior and anterior branch of spinal nerves.
Superior view

1. 脊髓 spinal cord
2. 后根 posterior root
3. 脊神经节 spinal ganglia
4. 椎动、静脉 vertebral a.and v.
5. 横突 transverse process
6. 前纵韧带 anterior longitudinal lig.
7. 脊神经前支 anterior branch of spinal n.
8. 脊神经 spinal n.
9. 脊神经后支 posterior branch of spinal n.
10. 前根 anterior root
11. 后纵韧带 posterio longitudinal lig.

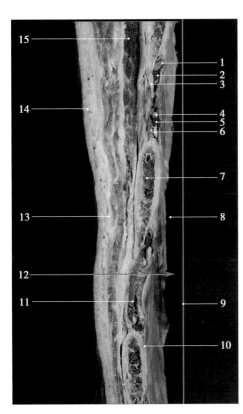

▲ 图 130　胸壁层次及胸膜腔穿刺部位
（胸前外侧壁 肩胛线外侧）
Different layers of thoracic wall and position for puncturing
pleural cavity.Lateral side of scapular line

1. 肋间后静脉上支 superior branch of posterior intercostal v.
2. 肋间后动脉上支 superior branch of posterior intercostal a.
3. 肋间神经上支 superior branch of intercostal n.
4. 肋间后静脉下支 inferior branch of posterior intercostal v.
5. 肋间后动脉下支 inferior branch of posterior intercostal a.
6. 肋间神经下支 inferior branch of intercostal n.
7. 肋骨 costal bone
8. 胸膜腔 pleural cavity
9. 脏胸膜 visceral pleura
10. 壁胸膜 parietal pleura
11. 肋间内肌 intercostales interni
12. 穿刺部位（肋间隙中部） position for puncture
13. 浅筋膜 superficial fascia
14. 皮肤 skin
15. 胸壁肌 muscles of thoracic wall

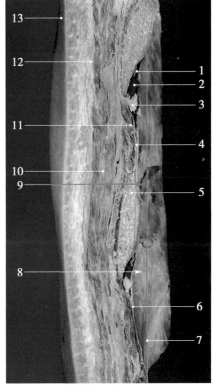

▲ 图 131　胸壁层次及胸膜腔穿刺部位
（胸后壁 肩胛线内侧）
Different layers of thoracic wall and position for puncturing
pleural cavity.Midial side of scapular line

1. 肋间后静脉 posterior intercostal v.
2. 肋间后动脉 posterior intercostal a.
3. 肋间神经 intercostal n.
4. 胸内筋膜 endothoracica fascia
5. 肋骨上缘 superior border of costal bone
6. 壁胸膜 parietal pleura
7. 脏胸膜 visceral pleura
8. 胸膜腔 pleural cavity
9. 穿刺部位（肋骨上缘部） postition for puncture
10. 胸壁肌 muscles of thoracic wall
11. 肋间内肌 intercostales interni
12. 浅筋膜 superficial fascia
13. 皮肤 skin

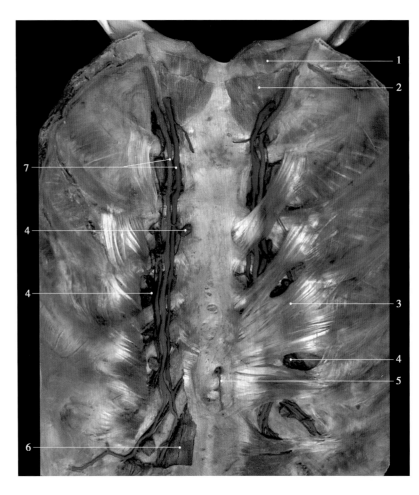

◀ 图 132 胸廓内动脉、静脉和胸骨旁淋巴结
Internal thoracic arteries，veins and parasternal lymph nodes

1. 胸骨舌骨肌 sternohyoid
2. 胸骨甲状肌 sternothyroid
3. 胸横肌 transversus thoracis
4. 胸骨旁淋巴结 parasternal lymph nodes
5. 剑突 xiphoid process
6. 腹直肌 rectus abdominis
7. 胸廓内动、静脉 internal thoracic a.and v.

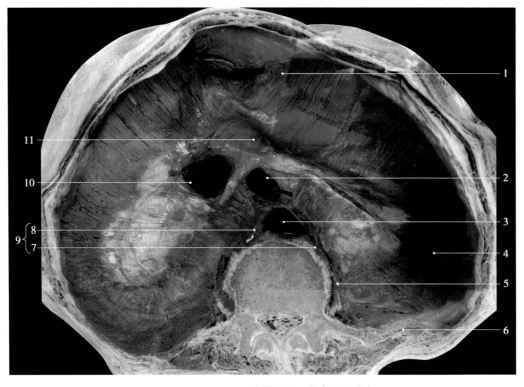

1. 胸骨部
   sternal part
2. 食管裂孔
   esophageal hiatus
3. 主动脉裂孔
   aortic hiatus
4. 肋部
   costal part
5. 腰大肌
   psoas major
6. 腰方肌
   quadratus lumborum
7. 左脚
   left crus
8. 右脚
   right crus
9. 腰部
   lumbar part
10. 腔静脉孔
    vena caval foramen
11. 中心腱
    central tendon

▲ 图 133 膈（下面观）
Diaphragm.Inferior view

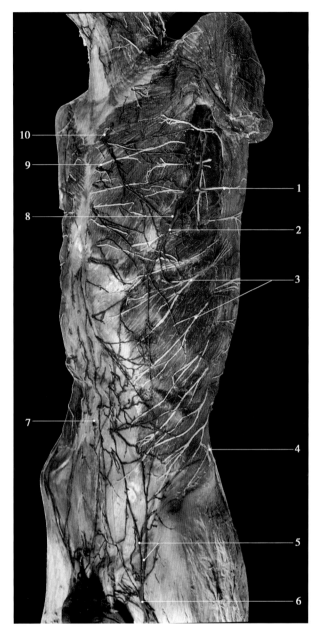

▲ 图 134　肋间神经外侧皮支及胸腹壁浅血管（前外侧面观）
Lateral cutaneous branches of intercostal nerves and superficial blood
vessels of thoraco abdominal wall.Anterolateral view

1. 肋间神经外侧皮支的后支 posterior branch of lateral cutaneous branch of intercostal n.
2. 胸腹壁静脉 thoracoepigastric v.
3. 肋间神经外侧皮支的前支 anterior branch of lateral cutaneous branch of intercostal n.
4. 髂腹下神经外侧皮支 lateral cutaneous branch of iliohypogastric n.
5. 腹壁浅静脉 superficial epigastric v.
6. 大隐静脉 great saphenous v.
7. 脐 omphalos
8. 肱胸皮动脉 brachii thoracic cutaneous a.
9. 肋间神经前皮支的外侧支 lateral branch of anterior cutaneous branch of intercostal n.
10. 胸廓内动脉穿支 perforator branches of interal thoracic a.

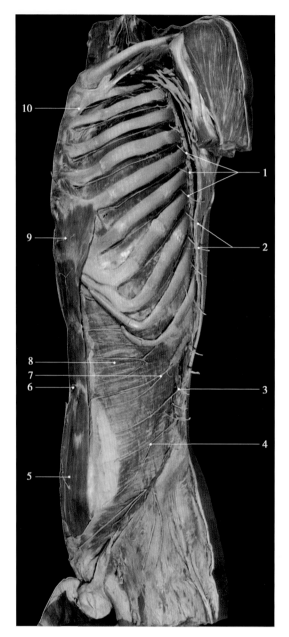

▲ 图 135　肋间神经的分布
Distribution of intercostal nerves

1. 第 4、5、6 肋间神经外侧皮支（女性乳腺外侧支）lateral cutaneous
   branches of the 4th、5th and 6th intercostal n.
2. 肋间神经外侧皮支 lateral cutaneous branch of intercostal n.
3. 肋下神经 subcostal n.
4. 髂腹下神经 iliohypogastric n.
5. 腹直肌 rectus abdominis
6. 脐 umbilicus
7. 第 11 肋间神经前皮支 anterior cutaneous branch of the 11th intercostal n.
8. 腹横肌 transversus abdominis
9. 第 5 肋间神经前皮支 anterior cutaneous branch of the 5th intercostal n.
10. 第 1 肋间神经前皮支 anterior cutaneous branch of the 1st intercostal n.

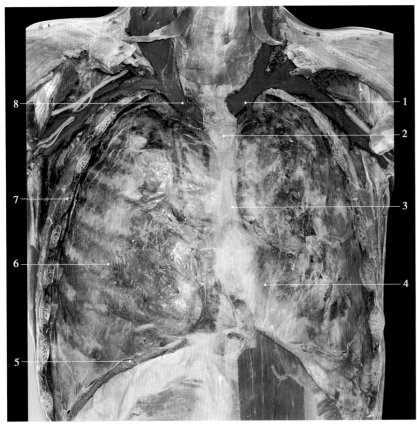

1. 左头臂静脉 left brachiocephalic v.
2. 胸腺 thymus
3. 前纵隔 anterior mediastinum
4. 心包 pericardium
5. 膈 diaphragm
6. 壁胸膜 parietal pleura
7. 肋骨 costal bone
8. 右头臂静脉 right brachiocephalic v.

▲ 图 136 壁胸膜（前面观）
Parietal pleura.Anterior view

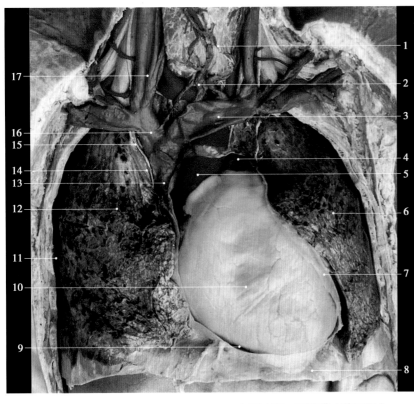

1. 甲状腺 thyroid gland
2. 甲状腺下静脉 inferior thyroid v.
3. 左头臂静脉 left brachiocephalic v.
4. 肺动脉干 pulmonary trunk
5. 升主动脉 ascending aorta
6. 左肺 left lung
7. 心包 pericardium
8. 膈 diaphragm
9. 心包腔 pericardial cavity
10. 心 heart
11. 胸膜腔 pleural cavity
12. 脏胸膜 visceral pleura
13. 上腔静脉 superior vena cava
14. 纵隔胸膜 mediastinal pleura
15. 膈神经 phrenic n.
16. 右头臂静脉 right brachiocephalic v.
17. 右颈内静脉 right internal jugular v.

▲ 图 137 脏胸膜（前面观）
Visceral pleura.Anterior view

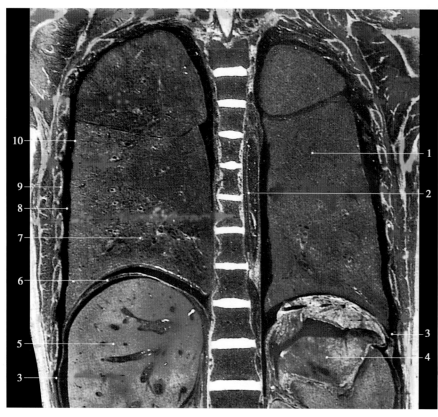

1. 左肺 left lung
2. 胸主动脉 thoracic aorta
3. 肋膈隐窝 costodiaphragmatic recess
4. 胃 stomach
5. 肝 liver
6. 膈 diaphragm
7. 右肺 right lung
8. 胸膜腔 pleural cavity
9. 壁胸膜 parietal pleura
10. 脏胸膜 visceral pleura

▲ 图 138　胸膜腔（冠状切面）
Pleural cavity.Coronal section

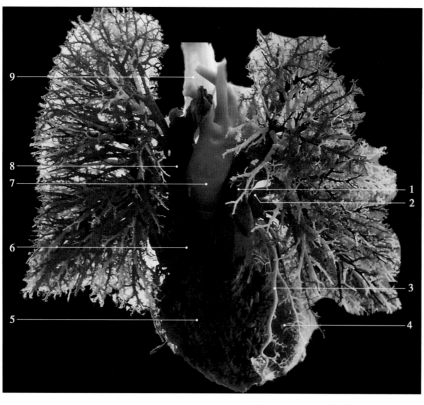

1. 肺动脉干 pulmonary trunk
2. 左肺静脉 left pulmonary v.
3. 前室间支 anterior interventricular branch
4. 左心室 left ventricle
5. 右心室 right ventricle
6. 右冠状动脉 right coronary a.
7. 升主动脉 ascending aorta
8. 上腔静脉 superior vena cava
9. 气管 trachea

▲ 图 139　心与肺的铸形
Cast of heard and lungs

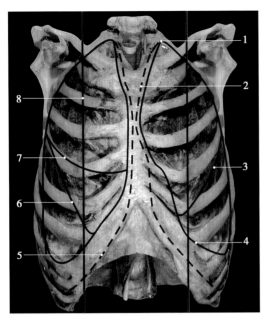

▲ 图 140　胸膜和肺的体表投影（前面观）
Surface projection of pleura and lung.Anterior view

1. 胸膜顶 cupula of pleura
2. 胸膜前线 anterior line of pleura
3. 左肺斜裂 oblique fissure of left lung
4. 肺下缘 inferior border of lung
5. 胸膜下线 inferior line of pleura
6. 右肺斜裂 oblique fissure of right lung
7. 水平裂 horizontal fissure
8. 锁骨中线 midclavicular line

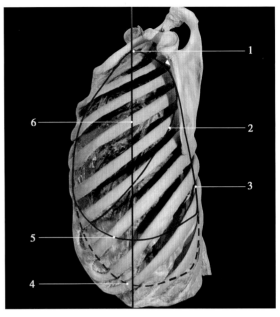

▲ 图 141　胸膜和肺体表投影（左侧面观）
Surface projection of pleura and lung.Left view

1. 胸膜顶 cupula of pleura
2. 斜裂 oblique fissure
3. 左肺后缘 inferior border of left lung
4. 胸膜下线 inferior line of pleura
5. 左肺下缘 inferior border of left lung
6. 腋中线 midaxillary line

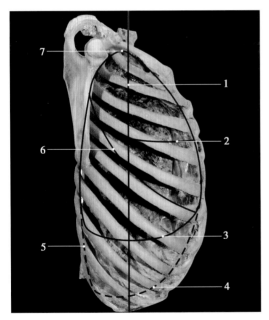

▲ 图 142　胸膜和肺体表投影（右侧面观）
Surface projection of pleura and lung.Right view

1. 腋中线 midaxillary line
2. 水平裂 horizontal fissure
3. 右肺下缘 inferior border of right lung
4. 胸膜下线 inferior line of pleura
5. 胸膜后线 posterior line of pleura
6. 斜裂 oblique fissure
7. 胸膜顶 cupula of pleura

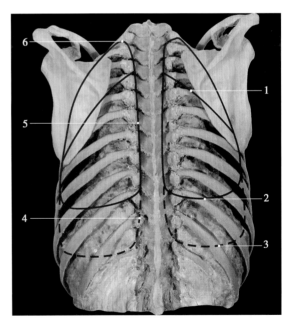

▲ 图 143　胸膜和肺体表投影（后面观）
Surface projection of pleura and lung.Posterior view

1. 斜裂 oblique fissure
2. 右肺下缘 inferior border of right lung
3. 胸膜下线 inferior line of pleura
4. 胸膜后线 posterior line of pleura
5. 左肺后缘 posterior border of left lung
6. 胸膜顶 cupula of pleura

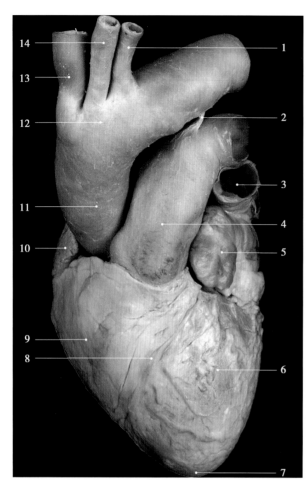

◀图 144　心（前面观）
Heart.Anterior view

1. 左锁骨下动脉 left subclavian a.
2. 动脉韧带 arterial lig.
3. 左肺静脉 left pulmonary v.
4. 肺动脉干 pulmonary trunk
5. 左心耳 left auricle
6. 左心室 left ventricle
7. 心尖 cardiac apex
8. 前室间沟 anterior interventricular groove
9. 右心室 right ventricle
10. 右心耳 right auricle
11. 升主动脉 ascending aorta
12. 主动脉弓 aortic arch
13. 头臂干 brachiocephalic trunk
14. 左颈总动脉 left common carotid a.

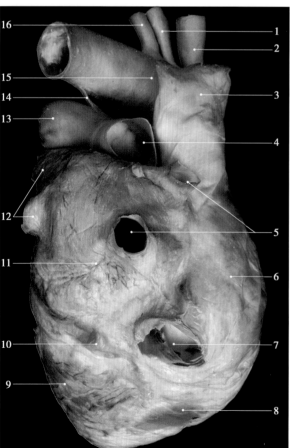

◀图 145　心（后面观）
Heart.Posterior view

1. 左颈总动脉 left common carotid a.
2. 头臂干 brachiocephalic trunk
3. 上腔静脉 superior vena cava
4. 右肺动脉 right pulmonary a.
5. 右肺静脉 right pulmonary v.
6. 右心房 right atrium
7. 下腔静脉 inferior vena cava
8. 右心室 right ventricle
9. 左心室 left ventricle
10. 冠状窦 coronary sinus
11. 左心房 left atrium
12. 左肺静脉 left pulmonary v.
13. 左肺动脉 left pulmonary a.
14. 动脉韧带 arterial lig.
15. 主动脉弓 aortic arch
16. 左锁骨下动脉 left subclavian a.

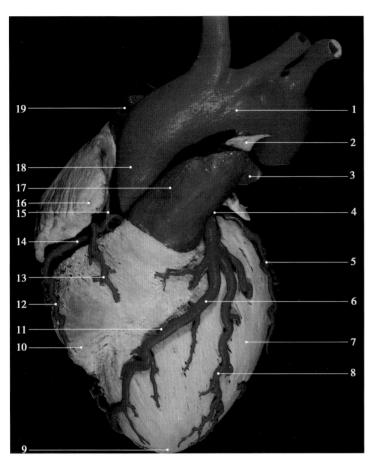

◀图 146　冠状动脉（前面观）
Coronary arteries.Anterior view

1. 主动脉弓 aortic arch
2. 动脉韧带 arterial lig.
3. 左肺动脉 left pulmonary a.
4. 左冠状动脉 left coronary a.
5. 左缘支 left marginal branch
6. 前室间支 anterior interventricular branch
7. 左心室 left ventricle
8. 左室前支 anterior branch of left ventricle
9. 心尖 cardiac apex
10. 右心室 right ventricle
11. 室间隔前支 anterior branches of interventricular septum
12. 右缘支 right marginal branch
13. 右室前支 anterior branch of right ventricle
14. 右冠状动脉 right coronary a.
15. 窦房结支 branch of sinuatrial node
16. 右心耳 right auricle
17. 肺动脉干 pulmonary trunk
18. 升主动脉 ascending aorta
19. 上腔静脉 superior vena cava

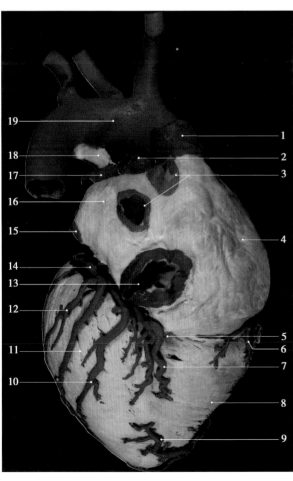

◀图 147　冠状动脉（后面观）
Coronary arteries.Posterior view

1. 上腔静脉 superior vena cava
2. 右肺动脉 right pulmonary a.
3. 右肺静脉 right pulmonary v.
4. 右心房 right atrium
5. 房室结支 branch of atrioventricular node
6. 右缘支 right marginal branch
7. 后室间支 posterior interventricular branch
8. 右心室 right ventricle
9. 前室间支 anterior interventricular branch
10. 左室后支 posterior branch of left ventricle
11. 左心室 left ventricle
12. 左缘支 left marginal branch
13. 下腔静脉 inferior vena cava
14. 旋支 circumflex branch
15. 左肺静脉 left pulmonary v.
16. 左心房 left atrium
17. 左肺动脉 left pulmonary a.
18. 动脉韧带 arterial lig.
19. 主动脉弓 aortic arch

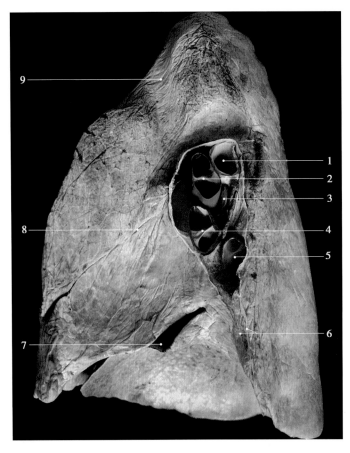

◀ 图 148　右肺门及肺根
Right hilum and root of lung

1. 右主支气管 right principal bronchus
2. 右肺动脉 right pulmonary a.
3. 支气管肺门淋巴结 bronchopulmonary hilar lymph nodes
4. 右上肺静脉 right superior pulmonary v.
5. 右下肺静脉 right inferior pulmonary v.
6. 肺韧带 pulmonary lig.
7. 斜裂 oblique fissure
8. 右肺水平裂 horizontal fissure of right lung
9. 锁骨下动脉沟 sulcus for subclavian a.

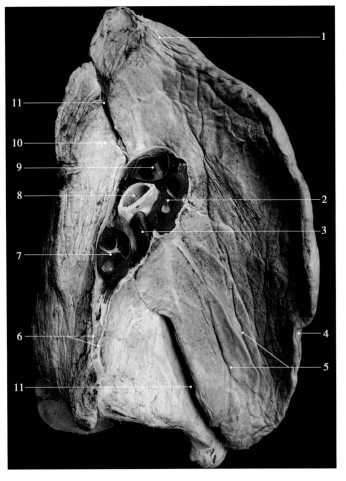

◀ 图 149　左肺门及肺根
Left hilum and root of lung

1. 锁骨下动脉沟 sulcus for subclavian a.
2. 左上肺静脉 left superior pulmonary v.
3. 支气管肺门淋巴结 bronchopulmonary hilar lymph nodes
4. 左肺心切迹 cardiac notch of left lung
5. 心压迹 cardiac impression
6. 肺韧带 pulmonary lig.
7. 左下肺静脉 left inferior pulmonary v.
8. 左主支气管 left principal bronchus
9. 左肺动脉 left pulmonary a.
10. 主动脉沟 sulcus for aorta
11. 斜裂 oblique fissure

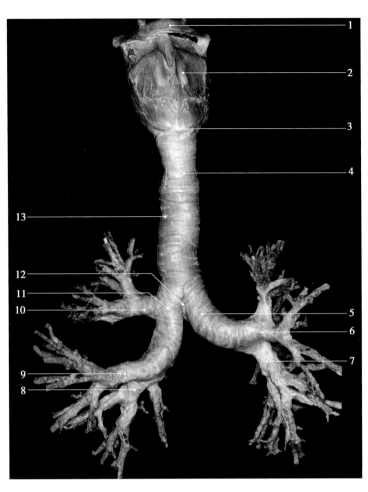

◀ 图 150　气管及支气管（前面观）
Trachea and bronchi.Anterior view

1. 舌骨 hyoid bone
2. 甲状软骨 thyroid cartilage
3. 环状软骨 cricoid cartilage
4. 气管软骨 tracheal cartilage
5. 左主支气管 left principal bronchus
6. 左肺上叶支气管 left superior lobar bronchus
7. 左肺下叶支气管 left inferior lobar bronchus
8. 右肺下叶支气管 right inferior lobar bronchus
9. 右肺中叶支气管 right middle lobar bronchus
10. 右肺上叶支气管 right superior lobar bronchus
11. 右主支气管 right principal bronchus
12. 气管杈 bifurcation of trachea
13. 环状韧带 annular lig.

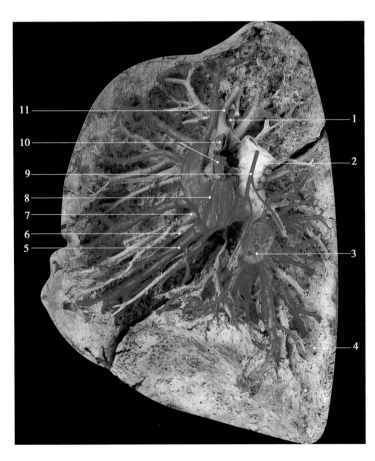

◀ 图 151　支气管肺段的结构
Structures inside bronchopulmonary segment

1. 肺段支气管 segmental bronchi
2. 右主支气管 right principal bronchus
3. 右下肺静脉 right inferior pulmonary v.
4. 右肺下叶 inferior lobe of right lung
5. 肺段静脉 segment v.
6. 肺段支气管 segmental bronchi
7. 肺段动脉 segment a.
8. 右上肺静脉 right superior pulmonary v.
9. 支气管动脉 bronchial a.
10. 右肺动脉 right pulmonary a.
11. 肺段动脉 segment a.

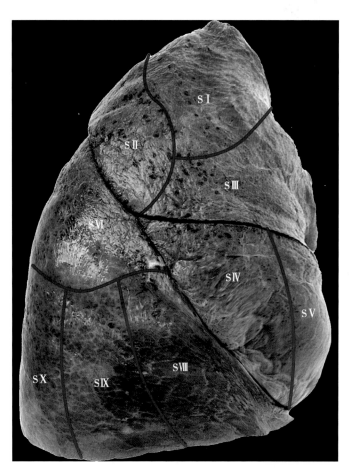

◀图 152 右肺支气管肺段（外侧面观）
Bronchopulmonary segment of right lung.
Lateral view

SⅠ. 尖段 apical segment
SⅡ. 后段 posterior segment
SⅢ. 前段 anterior segment
SⅣ. 外侧段 lateral segment
SⅤ. 内侧段 medial segment
SⅥ. 上段 superior segment
SⅧ. 前底段 anterior basal segment
SⅨ. 外侧底段 lateral basal segment
SⅩ. 后底段 posterior basal segment

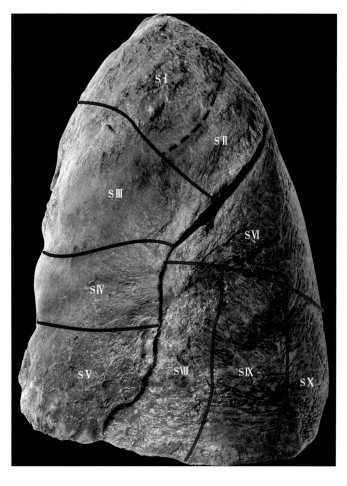

◀图 153 左肺支气管肺段（外侧面观）
Bronchopulmonary segment of left lung.
Lateral view

SⅠ. 尖段 apical segment
SⅡ. 后段 posterior segment
SⅢ. 前段 anterior segment
SⅣ. 上舌段 superior lingular segment
SⅤ. 下舌段 inferior lingular segment
SⅥ. 上段 superior segment
SⅧ. 前底段 anterior basal segment
SⅨ. 外侧底段 lateral basal segment
SⅩ. 后底段 posterior basal segment
SⅠ+SⅡ. 尖后段 apicoposterior segment
SⅦ+SⅧ. 内前底段 anteromedial basal segment

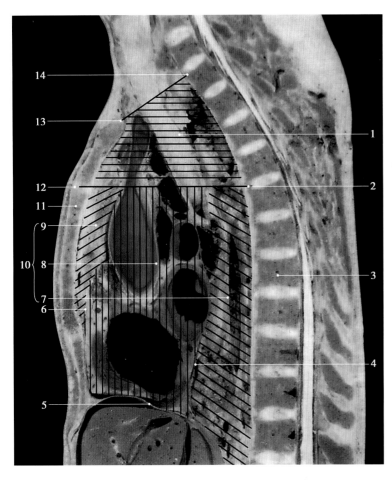

◀图 154　纵隔的分区（正中矢状切面）
Zonation of mediastinum.Median sagittal section

1. 上纵隔 superior mediastinum
2. 第 4 胸椎下缘 inferior border of the 4th thoracic vertebra
3. 脊柱 vertebral column
4. 心包后壁 posterior wall of pericardium
5. 膈 diaphragma
6. 心包前壁 anterior wall of pericardium
7. 后纵隔 posterior mediastinum
8. 中纵隔 middle mediastinum
9. 前纵隔 anterior mediastinum
10. 下纵隔 inferior mediastinum
11. 胸骨 sternum
12. 胸骨角 sternal angle
13. 颈静脉切迹 jugular notch
14. 第 1 胸椎上缘 superior border of the 1st thoracic vertebra

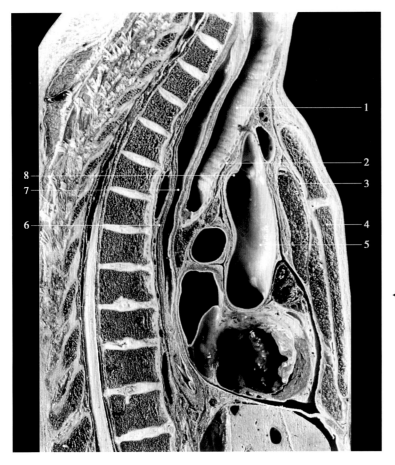

◀图 155　纵隔间隙
Mediastinum space

1. 气管 trachea
2. 气管前间隙 pretracheal space
3. 胸骨后间隙 retrosternal space
4. 胸骨 sternum
5. 升主动脉 ascending aorta
6. 食管后间隙 retroesophageal space
7. 食管 esophagus
8. 主动脉弓 aortic arch

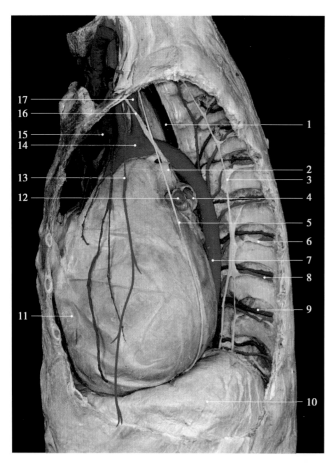

◀ 图 156　纵隔（左侧面观）
Mediastinum.Left view

1. 胸导管 thoracic duct
2. 左肺动脉 left pulmonary a.
3. 交感干 sympathetic trunk
4. 左主支气管 left principal bronchus
5. 膈神经 phrenic n.
6. 肋间神经 intercostal n.
7. 胸主动脉 thoracic aorta
8. 肋间后动脉 posterior intercostal a.
9. 肋间后静脉 posterior intercostal v.
10. 膈 diaphragm
11. 心包 pericardium
12. 左肺静脉 left pulmonary v.
13. 心包膈动脉 pericardiacophrenic a.
14. 主动脉弓 aortic arch
15. 左头臂静脉 left brachiocephalic v.
16. 迷走神经 vagus n.
17. 锁骨下动脉 subclavian a.

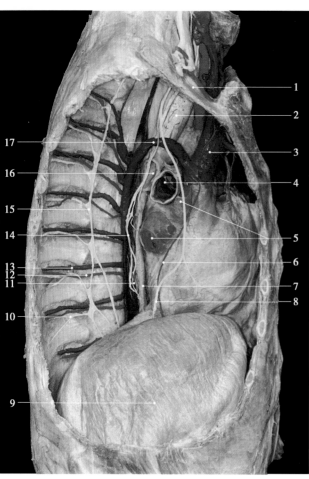

◀ 图 157　纵隔（右侧面观）
Mediastinum.Right view

1. 第 1 肋 the 1st rib
2. 气管 trachea
3. 上腔静脉 superior vena cava
4. 右肺动脉 right pulmonary a.
5. 右肺静脉 right pulmonary v.
6. 心包膈动脉 pericardiacophrenic a.
7. 食管 esophagus
8. 膈神经 phrenic n.
9. 膈 diaphragm
10. 肋间神经 intercostal n.
11. 胸导管 thoracic duct
12. 肋间后动脉 posterior intercostal a.
13. 肋间后静脉 posterior intercostal v.
14. 迷走神经 vagus n.
15. 交感干 sympathetic trunk
16. 右主支气管 right principal bronchus
17. 奇静脉 azygos v.

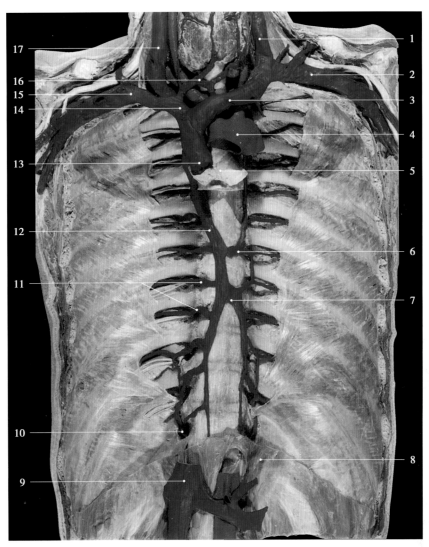

▲ 图 158　上腔静脉及其属支
Superior vena cava and its tributaries

1. 左颈内静脉 left internal jugular v.
2. 左锁骨下静脉 left subclavian v.
3. 左头臂静脉 left brachiocephalic v.
4. 主动脉弓 aortic arch
5. 气管 trachea
6. 副半奇静脉 accessory hemiazygos v.
7. 半奇静脉 hemiazygous v.
8. 膈 diaphragm
9. 下腔静脉 inferior vena cava
10. 腰升静脉 ascending lumbar v.
11. 肋间后静脉 posterior intercostal v.
12. 奇静脉 azygos v.
13. 上腔静脉 superior vena cava
14. 右头臂静脉 right brachiocephalic v.
15. 右锁骨下静脉 left subclavian v.
16. 甲状腺下静脉 inferior thyroid v.
17. 右颈内静脉 right internal jugular v.

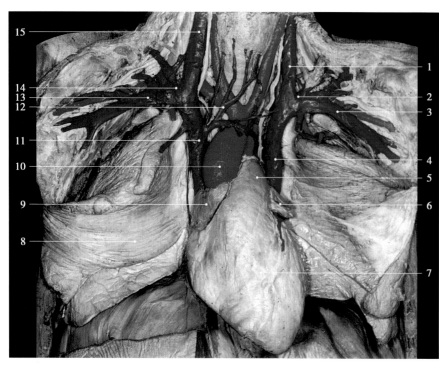

1. 左颈内静脉 left internal jugular v.
2. 左静脉角 left venous angle
3. 左锁骨下静脉 left subclavian v.
4. 左上腔静脉 left superior vena cava
5. 肺动脉干 pulmonary trunk
6. 左心耳 left auricle
7. 心 heart
8. 右肺 right lung
9. 右心耳 right auricle
10. 升主动脉 ascending aorta
11. 右上腔静脉 right superior vena cava
12. 甲状腺下静脉 inferior thyroid v.
13. 右锁骨下静脉 right subclavian v.
14. 右静脉角 right venous angle
15. 右颈内静脉 right internal jugular v.

▲ 图 159　双上腔静脉及其属支
Double superior vena cava and its tributaries

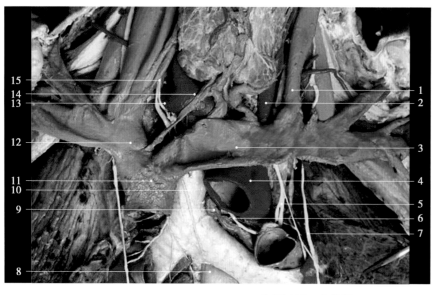

1. 左颈内静脉 left internal jugular v.
2. 左颈总动脉 left common carotid a.
3. 左头臂静脉 left brachiocephalic v.
4. 主动脉弓 aortic arch
5. 左迷走神经 left vagus n.
6. 左喉返神经 left recurrent laryngeal n.
7. 左膈神经 left phrenic n.
8. 食管 esophagus
9. 气管支气管上淋巴结 superior tracheobonchial lymph nodes
10. 气管 trachea
11. 上腔静脉 superior vena cava
12. 右头臂静脉 right brachiocephalic v.
13. 右锁骨下动脉 right subclavian a.
14. 头臂干 brachiocephalic trunk
15. 右迷走神经 right vagus n.

▲ 图 160　上纵隔
Superior mediastinum

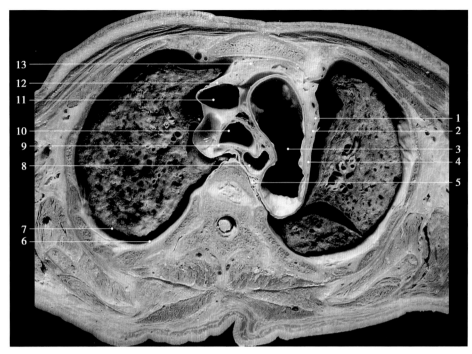

1. 左膈神经 left phrenic n.
2. 交感干 sympathetic trunk
3. 主动脉弓 aortic arch
4. 左迷走神经 left vagus n.
5. 胸导管 thoracic duct
6. 壁胸膜 parietal pleura
7. 脏胸膜 visceral pleura
8. 食管 esophagus
9. 右迷走神经 right vagus n.
10. 气管 trachea
11. 上腔静脉 superior vena cava
12. 右膈神经 right phrenic n.
13. 胸腺 thymus

▲ 图 161　上纵隔（横切面）
Superior mediastinum.Transverse section

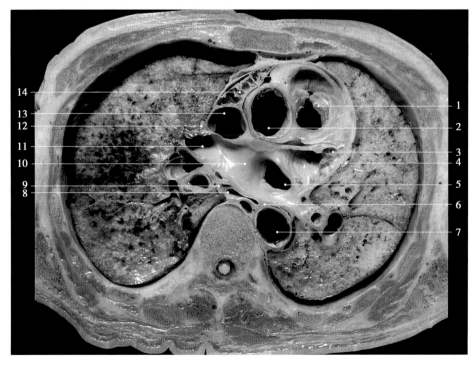

1. 肺动脉瓣 pulmonary valve
2. 升主动脉 ascending aorta
3. 左心耳 left auricle
4. 左膈神经 left phrenic n.
5. 左肺静脉 left pulmonary v.
6. 左迷走神经 left vagus n.
7. 胸主动脉 thoracic aorta
8. 食管 esophagus
9. 右迷走神经 right vagus n.
10. 左心房 left atrium
11. 右肺静脉 right pulmonary v.
12. 右膈神经 right phrenic n.
13. 上腔静脉 superior vena cava
14. 右心耳 right auricle

▲ 图 162　下纵隔（横切面）
Inferior mediastinum.Transverse section

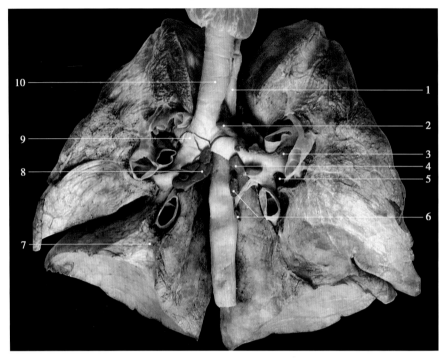

▲ 图 163 纵隔淋巴结（前面观）
Mediastinal lymph nodes.Anterior view

1. 食管 esophagus
2. 气管旁淋巴结 paratracheal lymph nodes
3. 支气管肺门淋巴结 bronchopulmonary hilar lymph nodes
4. 支气管下淋巴结 inferior bronchial lymph nodes
5. 肺淋巴结 pulmonary lymph nodes
6. 纵隔后淋巴结 posterior mediastinal lymph nodes
7. 右肺 right lung
8. 气管支气管下淋巴结 inferior tracheobronchial lymph nodes
9. 右主支气管 right principal bronchus
10. 气管 trachea

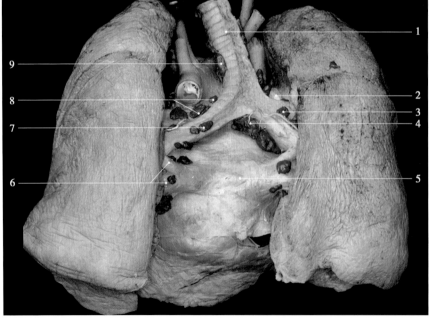

▲ 图 164 纵隔淋巴结（后面观）
Mediastinal lymph nodes.Posterior view

1. 气管 trachea
2. 奇静脉 azygos v.
3. 支气管肺门淋巴结 bronchopulmonary hilar lymph nodes
4. 气管支气管下淋巴结 inferior tracheobronchial lymph nodes
5. 心包 pericardium
6. 左肺静脉 right pulmonary v.
7. 左主支气管淋巴结 left principal bronchial lymph nodes
8. 气管支气管上淋巴结 superior tracheobronchial lymph nodes
9. 气管旁淋巴结 paratracheal lymph nodes

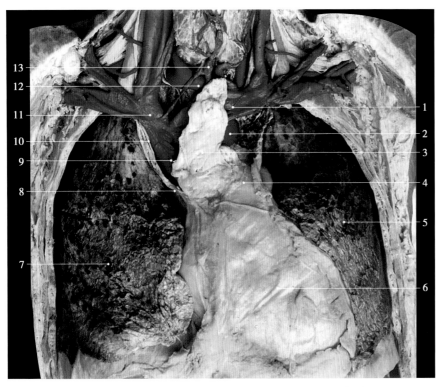

▲ 图 165　心包（1）
Pericardium（1）

1. 左头臂静脉 left brachiocephalic v.
2. 主动脉弓 aortic arch
3. 胸腺 thymus
4. 肺动脉干 pulmonary trunk
5. 左肺 left lung
6. 心包 pericardium
7. 右肺 right lung
8. 纵隔胸膜 mediastinal pleura
9. 上腔静脉 superior vena cava
10. 右膈神经 right phrenic n.
11. 右头臂静脉 right brachiocephalic v.
12. 头臂干 brachiocephalic trunk
13. 甲状腺下静脉 inferior thyroid v.

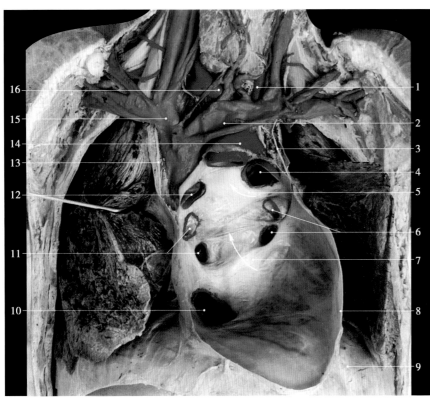

▲ 图 166　心包（2）
Pericardium（2）

1. 左颈总动脉 left common carotid a.
2. 左头臂静脉 left brachiocephalic v.
3. 左膈神经 left phrenic n.
4. 肺动脉干 pulmonary trunk
5. 心包横窦 transverse sinus of pericardium
6. 左肺静脉 left pulmonary v.
7. 心包斜窦 oblique sinus of pericardium
8. 心包 pericardium
9. 膈 diaphragm
10. 下腔静脉 inferior vena cava
11. 右肺静脉 right pulmonary v.
12. 上腔静脉 superior vena cava
13. 右膈神经 right phrenic n.
14. 主动脉弓 aortic arch
15. 右头臂静脉 right brachiocephalic v.
16. 头臂干 brachiocephalic trunk

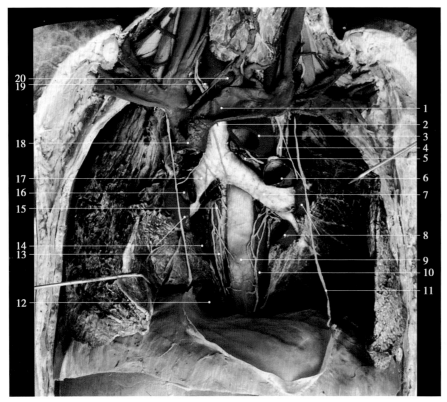

1. 左头臂静脉 left brachiocephalic v.
2. 气管 trachea
3. 主动脉弓 aortic arch
4. 左迷走神经 left vagus n.
5. 气管支气管上淋巴结 superior tracheobronchial lymph nodes
6. 左肺动脉 left pulmonary a.
7. 左主支气管 left principal bronchus
8. 左肺静脉 left pulmonary v.
9. 食管 esophagus
10. 胸主动脉 thoracic aorta
11. 左膈神经 left phrenic n.
12. 下腔静脉 inferior vena cava
13. 奇静脉 azygos v.
14. 右肺静脉 right pulmonary v.
15. 右迷走神经 right vagus n.
16. 右肺动脉 right pulmonary a.
17. 右主支气管 right principal bronchus
18. 上腔静脉 superior vena cava
19. 右喉返神经 right recurrent laryngeal n.
20. 头臂干 brachiocephalic trunk

▲ 图 167　后纵隔及肺根
Posterior mediastinum and roots of lung

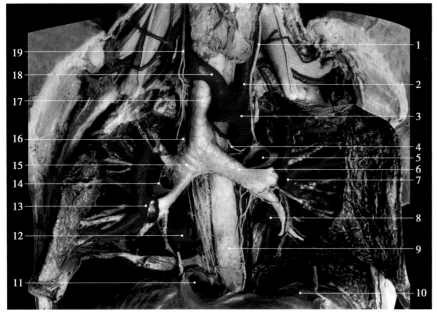

1. 左迷走神经 left vagus n.
2. 左颈总动脉 left common carotid a.
3. 主动脉弓 aortic arch
4. 左喉返神经 left recurrent laryngeal n.
5. 左肺动脉 left pulmonary a.
6. 左主支气管 left principal bronchus
7. 左上肺静脉 left superior pulmonary v.
8. 左下肺静脉 left inferior pulmonary v.
9. 食管 esophagus
10. 膈 diaphragm
11. 下腔静脉 inferior vena cava
12. 右下肺静脉 right inferior pulmonary v.
13. 右上肺静脉 right superior pulmonary v.
14. 右肺动脉 right pulmonary a.
15. 右主支气管 right principal bronchus
16. 奇静脉 azygos v.
17. 气管 trachea
18. 头臂干 brachiocephalic trunk
19. 右迷走神经 right vagus n.

▲ 图 168　后纵隔及肺的血管
Posterior mediastinum and blood vessels of lung

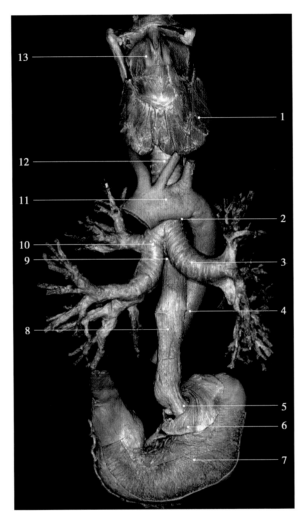

▲ 图 169　食管、气管和胸主动脉的毗邻
Adjacence of esophagus，trachea and thoracic aorta

1. 甲状腺 thyroid gland
2. 主动脉压迹 aortic impression
3. 左主支气管 left principal bronchus
4. 胸主动脉 thoracic aorta
5. 第 3 狭窄 the 3rd narrow
6. 膈 diaphragm
7. 胃 stomach
8. 左心房压迹 left atrial impression
9. 第 2 狭窄 the 2nd narrow
10. 右主支气管 right principal bronchus
11. 主动脉弓 aortic arch
12. 气管 trachea
13. 甲状软骨 thyroid cartilage

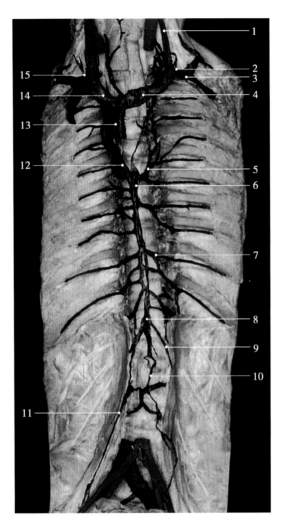

▲ 图 170　奇静脉和胸导管
Azygos vein and thoracic duct

1. 左颈内静脉 left internal jugular v.
2. 左静脉角 left venous angle
3. 左锁骨下静脉 left subclavian v.
4. 左头臂静脉 left brachiocephalic v.
5. 副半奇静脉 accessory hemiazygos v.
6. 胸导管 thoracic duct
7. 半奇静脉 hemiazygous v.
8. 乳糜池 cisterna chyli
9. 肠干 interstinal trunk
10. 左腰干 left lumbar trunk
11. 右腰干 right lumbar trunk
12. 奇静脉 azygos v.
13. 上腔静脉 superior vena cava
14. 右头臂静脉 right brachiocephalic v.
15. 右淋巴导管 right lymphatic duct

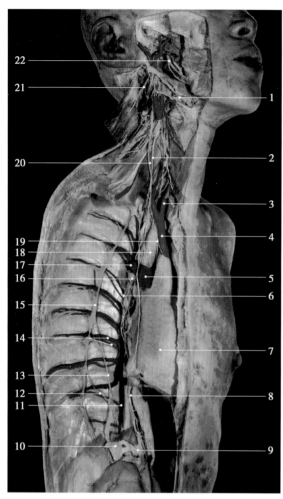

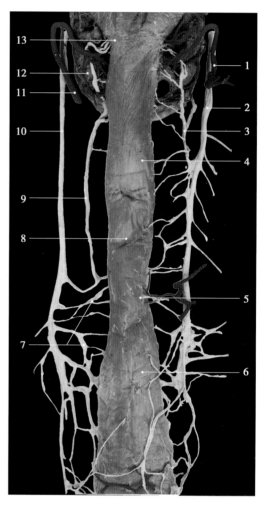

▲ 图 171　迷走神经和胸部交感神经
Vagus nerve and thoracic sympathetic nerve

1. 舌下神经 sublingual n.
2. 膈神经 phrenic n.
3. 右颈总动脉 right common carotid a.
4. 头臂干 brachiocephalic trunk
5. 上腔静脉 superior vena cava
6. 食管丛 esophageal plexus
7. 心 heart
8. 迷走神经后干 posterior vagal trunk
9. 腹腔神经节 celiac ganglia
10. 主动脉肾神经节 aorticorenal ganglia
11. 胸导管 thoracic duct
12. 内脏小神经 lesser splanchnic n.
13. 内脏大神经 greater splanchnic n.
14. 肋间后动、静脉 posterior intercostal a. and v.
15. 胸交感干 thoracic sympathetic trunk
16. 右主支气管 right principal bronchus
17. 奇静脉 azygos v.
18. 气管 trachea
19. 心丛 cardiac plexus
20. 右迷走神经 right vagus n.
21. 副神经 accessory n.
22. 下牙槽神经 inferior alveolar n.

▲ 图 172　迷走神经食管丛
Esophageal plexus of vagus nerve

1. 右甲状腺下动脉 right inferior thyroid a.
2. 右迷走神经 right vagus n.
3. 右喉返神经 right recurrent laryngeal n.
4. 食管颈部 cervical part of esophagus
5. 第 2 狭窄 the 2nd narrow
6. 食管胸部 thoracic part of esophagus
7. 食管丛 esophageal plexus
8. 食管 esophagus
9. 左喉返神经 left recurrent laryngeal n.
10. 左迷走神经 left vagus n.
11. 左甲状腺下动脉 left inferior thyroid a.
12. 甲状腺左叶 left lobe of thyroid gland
13. 第 1 狭窄 the 1st narrow

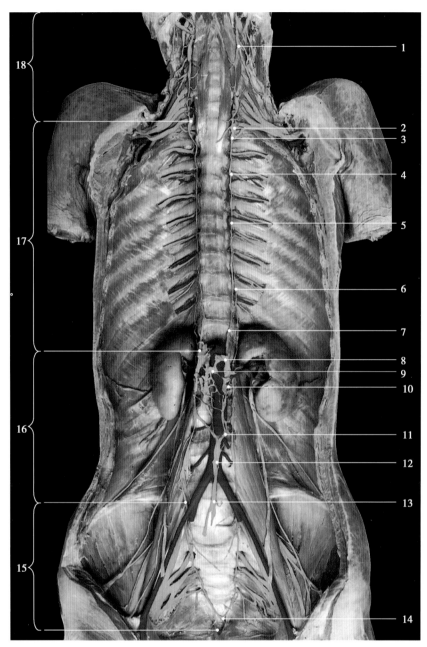

▲ 图 173　交感干及交感干神经节
Sympathetic trunk and ganglia

1. 颈上神经节 superior cervical ganglion
2. 颈中神经节 middle cervical ganglion
3. 颈下神经节 inferior cervical ganglion
4. 胸神经节 thoracic ganglia
5. 交感干 sympathetic trunk
6. 内脏小神经 lesser splanchnic n.
7. 内脏大神经 greater splanchnic n.
8. 腹腔神经节 celiac ganglia
9. 肠系膜上神经节 superior mesenteric ganglion
10. 主动脉肾神经节 aorticorenal ganglia
11. 肠系膜下神经节 inferior mesenteric ganglion
12. 腹主动脉丛 abdominal aortic plexus
13. 上腹下丛 superior hypogastric plexus
14. 奇神经节 ganglion impar
15. 交感神经盆部 pelvic sympathetic nerve
16. 交感神经腰部 lumbar sympathetic nerve
17. 交感神经胸部 thoracic sympathetic nerve
18. 交感神经颈部 cervical sympathetic nerve

连续层次局部解剖

彩色图谱

第四章

腹　　部

Chapter 4　Abdomen

　　腹部上界为剑胸结合、两侧肋弓下缘、第 11 肋前端、12 肋下缘直至第 12 胸椎棘突的连线；下界为耻骨联合上缘、两侧的耻骨嵴、耻骨结节、腹股沟韧带、髂前上棘、循髂嵴至第 5 腰椎棘突的连线。腹壁在两侧以腋后线为界，分为腹前外侧壁及腹后壁。

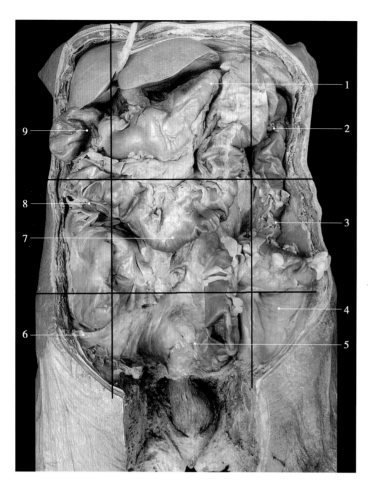

◀图 174 腹部的分区及主要器官的投影
Region of abdomen and projection of main organs

1. 腹上区 epigastric region
2. 左季肋区 left hypochondric region
3. 左腹外侧区 left lateral region of abdomen
4. 左腹股沟区（左髂区）left inguinal region
5. 腹下区 hypogastric region
6. 右腹股沟区（右髂区）right inguinal region
7. 脐区 umbilical region
8. 右腹外侧区 right lateral region of abdomen
9. 右季肋区 right hypochondric region

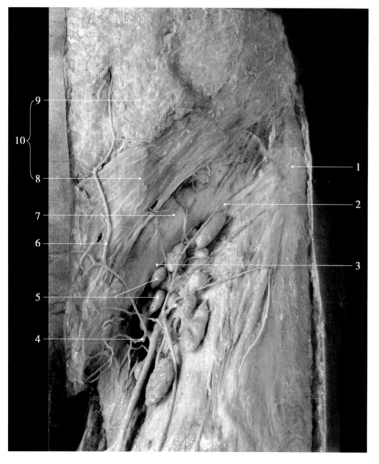

◀图 175 腹部浅筋膜及腹股沟浅淋巴结
Superficial fascia of abdomen and superficial inguinal lymph nodes

1. 髂前上棘 anterior superior iliac spine
2. 旋髂浅静脉 superficial iliac circumflex v.
3. 腹股沟韧带 inguinal lig.
4. 阴部外静脉 external pudendal v.
5. 腹股沟淋巴结 inguinal lymph nodes
6. 腹壁浅静脉 superficial epigastric v.
7. 腹外斜肌腱膜 aponeurosis of obliquus externus abdominis
8. Scarpa 筋膜（膜性层）Scarpa fascia
9. Camper 筋膜（脂肪层）Camper fascia
10. 浅筋膜 superficial fascia

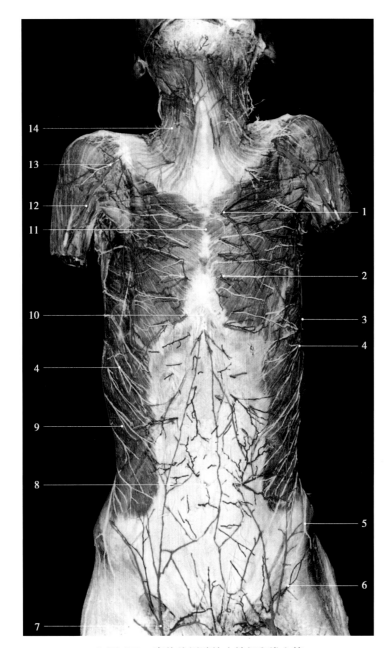

▲ 图 176 腹前外侧壁的皮神经和浅血管
Cutaneous nerves and superficial blood vessels of anterolateral abdominal wall

1. 胸廓内动脉穿支 perforating branches of internal thoracic a.
2. 肋间神经前皮支 anterior cutaneous branch of intercostal n.
3. 胸腹壁静脉 thoracoepigastric v.
4. 肋间神经外侧皮支 lateral cutaneous branch of intercostal n.
5. 髂腹下神经外侧皮支 lateral cutaneous branch of iliohypogastric n.
6. 旋髂浅动脉 superficial iliac circumflex a.
7. 腹壁浅静脉 superficial epigastric v.
8. 脐 umbilicus
9. 腹外斜肌 obliquus externus abdominis
10. 剑突 xiphoid process
11. 胸骨角 sternal angle
12. 头静脉 cephalic v.
13. 锁骨上神经 supraclavicular n.
14. 颈阔肌 platysma

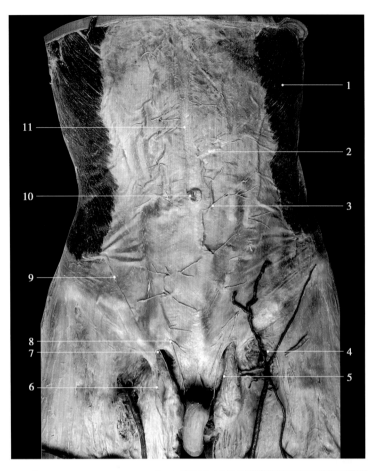

◀图 177　腹前外侧壁的肌肉（1）
Muscles of anterolateral abdominal wall（1）

1. 腹外斜肌 obliquus externus abdominis
2. 腹直肌鞘前层 anterior layer of sheath of rectus abdominis
3. 肋间神经前皮支 anterior cutaneous branch of intercostal n.
4. 筛筋膜 cribriform fascia
5. 髂腹股沟神经 ilioinguinal n.
6. 生殖股神经生殖支 genital branch of genitofemoral n.
7. 腹股沟管浅环 superficial inguinal ring
8. 髂腹下神经前皮支 anterior cutaneous branch of iliohypogastric n.
9. 腹外斜肌腱膜 aponeurosis of obliquus externus abdominis
10. 脐 umbilicus
11. 白线 linea alba

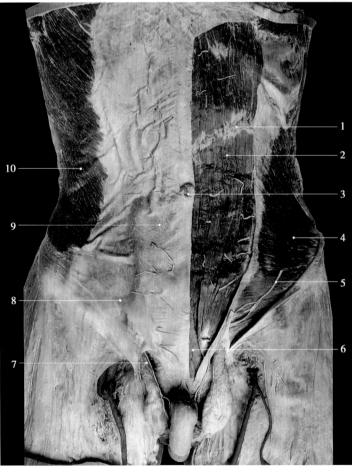

◀图 178　腹前外侧壁的肌肉（2）
Muscles of anterolateral abdominal wall（2）

1. 腱划 tendinous intersection
2. 腹直肌 rectus abdominis
3. 脐 umbilicus
4. 腹内斜肌 obliquus internus abdominis
5. 髂腹下神经 iliohypogastric n.
6. 锥状肌 pyramidalis
7. 精索 spermatic cord
8. 腹外斜肌腱膜 aponeurosis of obliquus externus abdominis
9. 腹直肌鞘前层 anterior layer of sheath of rectus abdominis
10. 腹外斜肌 obliquus externus abdominis

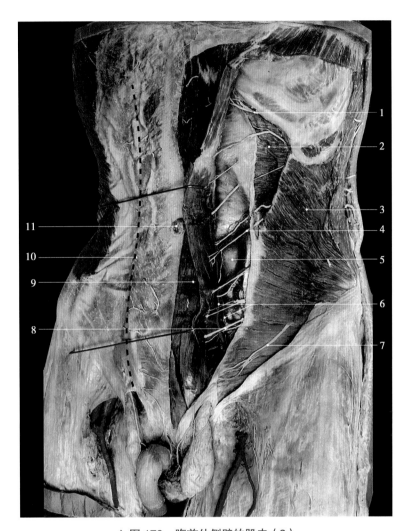

▲ 图 179　腹前外侧壁的肌肉（3）

Muscles of anterolateral abdominal wall（3）

1. 第 7 肋间神经 the 7th intercostal n.
2. 腹横肌 transverse abdominis
3. 腹内斜肌 obliquus internus abdominis
4. 第 10 肋间神经 the 10th intercostal n.
5. 腹直肌鞘后层 posterior layer of sheath of rectus abdominis
6. 腹壁下动、静脉 inferior epigastric a.and v.
7. 髂腹下神经 iliohypogastric n.
8. 肋下神经 subcostal n.
9. 腹直肌 rectus abdominis
10. 半月线 linea semilunaris
11. 脐 umbilicus

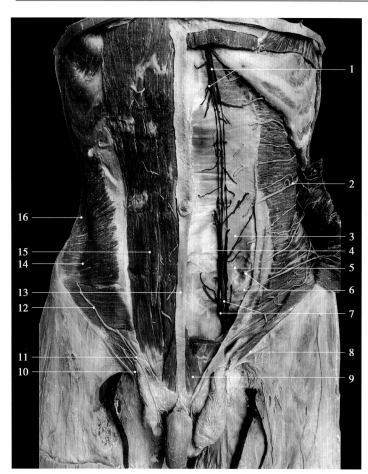

◀ 图 180　腹前外侧壁的肌肉（4）
Muscles of anterolateral abdominal wall（4）

1. 腹壁上动、静脉 superior epigastric a.and v.
2. 第 10 肋间神经 the10th intercostal n.
3. 腹直肌鞘后层 posterior layer of sheath of rectus abdominis
4. 弓状线 arcuate line
5. 腹横筋膜 transverse fascia
6. 肋下神经 subcostal n.
7. 腹壁下动、静脉 inferior epigastric a.and v.
8. 腹股沟韧带 inguinal lig.
9. 锥状肌 pyramidalis
10. 生殖股神经生殖支 genital branch of genitofemoral n.
11. 髂腹股沟神经 ilioinguinal n.
12. 髂腹下神经 iliohypogastric n.
13. 白线 linea alba
14. 腹内斜肌 obliquus internus abdominis
15. 腹直肌 rectus abdominis
16. 腹外斜肌 obliquus externus abdominis

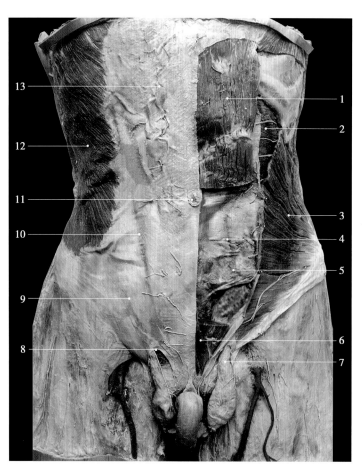

◀ 图 181　腹前外侧壁的肌肉（5）
Muscles of anterolateral abdominal wall（5）

1. 腹直肌 rectus abdominis
2. 腹横肌 transverse abdominis
3. 腹内斜肌 obliquus internus abdominis
4. 弓状线 arcuate line
5. 腹横筋膜 transverse fascia
6. 锥状肌 pyramidalis
7. 精索 spermatic cord
8. 腹股沟管浅环 superficial inguinal ring
9. 腹外斜肌腱膜 aponeurosis of obliquus externus abdominis
10. 半月线 semilunar line
11. 脐 umbilicus
12. 腹外斜肌 obliquus externus abdominis
13. 腹直肌鞘前层 anterior layer of sheath of rectus abdominis

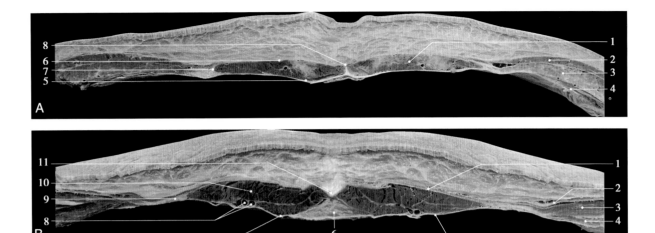

▲ 图 182 腹直肌鞘（横切面）
Sheath of rectus abdominis.Transverse section

A. 弓状线以上横断面 Cross section above arcuate line

1. 腹直肌 rectus abdominis
2. 腹外斜肌 obliquus externus abdominis
3. 腹内斜肌 obliquus internus abdominis
4. 腹横肌 transverse abdominis
5. 腹直肌鞘后层 posterior layer of sheath of rectus abdominis
6. 腹直肌鞘前层 anterior layer of sheath of rectus abdominis
7. 半月线 semilunar line
8. 白线 linea alba

B. 弓状线以下横断面 Cross section below arcuate line

1. 腹直肌鞘前层 anterior layer of sheath of rectus abdominis
2. 腹外斜肌腱膜 aponeurosis of obliquus externus abdominis
3. 腹内斜肌 obliquus internus abdominis
4. 腹横肌 transverse abdominis
5. 腹横筋膜 transverse fascia
6. 脂肪 fat
7. 腹膜 peritoneum
8. 腹壁下动、静脉 inferior epigastric a.and v.
9. 半月线 semilunar line
10. 腹直肌 rectus abdominis
11. 白线 linea alba

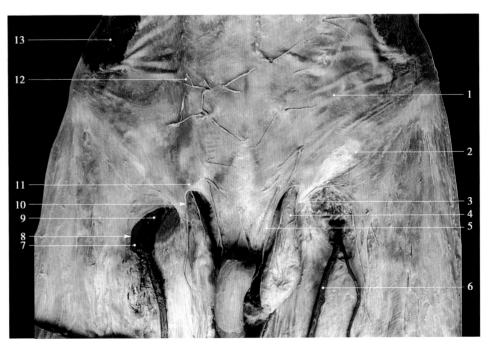

◀ 图 183 腹外斜肌腱膜
Aponeurosis of obliquus externus abdominis

1. 腹外斜肌腱膜 aponeurosis of obliquus externus abdominis
2. 腹股沟韧带 inguinal lig.
3. 外侧脚 lateral crus
4. 精索 spermatic cord
5. 内侧脚 medial crus
6. 大隐静脉 great saphenous v.
7. 股动脉 femoral a.
8. 隐静脉裂孔 saphenous hiatus
9. 股静脉 femoral v.
10. 腹股沟管浅环 superficial inguinal ring
11. 脚间纤维 intercrural fibers
12. 半月线 semilunar line
13. 腹外斜肌 obliquus externus abdominis

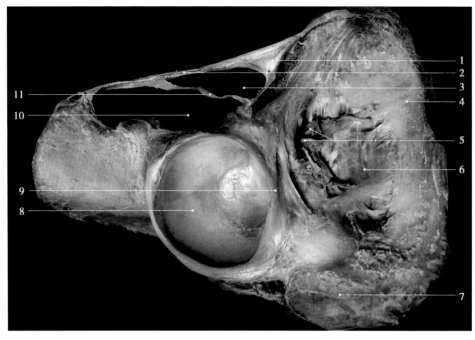

▲ 图 184 腹股沟区的韧带（1）
Ligaments of inguinal region（1）

1. 腔隙韧带 lacunar lig.
2. 腹股沟韧带 inguinal lig.
3. 血管腔隙 lacuna vasorum
4. 耻骨 pubis
5. 闭孔动、静脉 obturator a. and v.
6. 闭孔膜 obturator membrane
7. 坐骨 ischium
8. 髋臼 acetbalum
9. 髋臼横韧带 transverse acetabular lig.
10. 肌腔隙 lacuna musculorum
11. 髂耻弓 iliopectineal arch

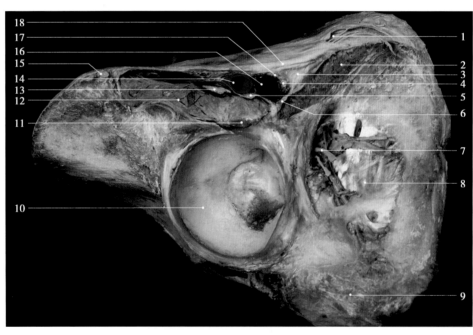

▲ 图 185 腹股沟区的韧带（2）
Ligaments of inguinal region（2）

1. 腹股沟管浅环 superficial inguinal ring
2. 耻骨肌 pectineus
3. 腔隙韧带 lacunar lig.
4. 股环淋巴结 lymph node in femoral ring
5. 髂耻弓 iliopectineal arch
6. 耻骨梳韧带 pectineal lig.
7. 闭孔神经 obturator n.
8. 闭孔膜 obturator membrane
9. 坐骨 ischium
10. 髋臼 acetbalum
11. 腰大肌腱 tendon of psoas major
12. 髂肌 iliacus
13. 股神经 femoral n.
14. 股动脉 femoral a.
15. 股外侧皮神经 lateral femoral cutaneous n.
16. 股静脉 femoral v.
17. 股鞘 femoral sheath
18. 腹股沟韧带 inguinal lig.

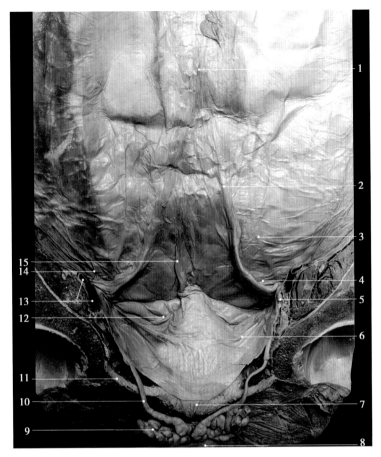

◀图 186　腹前外侧壁内面的皱襞和凹窝（1）
Peritoneal folds and fossae on inner surface
of anterolateral abdominal wall（1）

1. 脐 umbilicus
2. 脐内侧襞 medial umbilical fold
3. 脐外侧襞 lateral umbilical fold
4. 腹股沟内侧窝 medial inguinal fossa
5. 脐动脉 umbilical a.
6. 膀胱横襞 transverse vesical fold
7. 膀胱 urinary bladder
8. 前列腺 prostate
9. 精囊 seminal vesicle
10. 输精管 ductus deferens
11. 输尿管 ureter
12. 膀胱上窝 supravesical fossa
13. 髂外动、静脉 external iliac a.and v.
14. 腹股沟外侧窝 lateral inguinal fossa
15. 脐正中襞 median umbilical fold

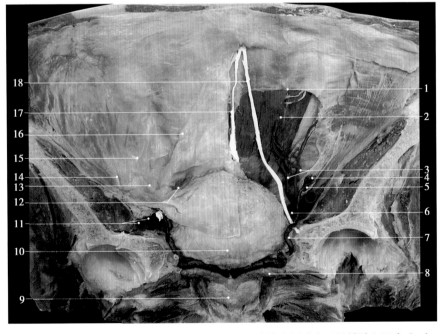

1. 弓状线 arcuate line
2. 腹直肌 rectus abdominis
3. 腹壁下动、静脉 inferior epigastric a.
and v.
4. 睾丸静脉 testicular v.
5. 腹股沟管深环 deep inguinal ring
6. 股环 femoral ring
7. 输精管 ductus deferens
8. 精囊 seminal vesicle
9. 前列腺 prostate
10. 膀胱 urinary bladder
11. 股动、静脉 femoral a.and v.
12. 膀胱上窝 supravesical fossa
13. 腹股沟内侧窝 medial inguinal fossa
14. 腹股沟外侧窝 lateral inguinal fossa
15. 脐外侧襞 lateral umbilical fold
16. 脐内侧襞 medial umbilical fold
17. 脐正中韧带 median umbilical lig.
18. 脐动脉闭锁部 occluded part of
umbilical a.

▲图 187　腹前外侧壁内面的皱襞和凹窝（2）
Peritoneal folds and fossae on inner surface of anterolateral abdominal wall（2）

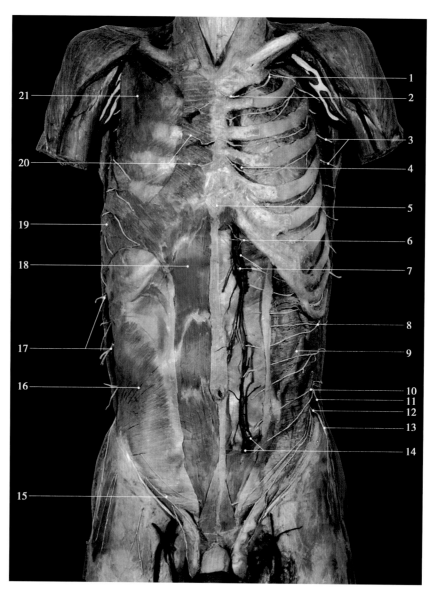

▲ 图 188 腹前外侧壁的神经
Nerves of anterolateral abdominal wall

1. 第 1 肋间神经 the 1st intercostal n.
2. 第 1 肋间神经前皮支 anterior cutaneous branch of the 1st intercostal n.
3. 肋间神经外侧皮支 lateral cutaneous branch of intercostal n.
4. 胸廓内动脉 internal thoracic a.
5. 剑突 xiphoid process
6. 第 6 肋间神经前皮支 anterior cutaneous branch of the 6th intercostal n.
7. 腹壁上动、静脉 superior epigastric a.and v.
8. 第 10 肋间神经 the10th intercostal n.
9. 腹横肌 transverse abdominis
10. 肋下神经 subcostal n.
11. 肋下神经外侧皮支 lateral cutaneous branch of subcostal n.
12. 髂腹下神经 iliohypogastric n.
13. 髂腹下神经外侧皮支 lateral cutaneous branch of iliohypogastric n.
14. 腹壁下动、静脉 inferior epigastric a.and v.
15. 髂腹股沟神经 ilioinguinal n.
16. 腹内斜肌 obliquus internus abdominis
17. 外侧皮支 lateral cutaneous branch
18. 腹直肌 rectus abdominis
19. 前锯肌 serratus anterior
20. 前皮支 anterior cutaneous branch（女性乳腺内侧支）
21. 胸小肌 pectoralis minor

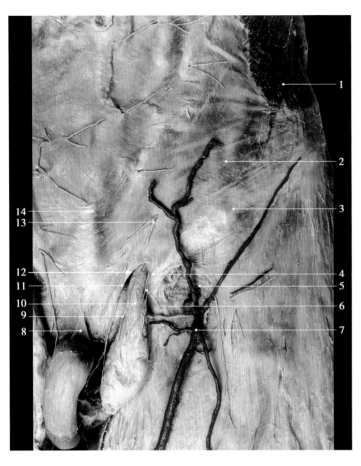

◀ 图 189　腹股沟管（1）
Inguinal canal（1）

1. 腹外斜肌 obliquus externus abdominis
2. 腹外斜肌腱膜 aponeurosis of obliquus externus abdominis
3. 腹股沟韧带 inguinal lig.
4. 外侧脚 lateral crus
5. 筛筋膜 cribriform fascia
6. 生殖股神经生殖支 genital branch of genitofemoral n.
7. 大隐静脉 great saphenous v.
8. 白线支座 stay of white line
9. 髂腹股沟神经 ilioinguinal n.
10. 精索 spermatic cord
11. 内侧脚 medial crus
12. 腹股沟管浅环 superficial inguinal ring
13. 髂腹下神经前皮支 anterior cutaneous branch of iliohypogastric n.
14. 白线 white line

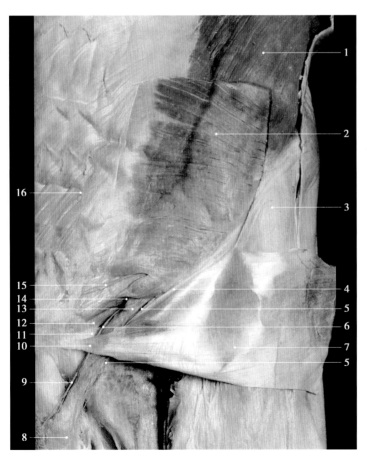

◀ 图 190　腹股沟管（2）
Inguinal canal（2）

1. 腹外斜肌 obliquus externus abdominis
2. 腹内斜肌 obliquus internus abdominis
3. 髂前上棘 anterior superior iliac spine
4. 腹股沟韧带 inguinal lig.
5. 生殖股神经生殖支 genital branch of genitofemoral n.
6. 髂腹股沟神经 ilioinguinal n.
7. 腹外斜肌腱膜 aponeurosis of obliquus externus abdominis
8. 睾丸 testis
9. 阴囊前神经 anterior scrotal n.
10. 内侧脚 medial crus
11. 反转韧带 reflected lig.
12. 腹股沟镰 inguinal falx
13. 精索 spermatic cord
14. 腹股沟管 inguinal canal
15. 髂腹下神经前皮支 anterior cutaneous branch of iliohypogastric n.
16. 腹直肌鞘前层 anterior layer of sheath of rectus abdominis

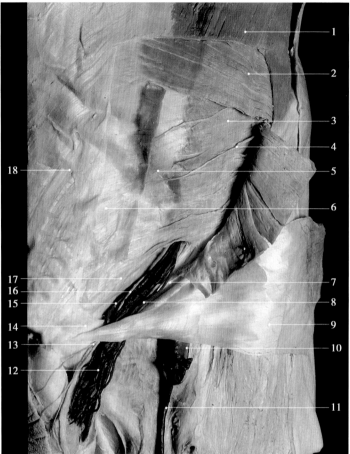

◀ 图 191 腹股沟管（3）
Inguinal canal（3）

1. 腹外斜肌 obliquus externus abdominis
2. 腹内斜肌 obliquus internus abdominis
3. 腹横肌 transversus abdominis
4. 髂腹下神经 iliohypogastric n.
5. 腹横肌腱膜 aponeurosis of transversus abdominis
6. 腹内斜肌腱膜 aponeurosis of obliquus internus abdominis
7. 腹股沟韧带 inguinal lig.
8. 睾丸动脉 testicular a.
9. 腹外斜肌腱膜 aponeurosis of obliquus externus abdominis
10. 股静脉 femoral v.
11. 大隐静脉 great saphenous v.
12. 蔓状静脉丛 pampiniform plexus
13. 阴囊前神经 anterior scrotal n.
14. 反转韧带 reflected lig.
15. 输精管 ductus deferens
16. 髂腹股沟神经 ilioinguinal n.
17. 腹股沟镰 inguinal falx
18. 腹直肌鞘前层 anterior layer of sheath of rectus abdominis

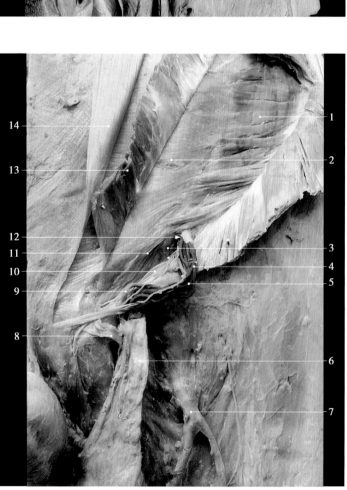

◀ 图 192 腹股沟管（4）
Inguinal canal（4）

1. 腹横肌 transversus abdominis
2. 腹横肌腱膜 aponeurosis of transversus abdominis
3. 腹壁下动、静脉 inferior epigastric a.and v.
4. 蔓状静脉丛 pampiniform plexus
5. 睾丸动脉 testicular a.
6. 精索 spermatic cord
7. 大隐静脉 great saphenous v.
8. 提睾肌（耻骨头）cremaster
9. 输精管 ductus deferens
10. 腹股沟韧带 inguinal lig.
11. 腹股沟镰 inguinal falx
12. 腹股沟管深环 deep inguinal ring
13. 腹内斜肌 obliquus internus abdominis
14. 腹外斜肌腱膜 aponeurosis of obliquus externus abdominis

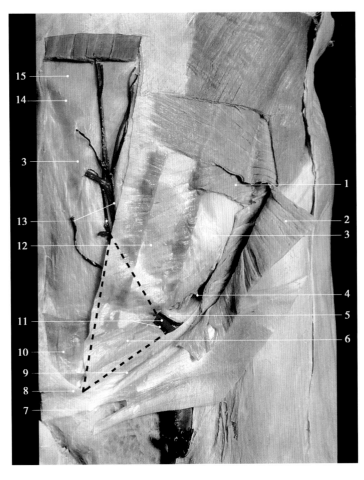

◀图 193 腹股沟管（5）
Inguinal canal（5）

1. 腹横肌 transversus abdominis
2. 腹内斜肌 obliquus internus abdominis
3. 腹横筋膜 transverse fascia
4. 腹股沟管深环 deep inguinal ring
5. 凹间韧带 interfoveolar lig.
6. 腹股沟三角 inguinal triangle
7. 腔隙韧带 lacunar lig.
8. 反转韧带 reflected lig.
9. 腹股沟韧带 inguinal lig.
10. 腹直肌 rectus abdominis
11. 腹壁下动、静脉 inferior epigastric a. and v.
12. 腹横肌腱膜 aponeurosis of transversus abdominis
13. 腹壁下静脉 inferior epigastric v.
14. 弓状线 arcuate line
15. 腹直肌鞘后层 posterior layer of sheath of rectus abdominis

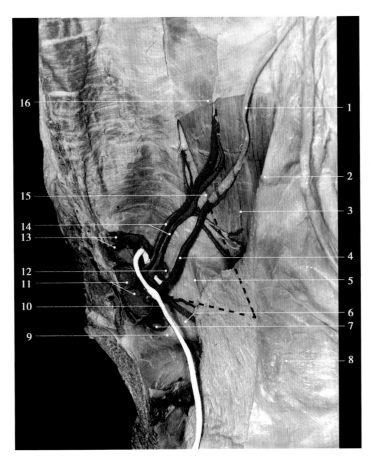

◀图 194 腹股沟三角（内面观）
Inguinal triangle.Internal view

1. 脐内侧韧带 medial umbilical lig.
2. 脐正中襞 median umbilical fold
3. 腹直肌 rectus abdominis
4. 脐动脉 umbilical a.
5. 腹股沟三角 inguinal triangle
6. 腹股沟韧带 inguinal lig.
7. 股管 femoral canal
8. 膀胱 urinary bladder
9. 腔隙韧带 lacunar lig.
10. 输精管 ductus deferens
11. 髂外动、静脉 external iliac a. and v.
12. 腹股沟管深环 deep inguinal ring
13. 睾丸动、静脉 testicular a.and v.
14. 腹壁下动、静脉 inferior epigastric a. and v.
15. 腹直肌外侧缘 lateral border of rectus abdominis
16. 弓状线 arcuate line

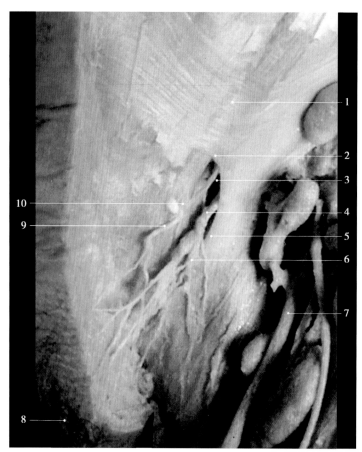

◀图 195 女性腹股沟管浅环
Superficial inguinal ring of female

1. 腹外斜肌腱膜 aponeurosis of obliquus externus abdominis
2. 脚间纤维 intercrural fibers
3. 腹股沟管浅环 superficial inguinal ring
4. 子宫圆韧带（皮下部）round ligament of uterus
5. 外侧脚 lateral crus
6. 生殖股神经生殖支 genital branch of genitofemoral n.
7. 大隐静脉 great saphenous v.
8. 阴阜 mons pubis
9. 阴唇前神经 anterior labial n.
10. 内侧脚 medial crus

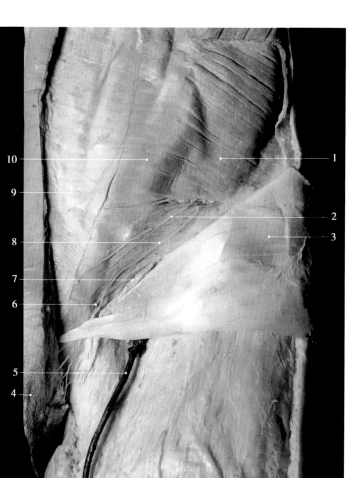

◀图 196 女性腹股沟管（1）
Inguinal canal of female（1）

1. 腹内斜肌 obliquus internus abdominis
2. 髂腹下神经 iliohypogastric n.
3. 腹外斜肌腱膜 aponeurosis of obliquus externus abdominis
4. 阴阜 mons pubis
5. 大隐静脉 great saphenous v.
6. 腹股沟镰 inguinal falx
7. 子宫圆韧带（腹股沟管部）round ligament of uterus
8. 髂腹股沟神经 ilioinguinal n.
9. 腹直肌鞘前层 anterior layer of sheath of rectus abdominis
10. 腹内斜肌腱膜 aponeurosis of obliquus internus abdominis

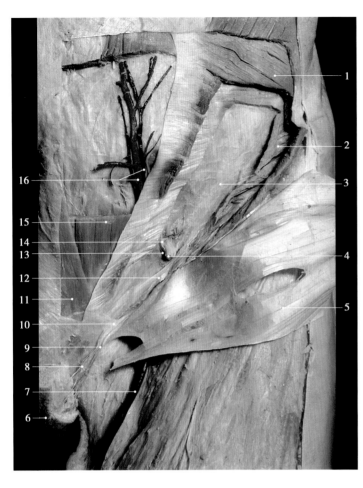

◀ 图 197　女性腹股沟管（2）
Inguinal canal of female（2）

1. 腹内斜肌 obliquus internal abdominis
2. 腹横肌 transversus abdominis
3. 腹横筋膜 transverse fascia
4. 子宫圆韧带 round ligament of uterus
5. 腹外斜肌腱膜 aponeurosis of obliquus externus abdominis
6. 阴阜 mons pubis
7. 大隐静脉 great saphenous v.
8. 阴唇前神经 anterior labial n.
9. 生殖股神经生殖支 genital branch of genitofemoral n.
10. 反转韧带 reflected lig.
11. 锥状肌 pyramidalis
12. 腹股沟韧带 inguinal lig.
13. 凹间韧带 interfoveolar lig.
14. 腹股沟管深环 deep inguinal ring
15. 腹直肌 rectus abdominis
16. 腹壁下动、静脉 inferior epigastric a. and v.

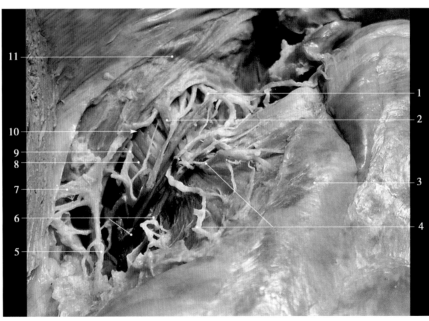

▲ 图 198　食管腹部
Abdominal part of esophagus

1. 迷走神经前干 anterior vagal trunk
2. 肌束 muscle bundle
3. 胃 stomach
4. 胃前支 anterior gastric branches
5. 胃后支 posterior gastric branches
6. 胃左动、静脉食管支 esophagus branches of left gastric a.and v.
7. 腹腔支 celiac branch
8. 食管腹部 abdominal part of esophagus
9. 迷走神经后干 posterior vagal trunk
10. 食管裂孔 esophageal hiatus
11. 膈 diaphragm

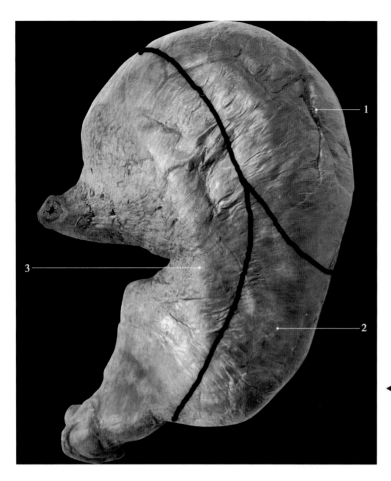

◀ 图 199　胃的毗邻（胃前壁）
Adjacence of stomach.Anterior gastric wall

1. 膈区 diaphragmatic area
2. 游离区 free area
3. 肝区 hepatic area

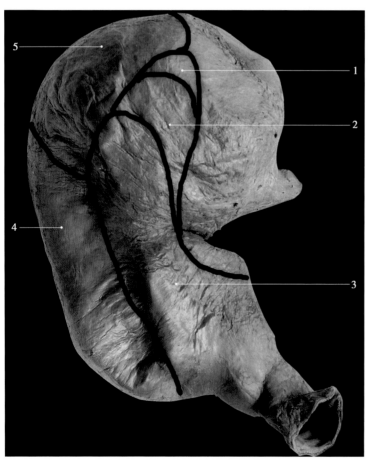

◀ 图 200　胃的毗邻（胃后壁）
Adjacence of stomach.Posterior gastric wall

1. 左肾上腺区 left suprarenal area
2. 左肾区 left renal area
3. 胰区 pancreatic area
4. 结肠区 colic area
5. 膈区 diaphragmatic area

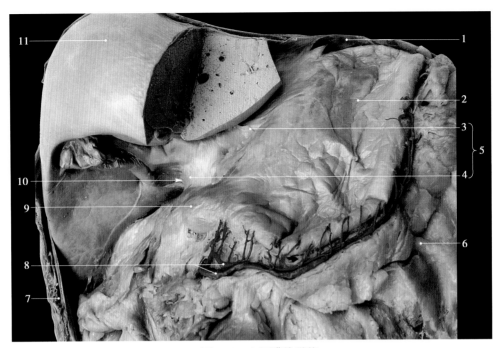

▲ 图 201 小网膜的附着
Coherence of lesser omentum

1. 膈 diaphragm
2. 胃 stomach
3. 肝胃韧带 hepatogastric lig.
4. 肝十二指肠韧带 hepatoduodenal lig.
5. 小网膜 lesser omentum
6. 大网膜 greater omentum
7. 肋膈隐窝 costodiaphragmatic recess
8. 胃网膜右动、静脉 right gastroepiploic a.and v.
9. 幽门 pylorus
10. 网膜孔 omental foramen
11. 肝右叶 right lobes of liver

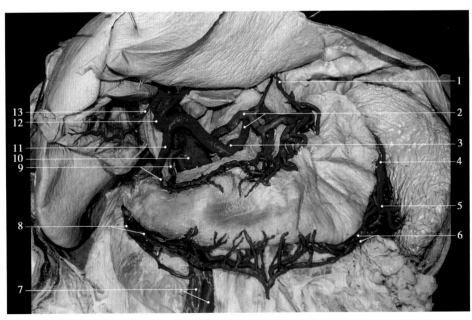

▲ 图 202 胃的血管（前面观）
Blood vessels of stomach.Anterior view

1. 胃左动脉食管支 esophageal branches of left gastric a.
2. 胃左动、静脉 left gastric a. and v.
3. 腹腔干 celiac trunk
4. 胃短动脉 short gastric a.
5. 脾动脉 splenic a.
6. 胃网膜左动、静脉 left gastroepiploic a.and v.
7. 肠系膜上动、静脉 superior mesenteric a. and v.
8. 胃网膜右动、静脉 right gastroepiploic a.and v.
9. 胃右动、静脉 right gastric a.and v.
10. 肝门静脉 hepatic portal v.
11. 胃十二指肠动脉 gastroduodenal a.
12. 肝固有动脉 proper hepatic a.
13. 胆囊动脉 cystic a.

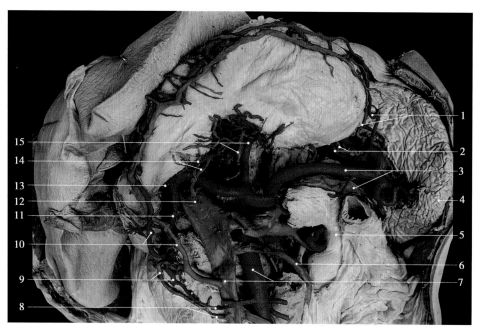

▲ 图 203　胃的血管（后面观）
Blood vessels of stomach.Posterior view

1. 胃网膜左动、静脉 left gastroepiploic a. and v.
2. 胃短动、静脉 short gastric a.and v.
3. 脾动、静脉 splenic a. and v.
4. 脾 spleen
5. 肾 kidney
6. 肠系膜下静脉 inferior mesenteric v.
7. 肠系膜上动、静脉 superior mesenteric a.and v.
8. 胰十二指肠下动、静脉 inferior pancreaticoduodenal a.and v.
9. 胰十二指肠上前动、静脉 anterior superior pancreaticoduodenal a.and v.
10. 胃网膜右动、静脉 right gastroepiploic a. and v.
11. 胃十二指肠动脉 gastroduodenal a.
12. 肝门静脉 hepatic portal v.
13. 肝固有动脉 proper hepatic a.
14. 胃右动、静脉 right gastric a.and v.
15. 胃左动、静脉 left gastric a.and v.

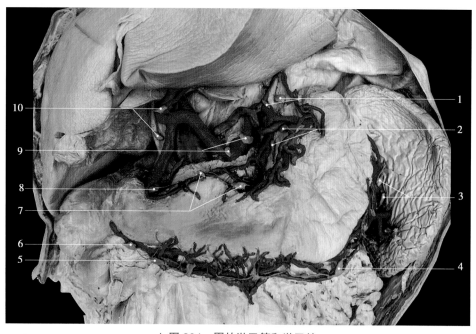

▲ 图 204　胃的淋巴管和淋巴结
Lymph vessels and nodes of stomach

1. 贲门淋巴结 cardiac lymph node
2. 胃左淋巴结 left gastric lymph node
3. 脾淋巴结 splenic lymph node
4. 胃网膜左淋巴结 left gastroomental lymph nodes
5. 胃网膜右淋巴结 right gastroomental lymph nodes
6. 幽门下淋巴结 subpyloric lymph node
7. 胃右淋巴结 right gastric lymph nodes
8. 幽门上淋巴结 suprapyloric lymph node
9. 腹腔淋巴结 celiac lymph nodes
10. 肝淋巴结 hepatic lymph nodes

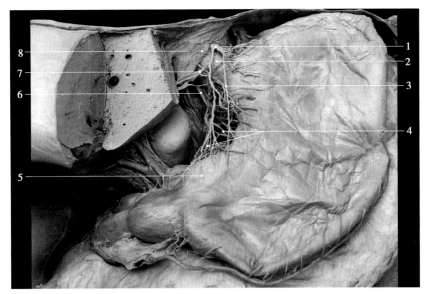

▲ 图 205　胃的迷走神经
Vagus nerves of stomach

1. 迷走神经前干 anterior vagal trunk
2. 食管腹部 abdominal part of esophagus
3. 前胃壁支 branches of anterior wall of stomach
4. 后胃壁支 branches of posterior wall of stomach
5. "鸦爪"形分支 Grow's claw branch
6. 迷走神经后干 posterior vagal trunk
7. 肝支 hepatic branches
8. 膈 diaphragm

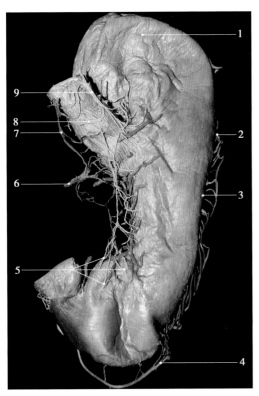

▲ 图 206　迷走神经前干
Anterior vagal trunk

1. 胃底 fundus of stomach
2. 胃网膜左动脉 left gastroepiploic a.
3. 胃大弯 greater curvature of stomach
4. 胃网膜右动脉 right gastroepiploic a.
5. "鸦爪"形分支 Grow's claw branch
6. 腹腔支 celiac branch
7. 迷走神经后干 posterior vagal trunk
8. 肝支 hepatic branches
9. 迷走神经前干 anterior vagal trunk

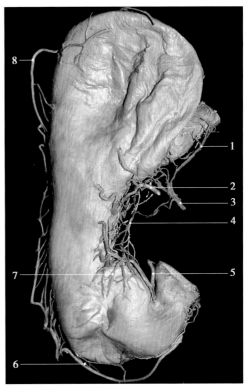

▲ 图 207　迷走神经后干
Posterior vagal trunk

1. 迷走神经后干 posterior vagal trunk
2. 胃左动脉 left gastric a.
3. 腹腔支 celiac branch
4. 后胃壁支 branches of posterior wall of stomach
5. 胃右动脉 right gastric a.
6. 胃网膜右动脉 right gastroepiploic a.
7. "鸦爪"形分支 Grow's claw branch
8. 胃网膜左动脉 left gastroepiploic a.

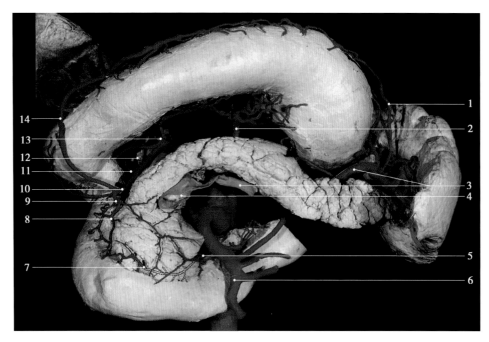

▲ 图 208　十二指肠动脉（前面观）
Arteries of duodenum.Anterior view

1. 胃网膜左动脉 left gastroepiploic a.
2. 胃左动脉 left gastric a.
3. 脾动、静脉 splenic a.and v.
4. 肠系膜上静脉 superior mesenteric v.
5. 胰十二指肠下动脉 inferior pancreaticoduodenal a.
6. 肠系膜上动脉 superior mesenteric a.
7. 胰十二指肠下动脉前支 anterior branch of inferior pancreaticoduodenal a.
8. 胰十二指肠上前动脉 anterior superior pancreaticoduodenal a.
9. 十二指肠上动脉 supraduodenal a.
10. 胃十二指肠动脉 gastroduodenal a.
11. 十二指肠后动脉 retroduodenal a.
12. 胆总管 common bile duct
13. 肝固有动脉 proper hepatic a.
14. 胃网膜右动脉 right gastroepiploic a.

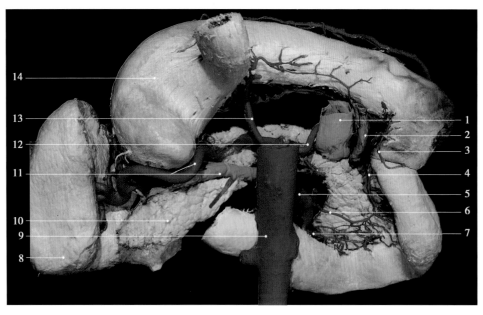

▲ 图 209　十二指肠动脉（后面观）
Arteries of duodenum.Posterior view

1. 肝门静脉 hepatic portal v.
2. 胆总管 common bile duct
3. 十二指肠后动脉 retroduodenal a.
4. 胰十二指肠上后动脉 superior posterior pancreaticoduodenal a.
5. 肠系膜上动脉 superior mesenteric a.
6. 胰十二指肠下动脉后支 posterior branch of inferior pancreaticoduodenal a.
7. 胰十二指肠下动脉前支 anterior branch of inforior pancreaticoduodenal a.
8. 脾 spleen
9. 腹主动脉 abdominal aorta
10. 胰 pancreas
11. 脾动、静脉 splenic a. and v.
12. 肝总动脉 common hepatic a.
13. 胃左动脉 left gastric a.
14. 胃 stomach

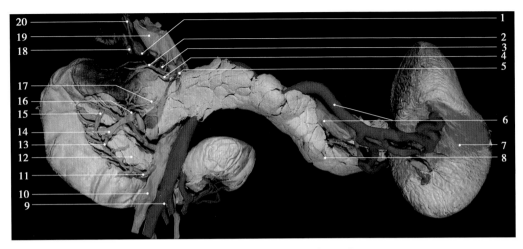

▲ 图 210 十二指肠静脉（前面观）
Veins of duodenum.Anterior view

1. 胆总管 common bile duct
2. 幽门上静脉 suprapyloric v.
3. 幽门后静脉 retropyloric v.
4. 幽门前静脉 prepyloric v.
5. 胃右静脉 right gastric v.
6. 脾动、静脉 splenic a.and v.
7. 脾 spleen
8. 胰 pancreas
9. 肠系膜上动脉 superior mesenteric a.
10. 肠系膜上静脉 superior mesenteric v.
11. 胰十二指肠下静脉前支 anterior branch of inferior pancreaticoduodenal v.
12. 胰头 head of pancreas
13. 胰十二指肠前静脉弓 venous arch of anterior pancreaticoduodenal
14. 中结肠静脉 middle colic v.
15. 胰十二指肠上前静脉 anterior superior pancreaticoduodenal v.
16. 胃网膜右静脉 right gastroepiploic v.
17. 幽门下静脉 subpyloric v.
18. 胆囊管 cystic duct
19. 肝门静脉 hepatic portal v.
20. 肝总管 common hepatic duct

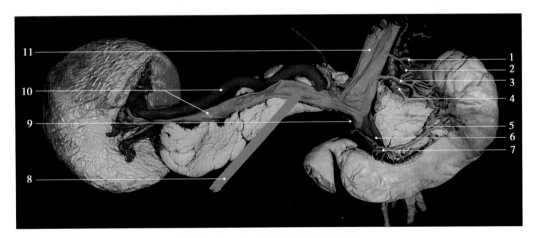

▲ 图 211 十二指肠静脉（后面观）
Veins of duodenum.Posterior view

1. 幽门上静脉 suprapyloric v.
2. 幽门后静脉 retropyloric v.
3. 胰十二指肠上后静脉 superior posterior pancreaticoduodenal v.
4. 胆总管 common bile duct
5. 胰十二指肠后静脉弓 venous arch of posterior pancreaticoduodenal
6. 肠系膜上静脉 superior mesenteric v.
7. 胰十二指肠下静脉后支 posterio branch of inferior pancreaticoduodenal v.
8. 肠系膜下静脉 inferior mesenteric v.
9. 肠系膜上动脉 superior mesenteric a.
10. 脾动、静脉 splenic a. and v.
11. 肝门静脉 hepatic portal v.

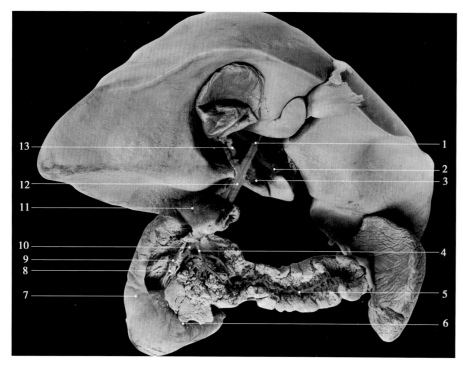

1. 肝总管 common hepatic duct
2. 肝固有动脉 proper hepatic a.
3. 肝门静脉 hepatic portal v.
4. 副胰管 accessory pancreatic duct
5. 胰管 pancreatic duct
6. 十二指肠下部 inferior part of duodenum
7. 十二指肠降部 descending part of duodenum
8. 十二指肠大乳头 major duodenal papilla
9. 十二指肠纵襞 longitudinal fold of duodenum
10. 胆总管（胰腺段）common bile duct
11. 十二指肠上部 superior part of duodenum
12. 胆总管（十二指肠上段）common bile duct
13. 胆囊管 cystic duct

▲ 图 212　十二指肠乳头
Duodenal papilla

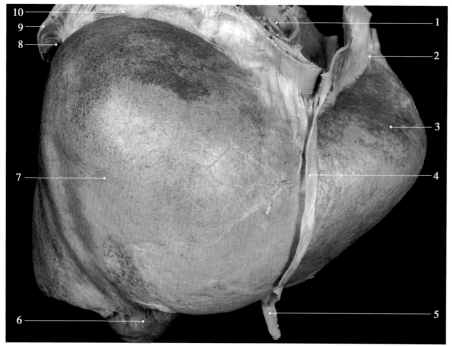

1. 下腔静脉 inferior vena cava
2. 左三角韧带 left triangular lig.
3. 肝左叶 left lobe of liver
4. 镰状韧带 falciform ligament of liver
5. 肝圆韧带 ligamentum teres hepatis
6. 胆囊 gallbladder
7. 肝右叶 right lobe of liver
8. 右三角韧带 right triangular lig.
9. 膈 diaphragm
10. 冠状韧带 coronary lig.

▲ 图 213　肝的前面
Anterior surface of liver

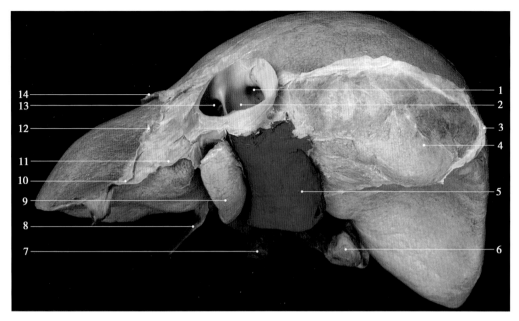

▲ 图 214 肝的膈面
Diaphragmatic surface of liver

1. 肝右静脉 right hepatic v.
2. 肝中间静脉 intermediate hepatic v.
3. 右三角韧带 right triangular lig.
4. 裸区（腹膜外间隙）bare area
5. 下腔静脉 inferior vena cava
6. 胆囊 gallbladder
7. 胆总管 common bile duct
8. 肝圆韧带 ligamentum teres hepatis
9. 尾状叶 caudate lobe
10. 左三角韧带 left triangular lig.
11. 冠状韧带下层 inferior layer of coronary lig.
12. 冠状韧带上层 superior layer of coronary lig.
13. 肝左静脉 left hepatic v.
14. 镰状韧带 falciform ligament of liver

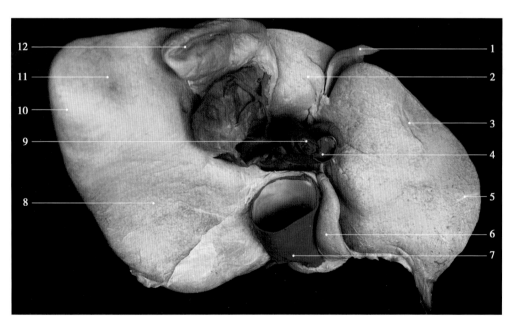

▲ 图 215 肝的脏面
Visceral surface of liver

1. 肝圆韧带 ligamentum teres hepatis
2. 方叶 quadrate lobe
3. 胃压迹 gastric impression
4. 肝门静脉 hepatic portal v.
5. 肝左叶 left lobe of liver
6. 尾状叶 caudate lobe
7. 下腔静脉 inferior vena cava
8. 肾压迹 renal impression
9. 胆总管 common bile duct
10. 肝右叶 right lobe of liver
11. 结肠压迹 colic impression
12. 胆囊 gallbladder

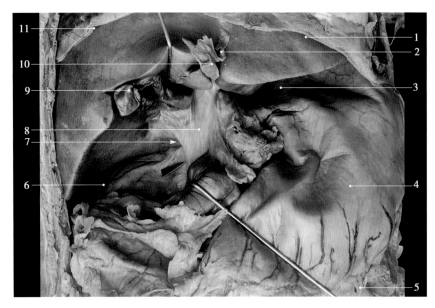

◀图 216　结肠上区
Superior region of colon

1. 左肝上前间隙 anterior superior space of
   left liver
2. 镰状韧带 falciform ligament of live
3. 左肝下前间隙 anterior inferior space of
   left liver
4. 胃 stomach
5. 大网膜 greater omentum
6. 右肝下间隙 inferior space of right liver
7. 网膜孔 omental foramen
8. 小网膜 lesser omentum
9. 胆囊 gallbladder
10. 肝圆韧带 ligamentum teres hepatis
11. 右肝上间隙 superior space of right liver

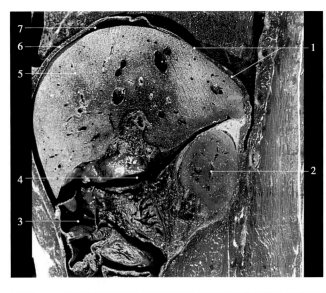

◀图 217　膈下间隙（矢状切面）
Subphrenic space.Sagittal section

经右肾的矢状切面 Sagittal section through right kidney
1. 裸区 bare area
2. 右肾 right kidney
3. 横结肠 transverse colon
4. 右肝下间隙 inferior space of right liver
5. 肝右叶 right lobe of liver
6. 膈 diaphragm
7. 右肝上间隙 superior space of right liver

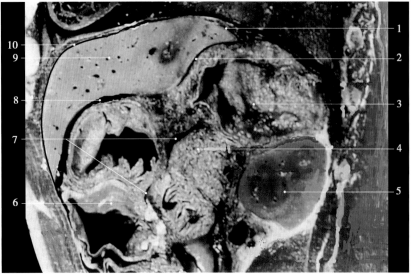

经左肾的矢状切面 Sagittal section through
left kidney
1. 左肝上后间隙 superior posterior space
   of left liver
2. 左肝下后间隙 inferior posterior space
   of left liver
3. 胃 stomach
4. 胰 pancreas
5. 左肾 left kidney
6. 横结肠 transverse colon
7. 网膜囊 omental bursa
8. 左肝下前间隙 anterior inferior space of
   left liver
9. 肝左叶 left lobe of liver
10. 左肝上前间隙 anterior superior space
    of left liver

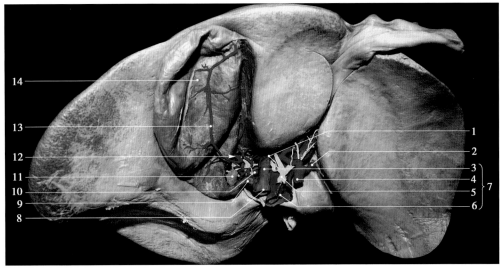

▲ 图 218　肝门及肝蒂
Porta hepatis and hepatic pedicle

1. 肝左管 left hepatic duct
2. 肝固有动脉左支 left branch of proper hepatic a.
3. 肝总管 common hepatic duct
4. 肝固有动脉 proper hepatic a.
5. 肝支 hepatic branches
6. 肝门静脉 hepatic portal v.
7. 肝蒂 hepatic pedicle

8. 胆总管 common duct
9. 胆囊管 cystic duct
10. 肝固有动脉右支 right branch of proper hepatic a.
11. 胆囊淋巴结 cystic lymph node
12. 肝门 porta hepatis
13. 胆囊动脉 cystic a.
14. 胆囊 gallbladder

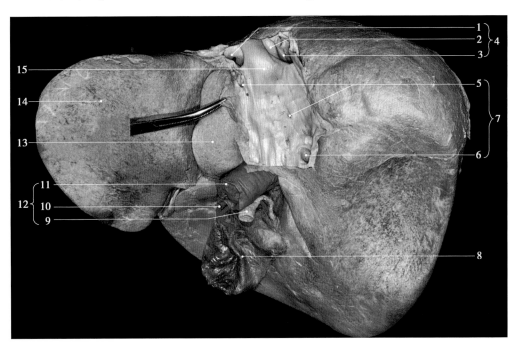

▲ 图 219　肝静脉（1）
Hepatic veins（1）

1. 肝左静脉 opening of left hepatic v.
2. 肝中间静脉 opening of intermediate hepatic v.
3. 肝右静脉 opening of right hepatic v.
4. 第二肝门 the 2nd porta hepatis
5. 尾状叶静脉口 vein orifice of caudate lobe
6. 肝右后下静脉 opening of right posterior inferior vein of liver
7. 第三肝门 the 3 rd porta hepatis

8. 胆囊 gallbladder
9. 胆总管 common bile duct
10. 肝固有动脉 proper hepatic a.
11. 肝门静脉 hepatic portal v.
12. 肝蒂 hepatic pedicle
13. 尾状叶 caudate lobe
14. 肝左叶 left lobe of liver
15. 下腔静脉 inferior vena cava

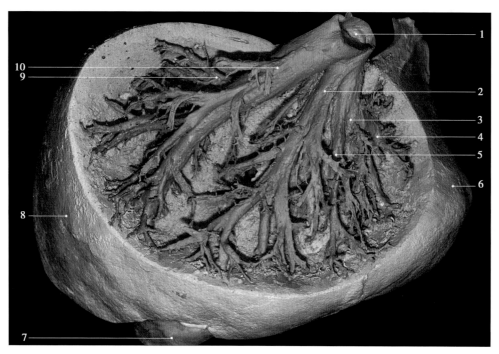

▲ 图 220　肝静脉（2）
Hepatic veins（2）

1. 下腔静脉 inferior vena cava
2. 肝中间静脉 intermediate hepatic v.
3. 肝左静脉 left hepatic v.
4. 左后上缘静脉 left posterior superior border v.
5. 左叶间静脉 left interlobar v.
6. 肝左叶 left lobe of liver
7. 胆囊 gallbladder
8. 肝右叶 right lobe of liver
9. 右后上缘静脉 right posterior superior border v.
10. 肝右静脉 right hepatic v.

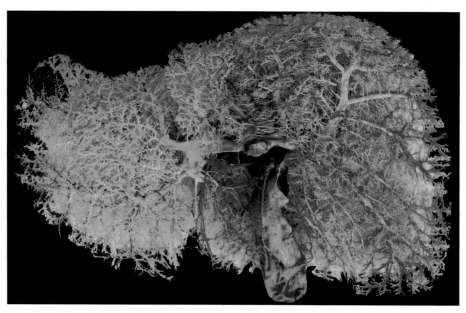

▲ 图 221　Glisson 系统肝内的分布
Distribution of Glisson system inside liver

黄色：肝门静脉 hepatic portal v.
红色：肝动脉（肝固有动脉右支）hepatic a.
绿色：胆囊和肝内胆管 gallbladder and intrahepatic bile duct

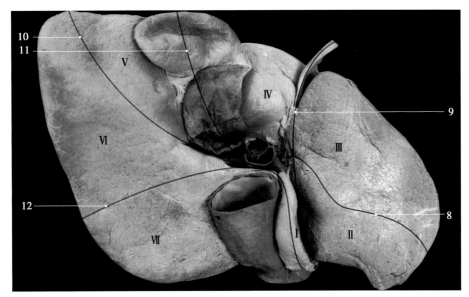

▲ 图 222　肝段划分（1）
Division of hepatic segments（1）

Ⅰ. 尾状叶 caudate lobe
Ⅱ. 左外叶上段 left lateral superior segment
Ⅲ. 左外叶下段 left lateral inferior segment
Ⅳ. 左内叶 right inner lobe
Ⅴ. 右前叶下段 right anterior inferior segment
Ⅵ. 右后叶下段 inferior segment of right posterior lobe

Ⅶ. 右后叶上段 superior segment of right posterior lobe
8. 左段间裂 left intersegmental fissure
9. 左叶间裂 left interlobar fissure
10. 右叶间裂 right interlobar fissure
11. 正中裂 middle hepatic fissure
12. 右段间裂 right intersegmental fissure

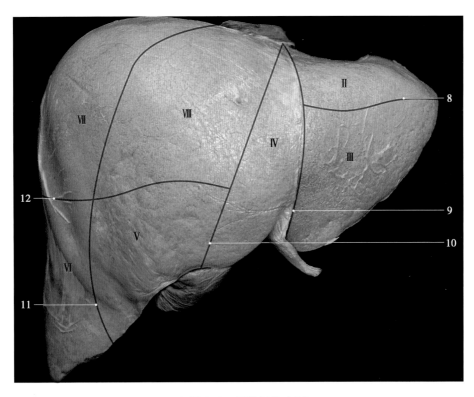

▲ 图 223　肝段划分（2）
Division of hepatic segments（2）

Ⅱ. 左外叶上段 left lateral superior segment
Ⅲ. 左外叶下段 left lateral inferior segment
Ⅳ. 左内叶 left inner lobe
Ⅴ. 右前叶下段 inferior segment of right anterior lobe
Ⅵ. 右后叶下段 inferior segment of right posterior lobe
Ⅶ. 右后叶上段 superior segment of right posterior lobe

Ⅷ. 右前叶上段 superior segment of right anterior lobe
8. 左段间裂 left intersegmental fissure
9. 左叶间裂 left interlobar fissure
10. 正中裂 middle hepatic fissure
11. 右叶间裂 right interlobar fissure
12. 右段间裂 right intersegmental fissure

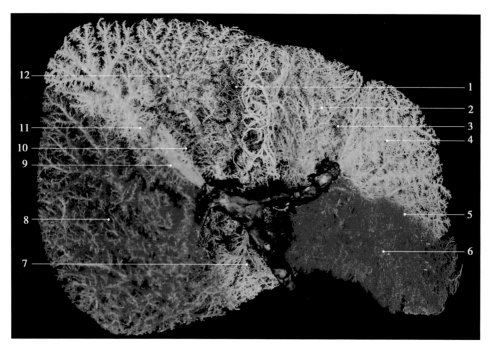

▲ 图 224　肝段铸形（下面观）
Cast of hepatic segments.Inferior aspect

1. 正中裂 middle hepatic fissure
2. 左内叶 left inner lobe
3. 左叶间裂 left interlobar fissure
4. 左外叶下段 inferior segment of left external lobe
5. 左段间裂 left intersegmental fissure
6. 左外叶上段 superior segment of left external lobe
7. 尾状叶 caudate lobe
8. 右后叶上段 superior segment of right posterior lobe
9. 右段间裂 right intersegmental fissure
10. 右叶间裂 right interlobar fissure
11. 右后叶下段 inferior segment of right posterior lobe
12. 右前叶下段 inferior segment of right anterior lobe

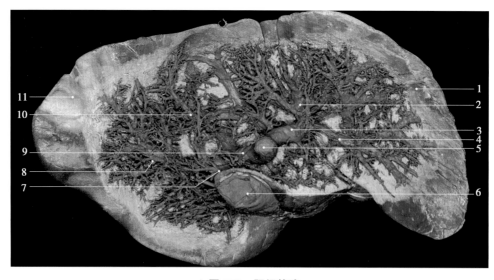

▲ 图 225　肝门静脉
Hepatic portal vein

1. 肝左叶 left lobe of liver
2. 肝门静脉左外下支 left lateral inferior branch of hepatic portal v.
3. 肝门静脉左支 left branch of hepatic portal v.
4. 肝门静脉左外上支 left lateral superior branch of hepatic portal v.
5. 肝门静脉 hepatic portal v.
6. 下腔静脉 inferior vena cava
7. 肝门静脉右后上支 right posterior superior branch of hepatic portal v.
8. 肝门静脉右后下支 right posterior inferior branch of hepatic portal v.
9. 肝门静脉右支 right branch of hepatic portal v.
10. 肝门静脉右前下支 right anterior inferior branch of hepatic portal v.
11. 肝右叶 right lobe of liver

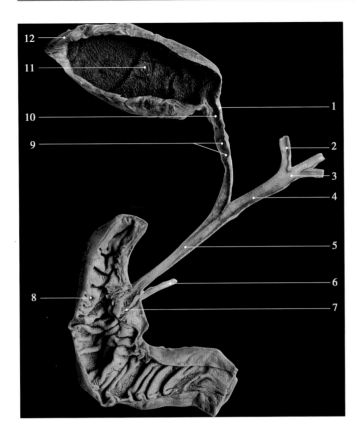

◀ 图 226 胆囊与肝外胆道
Gallbladder and extrahepatic biliary tract

1. Hartmann 囊 Hartmann capsule
2. 肝左管 left hepatic duct
3. 肝右管 right hepatic duct
4. 肝总管 common hepatic duct
5. 胆总管 common bile duct
6. 胰管 pancreatic duct
7. 肝胰壶腹 hepatopancreatic ampulla
8. 十二指肠 duodenum
9. 胆囊管与 Heister 瓣 cystic duct and Heister valve
10. 胆囊颈 neck of gallbladder
11. 胆囊体 body of gallbladder
12. 胆囊底 fundus of gallbladder

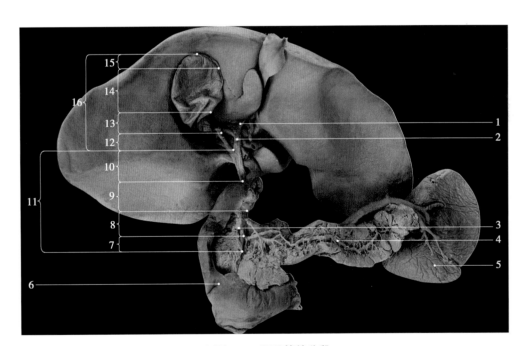

▲ 图 227 胆总管的分段
Segmentation of common bile duct

1. 左肝管 left hepatic duct
2. 肝总管 common hepatic duct
3. 十二指肠大乳头 major duodenal papilla
4. 胰管 pancreatic duct
5. 脾 spleen
6. 十二指肠 duodenum
7. 十二指肠壁段 portion inter duodenal wall
8. 胰腺段 pancreatic portion

9. 十二指肠后段 posterior portion of duodenum
10. 十二指肠上段 superior portion of duodenum
11. 胆总管 common bile duct
12. 胆囊管 cystic duct
13. 胆囊颈 neck of gallbladder
14. 胆囊体 body of gallbladder
15. 胆囊底 fundus of gallbladder
16. 胆囊 gallbladder

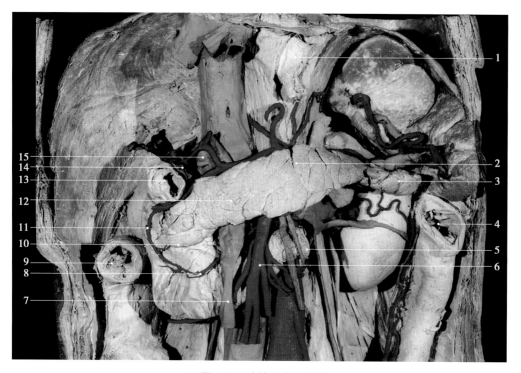

▲ 图 228　胰的分布及毗邻
Adjacent relations and distribution of pancreas

1. 食管 esophagus
2. 胰体 body of pancreas
3. 胰尾 tail of pancreas
4. 结肠左曲 left colic flexure
5. 十二指肠空肠曲 duodenojejunal flexure
6. 肠系膜上动脉 superior mesenteric a.
7. 肠系膜上静脉 superior mesenteric v.

8. 胰十二指肠下动脉前支 anterior branch of inferior pancreaticoduodenal a.
9. 结肠右曲 right colic flexure
10. 胰头 head of pancreas
11. 胰十二指肠上前动脉 anterior superior pancreaticoduodenal a.

12. 胰颈 neck of pancreas
13. 十二指肠上部 superior part of duodenum
14. 胆总管 common bile duct
15. 肝门静脉 hepatic portal v.

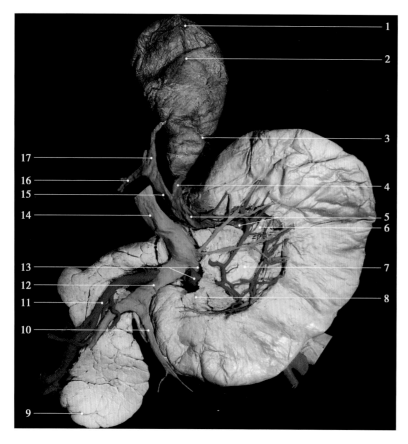

◀ 图 229　胰（后面观）
Pancreas.Posterior view

1. 胆囊底 fundus of gallbladder
2. 胆囊体 body of gallbladder
3. 胆囊颈 neck of gallbladder
4. 胆囊管 cystic duct
5. 胆总管 common bile duct
6. 胰管 pancreatic duct
7. 胰头 head of pancreas
8. 胰钩突 uncinate process of pancreas
9. 胰尾 tail of pancreas
10. 肠系膜下静脉 inferior mesenteric v.
11. 脾动脉 splenic a.
12. 脾静脉 splenic v.
13. 肠系膜上动、静脉 superior mesenteric a.and v.
14. 肝门静脉 hepatic portal v.
15. 肝总管 common hepatic duct
16. 肝左管 left hepatic duct
17. 肝右管 right hepatic duct

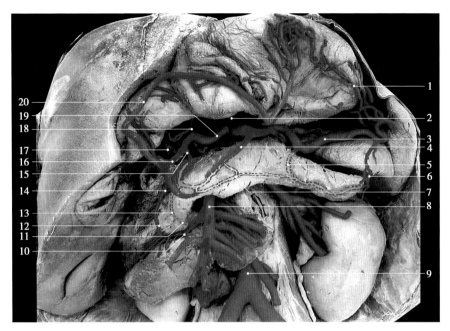

▲ 图 230 胰的动脉
Arteries of pancreas

1. 胃网膜左动脉 left gastroepiploic a.
2. 胃左动脉 left gastric a.
3. 脾动脉 splenic a.
4. 胰背动脉 dorsal pancreatic a.
5. 胰大动脉 great pancreatic a.
6. 胰尾动脉 caudal pancreatic a.
7. 胰下动脉 inferior pancreatic a.
8. 肠系膜上动脉 superior mesenteric a.
9. 腹主动脉 abdominal aorta
10. 胰十二指肠下动脉前支 anterior branch of inferior pancreaticoduodenal a.
11. 胰十二指肠下动脉后支 posterior branch of inferior pancreaticoduodenal a.
12. 胰十二指肠前动脉弓 artery arch of anterior pancreaticoduodenal
13. 胰十二指肠后动脉弓 artery arch of posterior pancreaticoduodenal
14. 胰十二指肠上前动脉 anterior superior pancreaticoduodenal a.
15. 胰十二指肠上后动脉 posterior superior pancreaticoduodenal a.
16. 胃十二指肠动脉 gastroduodenal a.
17. 胆总管 common bile duct
18. 肝固有动脉 proper hepatic a.
19. 肝总动脉 common hepatic a.
20. 胃网膜右动脉 right gastroepiploic a.

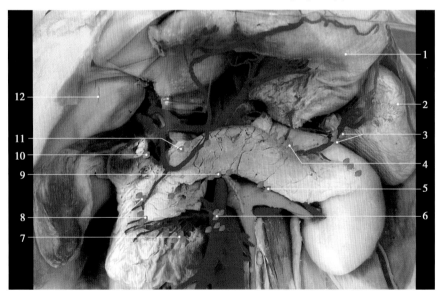

▲ 图 231 胰的淋巴结
Pancreatic lymph nodes

1. 胃 stomach
2. 脾 spleen
3. 脾淋巴结 splenic lymph nodes
4. 胰上淋巴结 superior pancreatic lymph nodes
5. 胰下淋巴结 inferior pancreatic lymph nodes
6. 肠系膜上淋巴结 superior mesenteric lymph nodes
7. 胰头下淋巴结 inferior head of pancreas lymph nodes
8. 胰十二指肠前淋巴结 anterior pancreaticoduodenal lymph nodes
9. 胰体下淋巴结 inferior body of pancreas lymph nodes
10. 幽门下淋巴结 subpyloric lymph nodes
11. 胰头上淋巴结 superior head of pancreas lymph nodes
12. 肝 liver

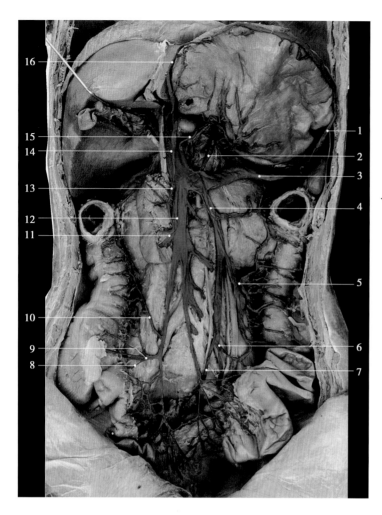

◀ 图 232 肝门静脉及其属支
Hepatic portal vein and its tributaries

1. 胃网膜左静脉 left gastroepiploic v.
2. 胃左静脉 left gastric v.
3. 脾静脉 splenic v.
4. 肠系膜下静脉 inferior mesenteric v.
5. 左结肠静脉 left colic v.
6. 乙状结肠静脉 sigmoid v.
7. 直肠上静脉 superior rectal v.
8. 阑尾静脉 appendicular v.
9. 回结肠静脉 ileocolic v.
10. 右结肠静脉 right colic v.
11. 中结肠静脉 middle colic v.
12. 肠系膜上静脉 superior mesenteric v.
13. 胰十二指肠上前静脉 anterior superior pancreaticoduodenal v.
14. 肝门静脉 hepatic portal v.
15. 胃右静脉 right gastric v.
16. 胃网膜右静脉 right gastroepiploic v.

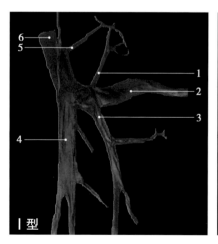 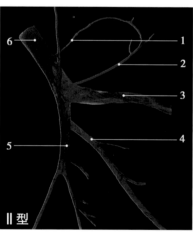 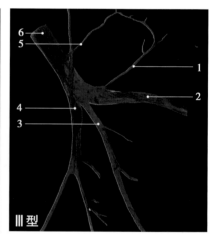

▲ 图 233 肠系膜下静脉汇入类型
Types of abouchement of inferior mesenteric vein

Ⅰ型 52.9%

1. 胃右静脉 right gastric v.
2. 脾静脉 splenic v.
3. 肠系膜下静脉 inferior mesenteric v.
4. 肠系膜上静脉 superior mesenteric v.
5. 胃左静脉 left gastric v.
6. 肝门静脉 hepatic portal v.

Ⅱ型 34.7%

1. 胃左静脉 left gastric v.
2. 胃右静脉 right gastric v.
3. 脾静脉 splenic v.
4. 肠系膜下静脉 inferior mesenteric v.
5. 肠系膜上静脉 superior mesenteric v.
6. 肝门静脉 hepatic portal v.

Ⅲ型 13.3%

1. 胃右静脉 right gastric v.
2. 脾静脉 splenic v.
3. 肠系膜下静脉 inferior mesenteric v.
4. 肠系膜上静脉 superior mesenteric v.
5. 胃左静脉 left gastric v.
6. 肝门静脉 hepatic portal v.

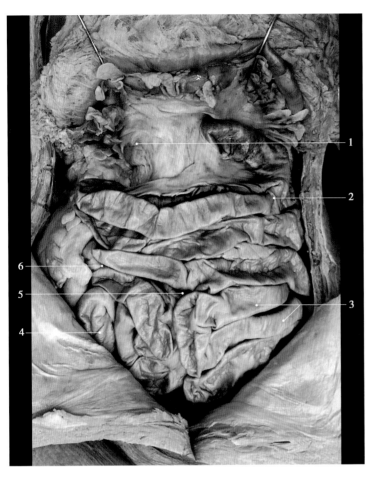

◀图 234　腹腔自然位置
Natural position of abdominal cavity

1. 十二指肠（上腹部）
   duodenum
2. 空肠上段肠襻（左腹外侧区）
   ansa interstinal of superior segment of jejunum
3. 空肠下段（左髂窝部）
   inferior segment of jejunum
4. 回肠下段（右髂窝部）
   inferior segment of ileum
5. 回肠上段（脐中部）
   superior segment of ileum
6. 回肠中段（右腹外侧区）
   midpiece of ileum

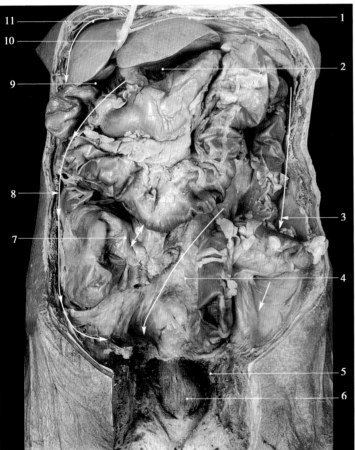

◀图 235　腹膜腔通道
Passage of peritoneal cavity

1. 左肝上前间隙 superoanterior space of left liver
2. 左肝下前间隙 inferoanterior space of left liver
3. 左结肠旁沟 left paracolic sulci
4. 左肠系膜窦 left mesenteric sinuses
5. 盆腔 pelvic cavity
6. 直肠 rectum
7. 右肠系膜窦 right mesenteric sinuses
8. 右结肠旁沟 right paracolic sulci
9. 右肝下间隙 inferior space of right liver
10. 肝圆韧带 ligamentum teres hepatis
11. 右肝上间隙 superior space of right liver

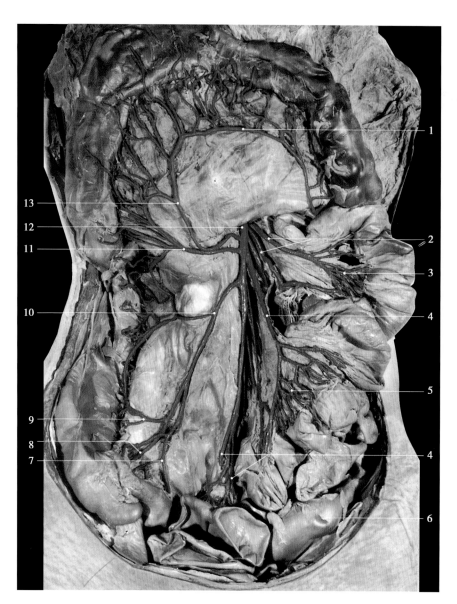

▲ 图 236　肠系膜上动脉
Superior mesenteric artery

1. 边缘动脉 marginal a.
2. 空肠动脉 jejunal a.
3. 空肠动脉弓 arterial arcades of jejunum
4. 回肠动脉 ileal a.
5. 回肠动脉弓 arterial arcades of ileum
6. 乙状结肠 sigmoid colon
7. 回肠支 ileal branch
8. 阑尾动脉 appendicular a.
9. 结肠支 colic branch
10. 回结肠动脉 ileocolic a.
11. 右结肠动脉 right colic a.
12. 肠系膜上动脉 superior mesenteric a.
13. 中结肠动脉 middle colic a.

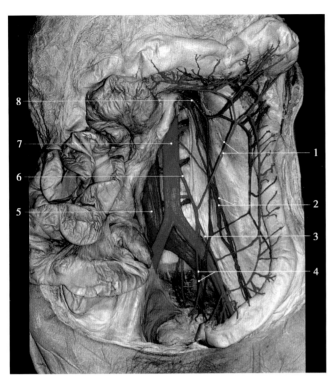

◀ 图 237　肠系膜下动脉
Inferior mesenteric artery

1. 左结肠动、静脉 left colic a.and v.
2. 睾丸动、静脉 testicular a.and v.
3. 乙状结肠动脉 sigmoid a.
4. 直肠上动、静脉 superior rectal a.and v.
5. 下腔静脉 inferior vena cava
6. 肠系膜下动脉 inferior mesenteric a.
7. 腹主动脉 abdominal aorta
8. 肠系膜下静脉 inferior mesenteric v.

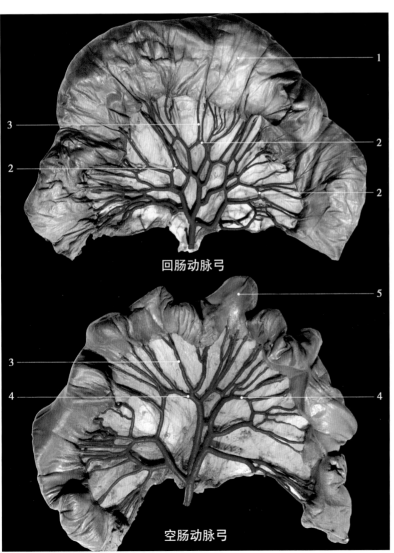

回肠动脉弓

空肠动脉弓

◀ 图 238　空、回肠动脉弓
Arterial arcades of jejunum and ileum

1. 回肠 ileum
2. 回肠动脉弓 arterial arcades of ileum
3. 直动脉 straight a.
4. 空肠动脉弓 arterial arcades of jejunum
5. 空肠 jeunum

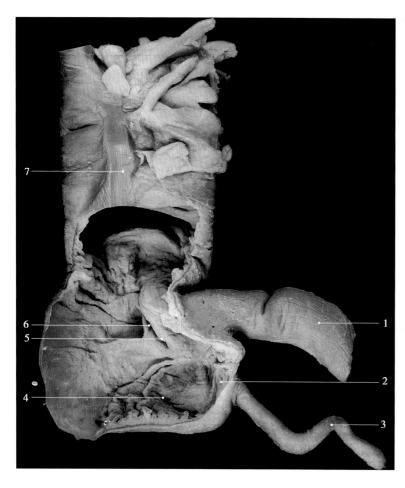

◀ 图 239 回盲部
Ileocecal junction

1. 回肠 ileum
2. 阑尾口 orifice of vermiform appendix
3. 阑尾 vermiform appendix
4. 盲肠 cecum
5. 回盲瓣 ileocecal valve
6. 回盲口 ileocecal orifice
7. 结肠带 colic bands

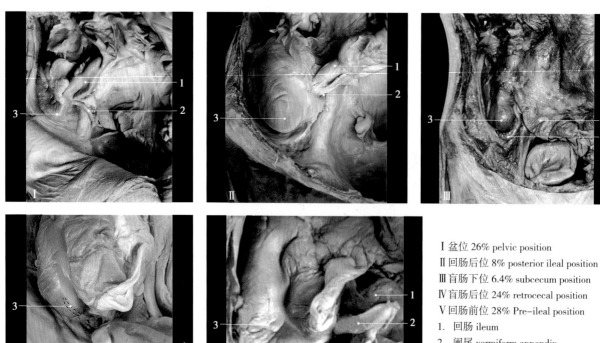

I 盆位 26% pelvic position
II 回肠后位 8% posterior ileal position
III 盲肠下位 6.4% subcecum position
IV 盲肠后位 24% retrocecal position
V 回肠前位 28% Pre-ileal position
1. 回肠 ileum
2. 阑尾 vermiform appendix
3. 盲肠 cecum

▲ 图 240 阑尾的常见位置
Common sites of vermiform appendix

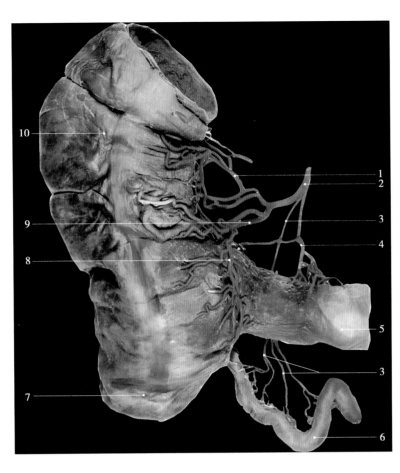

◀图 241 阑尾动脉
Appendicular artery

1. 结肠支 colic branch
2. 回结肠动脉 ileocolic a.
3. 阑尾动脉 appendicular a.
4. 回肠支 ileal branch
5. 回肠 ileum
6. 阑尾 vermiform appendix
7. 盲肠 cecum
8. 盲肠前动脉 anterior cecal a.
9. 盲肠后动脉 posterior cecal a.
10. 升结肠 ascending colon

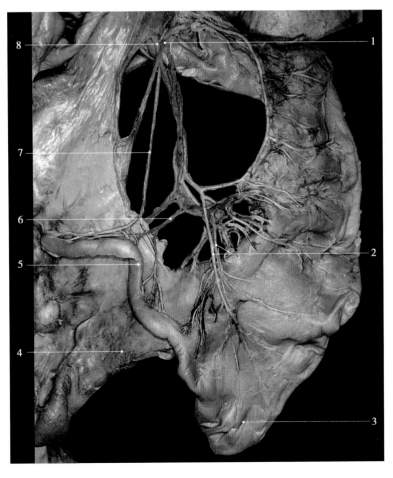

◀图 242 阑尾动、静脉（后面观）
Appendicular artery and vein.Posterior view

1. 回结肠静脉 ileocolic v.
2. 盲肠后动、静脉 posterior cecal a.and v.
3. 盲肠 cecum
4. 回肠 ileum
5. 阑尾 vermiform appendix
6. 阑尾静脉 appendicular v.
7. 阑尾动脉 appendicular a.
8. 回结肠动脉 ileocolic a.

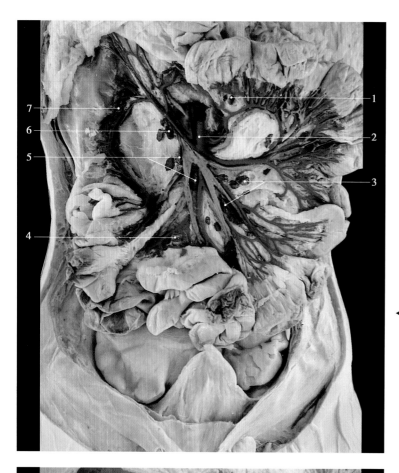

◀ 图 243 肠系膜上淋巴结
Superior mesenteric lymph nodes

1. 肠淋巴结 intestinal lymph nodes
2. 肠系膜上动脉 superior mesenteric a.
3. 肠系膜淋巴结 mesenteric lymph nodes
4. 回结肠淋巴结 ileocolic lymph nodes
5. 肠系膜上淋巴结 superior mesenteric lymph nodes
6. 中结肠淋巴结 middle colic lymph nodes
7. 右结肠淋巴结 right colic lymph nodes

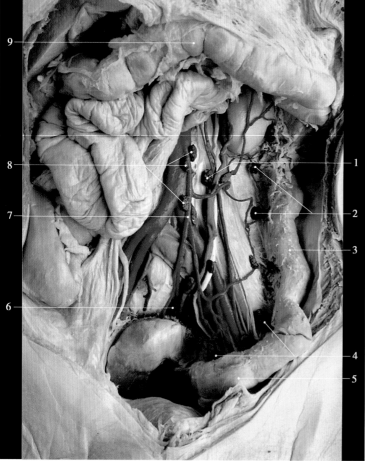

◀ 图 244 肠系膜下淋巴结
Inferior mesenteric lymph nodes

1. 中间淋巴结 intermediate lymph nodes
2. 左结肠淋巴结 left colic lymph nodes
3. 降结肠 descending colon
4. 乙状结肠淋巴结 sigmoid lymph nodes
5. 乙状结肠 sigmoid colon
6. 直肠上淋巴结 superior rectal lymph nodes
7. 肠系膜下动脉 inferior mesenteric a.
8. 肠系膜下淋巴结 inferior mesenteric lymph nodes
9. 横结肠 transverse colon

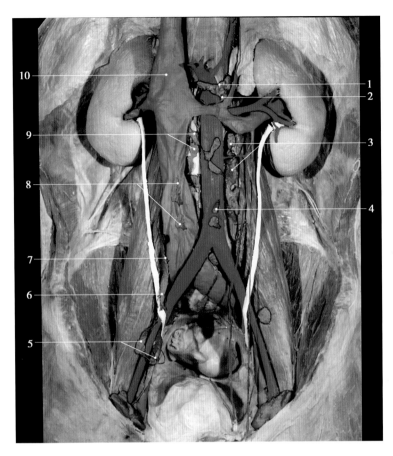

◀图 245 腹膜后隙的淋巴结
Lymph nodes in retroperitoneal space

1. 腹腔淋巴结 celiac lymph nodes
2. 肠系膜上淋巴结 superior mesenteric lymph nodes
3. 主动脉外淋巴结 lateral aortic lymph nodes
4. 肠系膜下淋巴结 inferior mesenteric lymph nodes
5. 髂外淋巴结 lateral iliac lymph nodes
6. 髂总淋巴结 common iliac lymph node
7. 腔静脉外侧淋巴结 lateral caval lymph node
8. 腔静脉前淋巴结 precaval lymph node
9. 中间腰淋巴结 intermediate lumbar lymph node
10. 下腔静脉 inferior vena cava

◀图 246 腹膜后隙的血管、神经
Blood vessels and nerves in retroperitoneal space

1. 膈 diaphragm
2. 腹腔神经节 celiac ganglia
3. 肠系膜上神经节 superior mesenteric ganglion
4. 腹主动脉丛 abdominal aortic plexus
5. 肋下神经 subcostal n.
6. 肠系膜下神经节 inferior mesenteric ganglia
7. 肠系膜下动脉 inferior mesenteric a.
8. 上腹下丛 superior hypogastric plexus
9. 髂总动脉 common iliac a.
10. 腰神经节 lumbar ganglia
11. 腰交感干 lumbar sympathetic trunk
12. 腹主动脉 abdominal aorta
13. 肠系膜上动脉 superior mesenteric a.
14. 主动脉肾神经节 aorticorenal ganglia
15. 右肾 right kidney

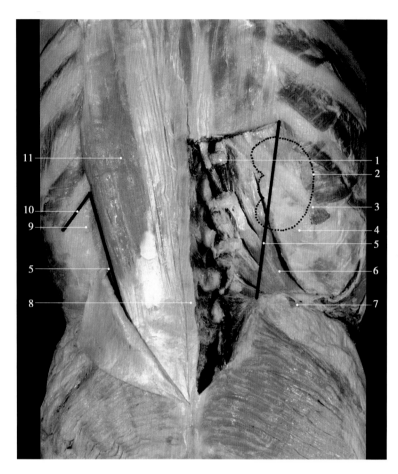

◀ 图 247　脊肋角
Costovertebral angle

1. 横突 transverse process
2. 右肾投影 projection of right kidney
3. 第 12 肋 the 12th rib
4. 腹横筋膜 transverse fascia
5. 竖脊肌外缘 lateral border of erector spinae
6. 腰方肌 quadratus lumborum
7. 髂嵴 iliac crest
8. 棘突 spinous process
9. 脊肋角（肾角）costovertebral angle
10. 第 12 肋下缘 inferior border of the 12th rib
11. 竖脊肌 erector spinae

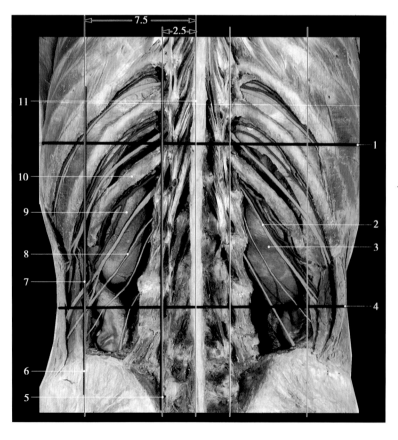

◀ 图 248　肾的体表投影（后面观）
Surface projection of kidney.Posterior view

1. 通过第 11 胸椎棘突水平线 horizontal line through spinous process of the11th thoracic vertebra
2. 肋下神经 subcostal n.
3. 右肾 right kidney
4. 通过第 3 腰椎棘突水平线 horizontal line through spinous process of the 3th lumbar vertebra
5. 内侧垂直线 medial vertical line
6. 外侧垂直线 lateral vertical line
7. 竖脊肌外侧缘 lateral border of erector spinae
8. 髂腹下神经 iliohypogastric n.
9. 左肾 left kidney
10. 第 12 肋 the 12th rib
11. 后正中线 posterior median line

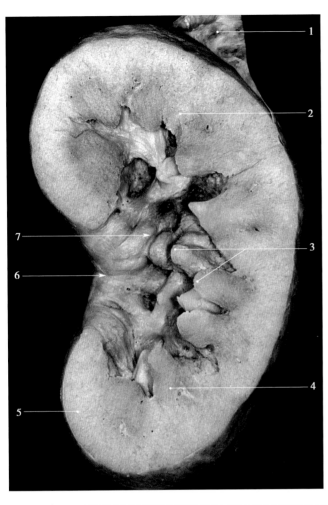

◀ 图 249　肾门与肾窦
Renal hilus and sinus

1. 纤维囊 fibrous capsule
2. 肾柱 renal columns
3. 肾乳头 renal papillae
4. 肾锥体 renal pyramid
5. 肾皮质 renal cortex
6. 肾门 renal hilus
7. 肾窦 renal sinus

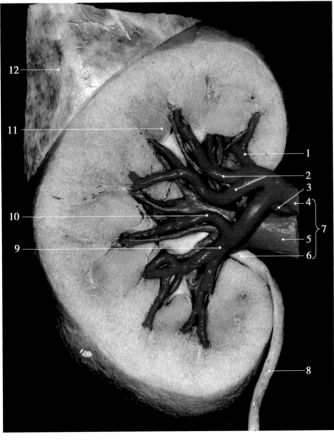

◀ 图 250　肾蒂
Renal pedicle

1. 上段动脉 superior segmental a.
2. 上前段动脉 superior anterior segmental a.
3. 后段动脉 posterior segmental a.
4. 肾动脉 renal a.
5. 肾静脉 renal v.
6. 肾盂 renal pelvis
7. 肾蒂 renal pedicle
8. 输尿管 ureter
9. 下段动脉 inferior segmental a.
10. 下前段动脉 inferior anterior segmental a.
11. 肾乳头 renal papillae
12. 纤维囊 fibrous capsule

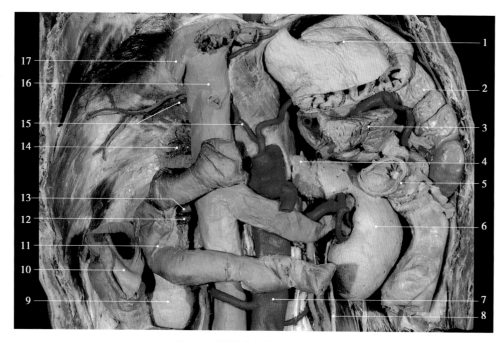

▲ 图 251　肾的毗邻关系（前面观）
Adjacent relationship of kidney with peripheral organs.Anterior view

1. 胃 stomach
2. 脾 spleen
3. 胰 pancreas
4. 左肾上腺 left suprarenal gland
5. 结肠左曲 left colic flexure
6. 左肾 left kidney
7. 腹主动脉 abdominal aorta
8. 左输尿管 left ureter
9. 右肾 right kidney
10. 结肠右曲 right colic flexure
11. 十二指肠 duodenum
12. 胰管 pancreatic duct
13. 胆总管 common bile duct
14. 右肾上腺 right suprarenal gland
15. 膈下动脉 inferior phrenic a.
16. 下腔静脉 inferior vena cava
17. 肝右静脉 right hepatic v.

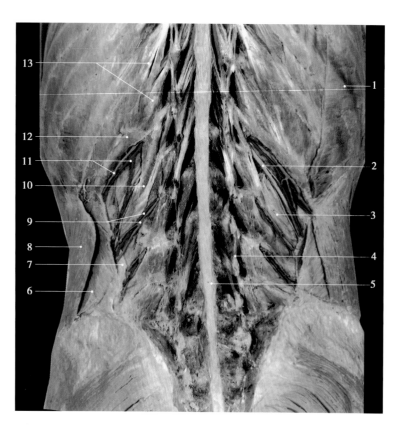

◀ 图 252　肾的毗邻关系（后面观 1）
Adjacent relationship of kidney with peripheral organs.Poterior view（1）

1. 下后锯肌 serratus posterior inferior
2. 肋下神经 subcostal n.
3. 胸腰筋膜中层 middle layer of thoracolumbar fascia
4. 横突间肌 intertransversarii
5. 棘突 spinous process
6. 腹内斜肌 obliquus internus abdominis
7. 腹横肌 transverse abdominis
8. 腹外斜肌 obliquus externus abdominis
9. 第 1 腰动、静脉 the 1st lumbar a.and v.
10. 腰方肌 quadratus lumborum
11. 肋下动、静脉 subcostal a.and v.
12. 第 12 肋 the 12th rib
13. 肋提肌 levatores costarum

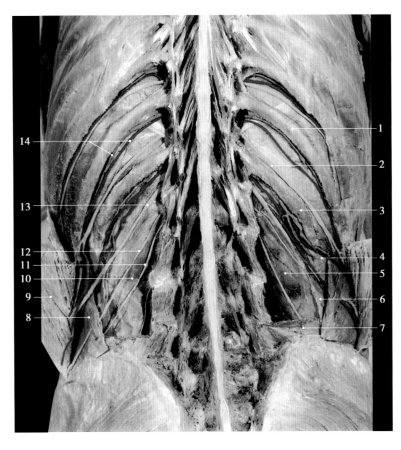

◀图 253 肾的毗邻关系（后面观 2）
Adjacent relationship of kidney with peripheral organs.Posterior view（2）

1. 第 11 肋 the 11th rib
2. 第 11 肋间神经 the 11th intercostal n.
3. 第 12 肋 the 12th rib
4. 膈 diaphragm
5. 肾后筋膜 posterior layer of renal fascia
6. 腹横肌 transverse abdominis
7. 腰方肌 quadratus lumborum
8. 腹内斜肌 obliquus internus abdominis
9. 腹外斜肌 obliquus externus abdominis
10. 肾下端 inferior extremity of kidney
11. 髂腹股沟神经 ilioinguinal n.
12. 髂腹下神经 iliohypogastric n.
13. 肋下神经 subcostal n.
14. 肋间后动、静脉 posterior intercostal a.and v.

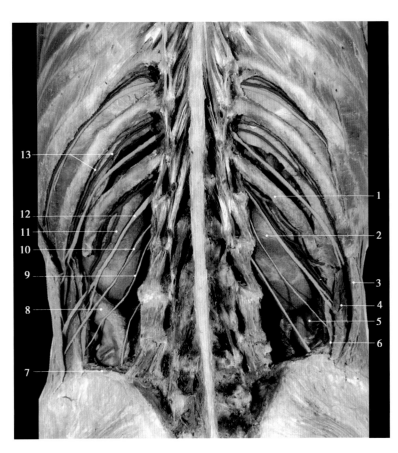

◀图 254 肾的毗邻关系（后面观 3）
Adjacent relationship of kidney with peripheral organs.Posterior view（3）

1. 第 12 肋 the 12th rib
2. 右肾 right kidney
3. 腹外斜肌 obliquus externus abdominis
4. 腹内斜肌 obliquus internus abdominis
5. 升结肠 ascending colon
6. 腹横肌 transverse abdominis
7. 髂嵴 iliac crest
8. 降结肠 descending colon
9. 髂腹股沟神经 ilioinguinal n.
10. 髂腹下神经 iliohypogastric n.
11. 左肾 left kidney
12. 肋下神经 subcostal n.
13. 第 11 肋间后动、静脉 the 11th posterior intercostal a.and v.

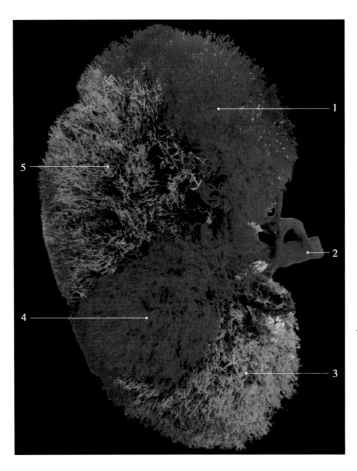

◀图 255　肾段与肾动脉的铸形（前面观）
Cast of renal segments and their arteries.
Anterior view

1. 上段 superior segment
2. 肾动脉 renal a.
3. 下段 inferior segment
4. 下前段 inferior anterior segment
5. 上前段 superior anterior segment

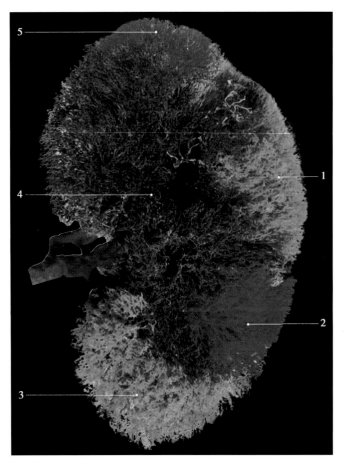

◀图 256　肾段与肾动脉的铸形（后面观）
Cast of renal segments and their arteries.
Posterior view

1. 上前段 superior anterior segment
2. 下前段 inferior anterior segment
3. 下段 inferior segment
4. 后段 posterior segment
5. 上段 superior segment

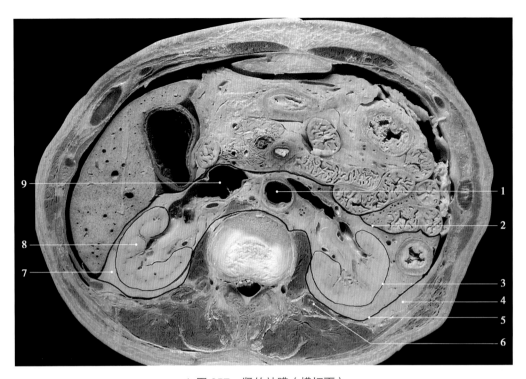

▲ 图 257　肾的被膜（横切面）
Coverings of kidney.Transverse section

1. 腹主动脉 abdominal aorta
2. 肾前筋膜 anterior layer of renal fascia
3. 纤维囊 fibrous capsule
4. 肾旁脂体 pararenal adipose body
5. 肾后筋膜 posterior layer of renal fascia
6. 腰方肌 quadratus lumborum
7. 脂肪囊 renal fat capsule
8. 右肾 right kidney
9. 下腔静脉 inferior vena cava

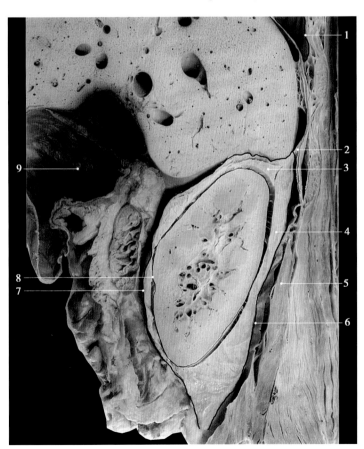

◀ 图 258　肾的被膜（纵切面）
Coverings of kidney.Longitudinal section

1. 壁胸膜 parietal pleura
2. 膈下筋膜 subdiaphragm fascia
3. 肾上腺 suprarenal gland
4. 脂肪囊 renal fat capsule
5. 腰方肌 quadratus lumborum
6. 肾后筋膜 posterior layer of renal fascia
7. 肾前筋膜 anterior layer of renal fascia
8. 纤维囊 fibrous capsule
9. 横结肠 transverse colon

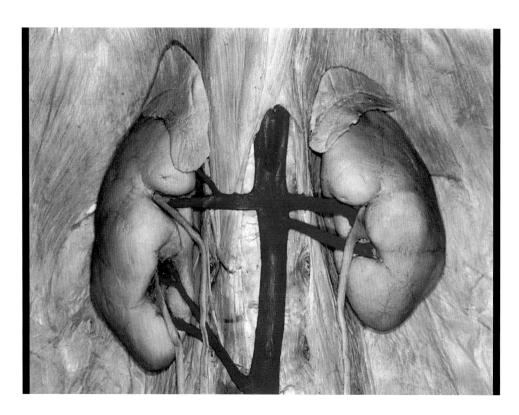

▲ 图 259 　肾动脉的变异
Variations of renal artery

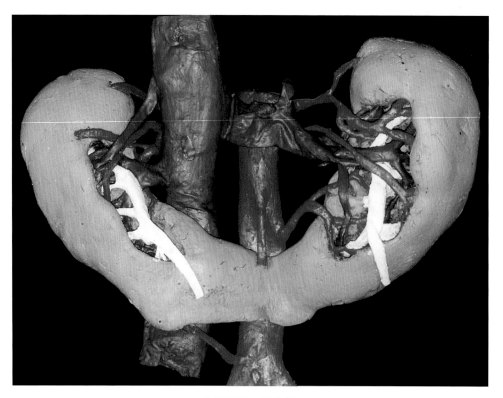

▲ 图 260 　马蹄肾
Horseshoe kidney

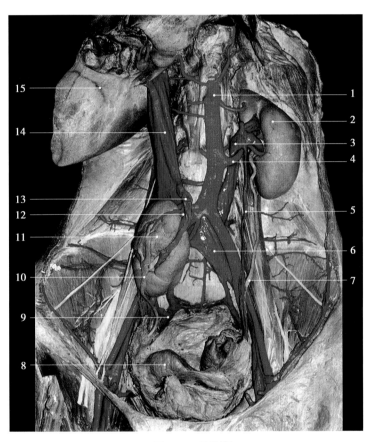

▲ 图 261　异位肾
Ectopic kidney

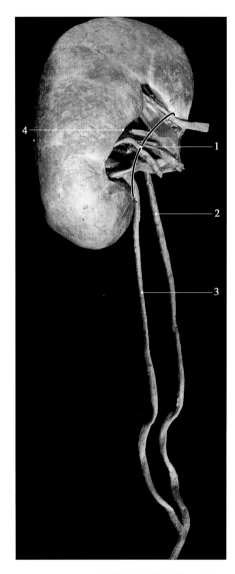

▲ 图 262　不完全性重复肾（前面观）
Incomplete renal duplication.Anterior view

1. 腹主动脉 abdominal aorta
2. 左肾 left kidney
3. 左肾静脉 left renal v.
4. 左肾动脉 left renal a.
5. 左卵巢静脉 left ovarian v.
6. 左髂总静脉 left common iliac v.
7. 左输尿管 left ureter
8. 子宫 uterus
9. 右髂内静脉 right internal iliac v.
10. 右输尿管 right ureter
11. 右异位肾 right ectopic kidney
12. 右肾动脉 right renal a.
13. 右肾静脉 right renal v.
14. 下腔静脉 inferior vena cava
15. 肝 liver

1. 肾蒂 renal pedicle
2. 上位输尿管 superior ureter
3. 下位输尿管 inferior ureter
4. 肾门 renal hilum

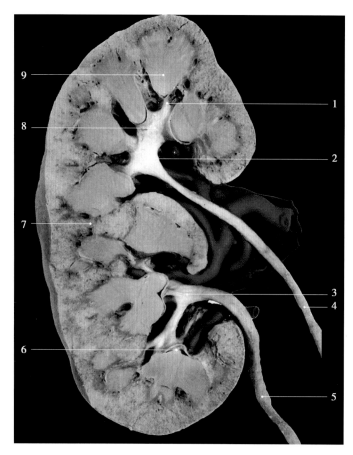

◀ 图 263　不完全性重复肾（冠状切面）
Incomplete renal duplication.Coronal section

1. 肾小盏 minor renal calices
2. 上位肾盂 superior renal pelvis
3. 下位肾盂 inferior renal pelvis
4. 上位输尿管 superior ureter
5. 下位输尿管 inferior ureter
6. 肾乳头 renal papillae
7. 肾柱 renal columns
8. 肾大盏 major renal calices
9. 肾锥体 renal pyramid

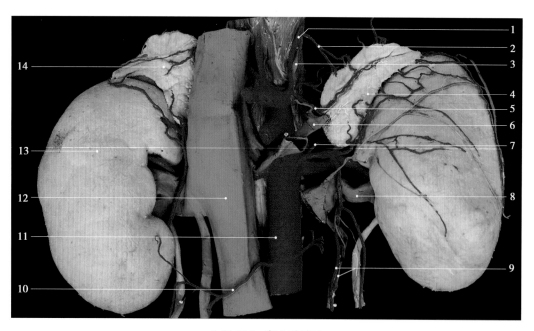

▲ 图 264　肾上腺动脉
Arteries of suprarenal glands

1. 膈下动脉 inferior phrenic a.
2. 肾上腺上动脉 superior suprarenal a.
3. 膈下静脉 inferior phrenic v.
4. 左肾上腺 left suprarenal gland
5. 肾上腺中动脉 middle suprarenal a.
6. 肾上腺静脉 suprarenal v.
7. 肾上腺下动脉 inferior suprarenal a.
8. 肾静脉（切断）renal v.
9. 睾丸动、静脉 testicular a. and v.
10. 睾丸动脉 testicular a.
11. 腹主动脉 abdominal aorta
12. 下腔静脉 inferior vena cava
13. 右肾 right kidney
14. 右肾上腺 right suprarenal gland

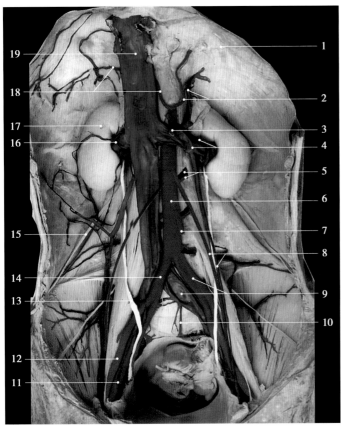

◀ 图 265　腹膜后隙的血管
Blood vessels in retroperitoneal space

1. 膈 diaphragm
2. 左膈下动、静脉 left inferior phrenic a.and v.
3. 肠系膜上动脉 superior mesenteric a.
4. 左肾动、静脉 left renal a.and v.
5. 腰动、静脉 lumbar a.and v.
6. 腹主动脉 abdominal aorta
7. 肠系膜下动脉 inferior mesenteric a.
8. 左睾丸动、静脉 left testicular a.and v.
9. 左髂总动、静脉 left common iliac a.and v.
10. 骶正中动脉 median sacral a.
11. 右髂外静脉 right external iliac v.
12. 右髂外动脉 right external iliac a.
13. 右输尿管 right ureter
14. 右髂总动脉 right common iliac a.
15. 髂腹下神经 iliohypogastric n.
16. 右肾静脉 right renal v.
17. 右肾 right kidney
18. 右膈下动脉 right inferior phrenic a.
19. 下腔静脉 inferior vena cava

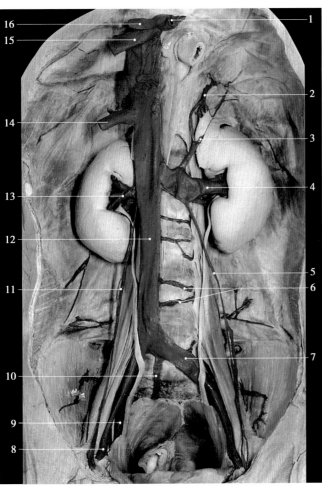

◀ 图 266　下腔静脉及其属支
Inferior vena cava and its tributaries

1. 肝左静脉 left hepatic v.
2. 膈下静脉 inferior phrenic v.
3. 左肾上腺静脉 left suprarenal v.
4. 左肾静脉 left renal v.
5. 左睾丸静脉 left testicular v.
6. 左腰静脉 left lumbar v.
7. 左髂总静脉 left common iliac v.
8. 髂外静脉 external iliac v.
9. 髂内静脉 internal iliac v.
10. 骶正中静脉 median sacral v.
11. 右睾丸静脉 right testicular v.
12. 下腔静脉 inferior vena cava
13. 右肾静脉 right renal v.
14. 肝右后静脉 right posterior hepatic v.
15. 肝右静脉 right hepatic v.
16. 肝中间静脉 intermediate hepatic v.

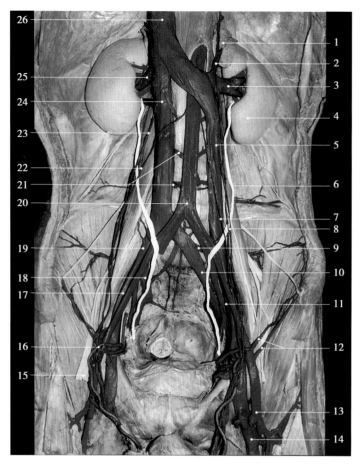

◀ 图 267 双下腔静脉及其属支
Double inferior vena cava and its tributaries

1. 左肾上腺 left suprarenal gland
2. 左肾上腺静脉 left suprarenal v.
3. 左肾静脉 left renal v.
4. 左肾 left kidney
5. 左下腔静脉 left inferior vena cava
6. 左输尿管 left ureter
7. 左睾丸动脉 left testicular a.
8. 左睾丸静脉 left testicular v.
9. 吻合支 anastomotic branch
10. 左髂内静脉 left internal iliac v.
11. 左髂外静脉 left external iliac v.
12. 旋髂深动、静脉 deep iliac circumflex a.and v.
13. 股动脉 femoral a.
14. 股静脉 femoral v.
15. 股神经 femoral n.
16. 输精管 ductus deferens
17. 右髂外静脉 right external iliac v.
18. 右髂内静脉 right internal iliac v.
19. 右髂总静脉 right common iliac v.
20. 腹主动脉 abdominal aorta
21. 腰动、静脉 lumbar a.and v.
22. 右睾丸动脉 right testicular a.
23. 右睾丸静脉 right testicular v.
24. 右下腔静脉 right inferior vena cava
25. 右肾静脉 right renal v.
26. 总下腔静脉 common inferior vena cava

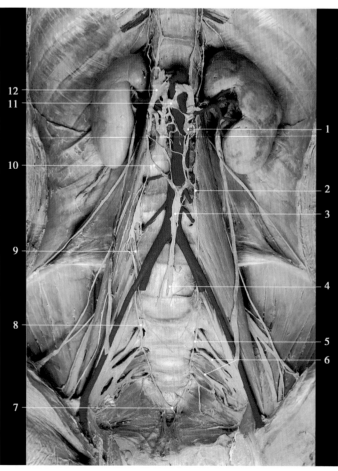

◀ 图 268 腹膜后隙的神经（1）
Nerves in retroperitoneal space（1）

1. 主动脉肾神经节 aorticorenal ganglia
2. 腰交感干 lumbar sympathetic trunk
3. 腹主动脉丛 abdominal aortic plexus
4. 上腹下丛 superior hypogastric plexus
5. 骶交感干 sacral sympathetic truck
6. 骶神经 sacral n.
7. 奇神经节 ganglion impar
8. 骶神经节 sacral ganglia
9. 灰交通支 gray communicating branches
10. 腰内脏神经 lumbar splanchnic n.
11. 肠系膜上神经节 superior mesenteric ganglion
12. 腹腔神经节 celiac ganglia

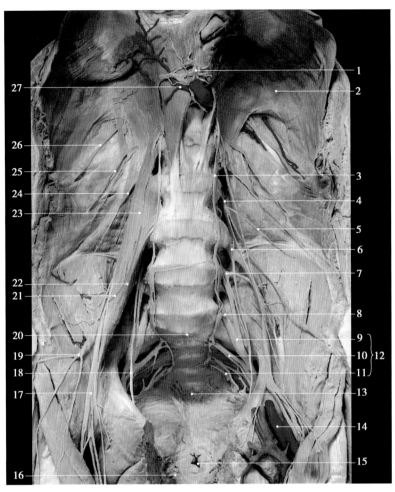

◀ 图 269　腹膜后隙的神经（2）
Nerves in retroperitoneal space（2）

1. 腹腔神经节 celiac ganglia
2. 膈 diaphragm
3. 交感干 sympathetic trunk
4. 第 2 腰神经前支 anterior branch of the 2nd lumbar n.
5. 生殖股神经 genitofemoral n.
6. 第 3 腰神经前支 anterior branch of the 3rd lumbar n.
7. 第 4 腰神经前支 anterior branch of 4th lumbar n.
8. 第 5 腰神经前支 anterior branch of the 5th lumbar n.
9. 腰骶干 lumbosacral trunk
10. 第 1 骶神经 the 1st sacral n.
11. 第 3 骶神经 the 3rd sacral n.
12. 骶丛 sacral plexus
13. 奇神经节 ganglion impar
14. 股动脉 femoral a.
15. 直肠 rectum
16. 肛门括约肌 anal sphincter
17. 股神经 femoral n.
18. 闭孔神经 obturator n.
19. 股外侧皮神经 lateral femoral cutaneous n.
20. 岬 promontory
21. 生殖支 genital branch
22. 股支 femoral branch
23. 腰大肌 psoas major
24. 髂腹股沟神经 ilioinguinal n.
25. 髂腹下神经 iliohypogastric n.
26. 肋下神经 subcostal n.
27. 膈下动脉 inferior phrenic a.

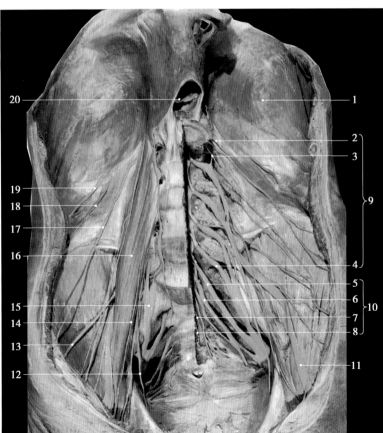

◀ 图 270　腰骶丛的组成
Component of lumbar and sacral plexus

1. 膈 diaphragm
2. 第 12 胸神经 the 12 th thoracic n.
3. 第 1 腰神经 the 1st lumbar n.
4. 第 5 腰神经 the 5th lumbar n.
5. 第 1 骶神经 the 1st sacral n.
6. 第 2 骶神经 the 2nd sacral n.
7. 第 5 骶神经 the 5th sacral n.
8. 尾神经 coccygeal n.
9. 腰丛 lumbar plexus
10. 骶丛 sacral plexus
11. 股神经 femoral n.
12. 闭孔神经 obturator n.
13. 股外侧皮神经 lateral femoral cutaneous n.
14. 生殖股神经 genitofemoral n.
15. 腰骶干 lumbosacral trunk
16. 腰大肌 psoas major
17. 髂腹股沟神经 ilioinguinal n.
18. 髂腹下神经 iliohypogastric n.
19. 肋下神经 subcostal n.
20. 主动脉裂孔 aortic hiatus

连续层次局部解剖

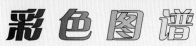

第五章

盆部和会阴

Chapter 5 Pelvis and perineum

盆部上界为耻骨联合上缘、两侧的耻骨嵴、耻骨结节、腹股沟韧带、髂前上棘，循髂嵴至第 5 腰椎棘突的连线。会阴是指盆膈以下封闭骨盆下口的全部软组织。会阴的外侧与股部相连，会阴可分为肛区和尿生殖区。

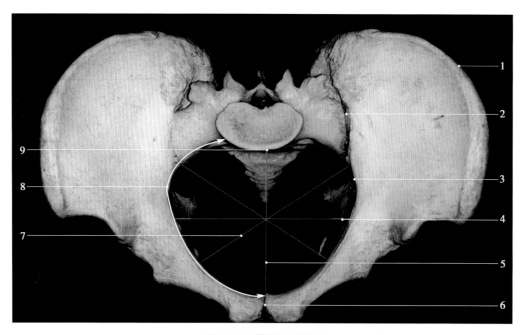

▲ 图 271　骨盆上口径线
Diameter of superior pelvic aperture

1. 髂嵴 iliac crest
2. 骶髂关节 sacroiliac joint
3. 弓状线 arcuate line
4. 横径 transverse diameter
5. 前后径 anteroposterior diameter
6. 耻骨联合 pubic symphysis
7. 斜径 oblique diameter
8. 界线 terminal line
9. 岬 promontory

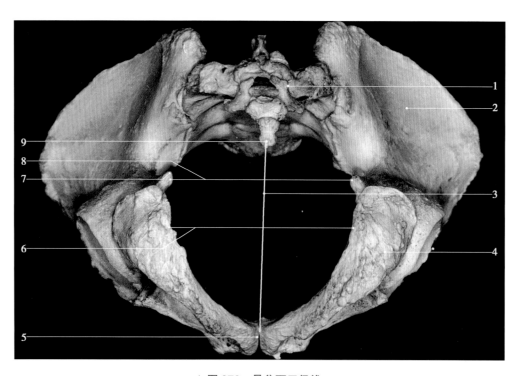

▲ 图 272　骨盆下口径线
Diameter of inferior pelvic aperture

1. 骶骨 sacrum
2. 髂骨 ilium
3. 骨盆出口前后径线 anteroposterior diameter of pelvic outlet
4. 坐骨结节 ischial tuberosity
5. 耻骨联合下缘 inferior border of pubic symphysis
6. 骨盆出口横径 transverse diameter of pelvic outlet
7. 坐骨棘 ischial spine
8. 坐骨棘间径 bi-ischial diameter
9. 尾骨 coccyx

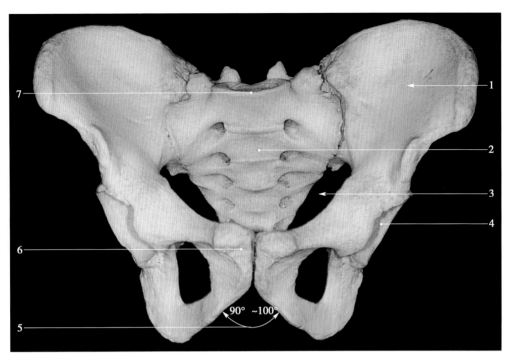

▲ 图 273　女性骨盆（前面观）
Pelvis of female.Anterior view

1. 大骨盆 greater pelvis　　5. 耻骨下角 subpubic angle
2. 骶骨 sacrum　　　　　　6. 耻骨 pubis
3. 小骨盆 lesser pelvis　　　7. 岬 promontory
4. 髋臼 acetabulum

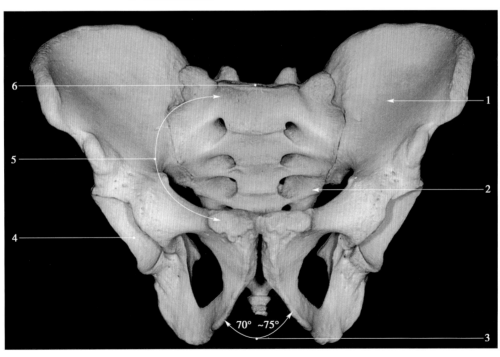

▲ 图 274　男性骨盆（前面观）
Pelvis of male.Anterior view

1. 大骨盆 greater pelvis　　4. 髋臼 acetabulum
2. 小骨盆 lesser pelvis　　　5. 界线 terminal line
3. 耻骨下角 subpubic angle　6. 岬 promontory

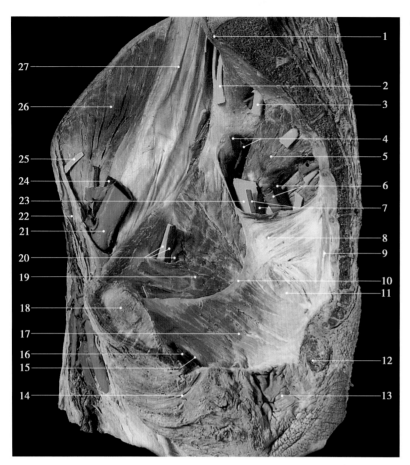

◀ 图 275　盆壁肌（1）
Muscles of pelvic wall（1）

1. 岬 promontory
2. 腰骶干 lumbosacral trunk
3. 第 1 骶 神 经 前 支 anterior branch of the 1st sacral n.
4. 臀上动、静脉 superior gluteal a.and v.
5. 梨状肌 piriformis
6. 臀下动、静脉 inferior gluteal a.and v.
7. 阴部内动、静脉 internal pudendal a.and v.
8. 尾骨肌 coccygeus
9. 直肠尾骨肌 rectococcygeal
10. 肛提肌腱弓 tendinous arch of levator ani
11. 髂尾肌 iliococcygeus
12. 肛门外括约肌 sphincter ani externus
13. 肛门 anus
14. 尿道 urethra
15. 前列腺提肌 levator prostatae
16. 阴茎背动脉吻合支 anastomotic branch with dorsal artery of penis
17. 耻尾肌 pubococcygeus
18. 耻骨联合面 symphysial surface
19. 闭孔内肌 obturator internus
20. 闭孔动、静脉和神经 obturator a.,v.and n.
21. 髂外静脉 external iliac v.
22. 腹股沟韧带 inguinal lig.
23. 坐骨神经 sciatic n.
24. 髂外动脉 exteral iliac a.
25. 股外侧皮神经 lateral femoral cutaneous n.
26. 髂肌 iliacus
27. 腰大肌 psoas major

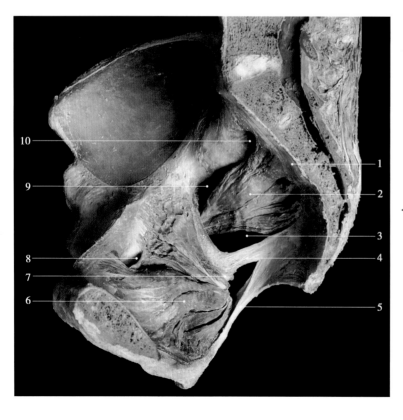

◀ 图 276　盆壁肌（2）
Muscles of pelvic wall（2）

1. 骶骨 sacrum
2. 梨状肌 piriformis
3. 梨状肌下孔 infrapiriformis foramen
4. 骶棘韧带 sacrospinous lig.
5. 骶结节韧带 sacrotuberous lig.
6. 闭孔内肌 obturator internus
7. 坐骨棘 ischial spine
8. 闭膜管 obturator canal
9. 梨状肌上孔 suprapiriformis foramen
10. 骶前孔 anterior sacral foramina

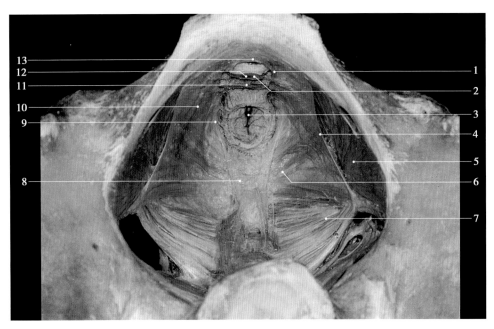

▲ 图 277 女性盆底肌
Muscles of female pelvic floor

1. 耻骨阴道肌 pubovaginalis
2. 尿道括约肌 sphincter of urethra
3. 直肠 rectum
4. 肛提肌腱弓 tendinous arch of levator ani
5. 闭孔内肌 obturator internus
6. 髂尾肌 iliococcygeus
7. 尾骨肌 coccygeus
8. 肛尾韧带 anococcygeal lig.
9. 耻骨直肠肌 puborectalis
10. 耻尾肌 pubococcygeus
11. 阴道 vagina
12. 尿道 urethra
13. 耻骨弓状韧带 arcuate pubic lig.

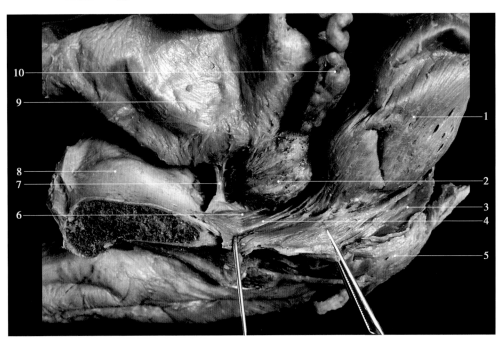

▲ 图 278 耻骨直肠肌
Puborectalis

1. 直肠 rectum
2. 前列腺 prostate
3. 肛提肌 levator ani
4. 耻骨直肠肌 puborectalis
5. 肛门外括约肌 sphincter ani externus
6. 耻骨前列腺肌 puboprostatic m.
7. 耻骨膀胱肌 pubovesical m.
8. 耻骨 pubis
9. 膀胱 urinary bladder
10. 精囊 seminal vesicle

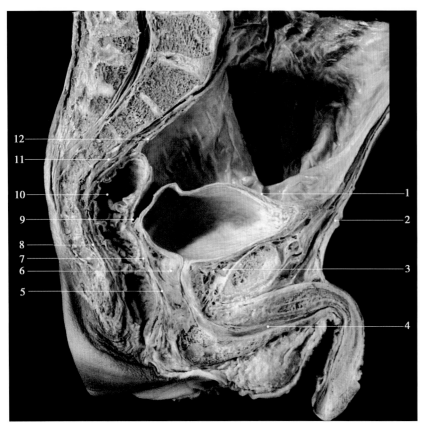

◀ 图 279　男性盆部筋膜（正中矢状切面）
Fascia of male pelvic cavity.Median
sagittal section

1. 膀胱筋膜 urocystic fascia
2. 腹壁浅筋膜 superficial fascia of abdominal wall
3. 耻骨后间隙 retropubic space
4. 尿道 urethra
5. 前列腺鞘 fascial sheath of prostate
6. 前列腺 prostate
7. 直肠膀胱隔 rectovesical septum
8. 直肠筋膜 rectal fascia
9. 直肠膀胱陷凹 rectovesical pouch
10. 直肠 rectum
11. 骶前筋膜 anterior sacral fascia
12. 腹膜 peritoneum

图 280　女性盆部筋膜（正中矢状切面）▶
Fascia of female pelvic cavity.Median
sagittal section

1. 腹膜 peritoneum
2. 膀胱筋膜 urocystic fascia
3. 膀胱子宫陷凹 vesicouterine pouch
4. 膀胱阴道隔 vesicovaginal septum
5. 耻骨后脂肪垫 retropubic fat pad
6. 尿道 urethra
7. 耻骨联合 pubic symphysis
8. 阴道 vagina
9. 直肠阴道隔 rectovaginal septum
10. 直肠子宫陷凹 rectouterine pouch
11. 直肠后隙 retrorectal space
12. 直肠筋膜 rectal fascia
13. 骶前筋膜 anterior sacral fascia

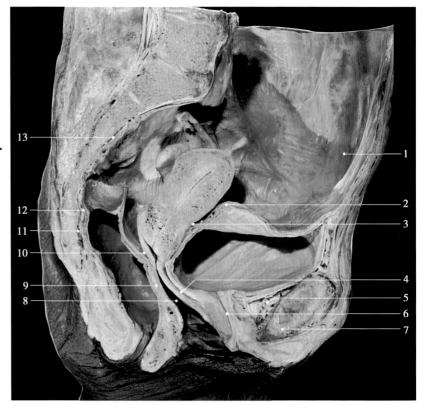

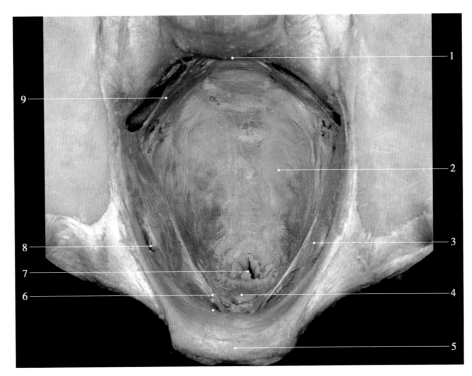

▲ 图 281　盆壁筋膜
Parietal pelvic fascia

1. 岬 promontory
2. 盆膈上筋膜 superior fascia of pelvis diaphragm
3. 闭孔筋膜 obturator fascia
4. 尿道 urethra
5. 耻骨联合 pubic symphysis
6. 肛提肌腱弓 tendinous arch of levator ani
7. 直肠 rectum
8. 闭膜管 obturator canal
9. 梨状肌筋膜 fascia of piriformis

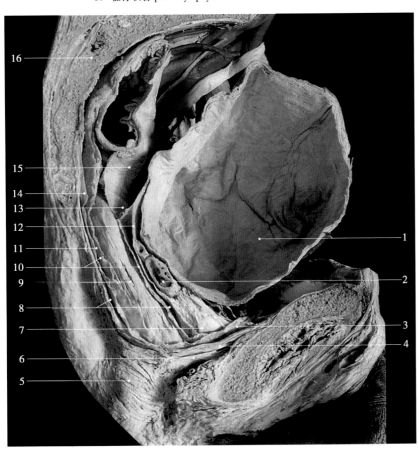

◀ 图 282　直肠周围间隙
Pararectal space

1. 膀胱 urinary bladder
2. 精囊 seminal vesicle
3. 盆膈上筋膜 superior fascia of pelvic diaphragm
4. 耻骨直肠肌 puborectalis
5. 肛门外括约肌 sphincter ani externus
6. 盆膈下筋膜 inferior fascia of pelvic diaphragm
7. 前列腺鞘 fascial sheath of prostate
8. 直肠周围间隙 pararectal space
9. 直肠 rectum
10. 直肠筋膜 rectal fascia
11. 直肠后隙 retrorectal space
12. 直肠膀胱隔 rectovesical septum
13. 直肠膀胱陷凹 rectovesical pouch
14. 骶前筋膜 anterior sacral fascia
15. 腹膜 peritoneum
16. 骶骨 sacrum

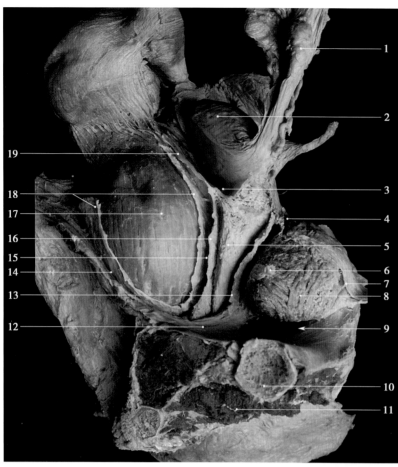

◀图 283　直肠阴道隔（侧面观）
Rectovaginal septum.Lateral view

1. 卵巢 ovary
2. 子宫 uterus
3. 直肠子宫陷凹 rectouterine pouch
4. 膀胱子宫陷凹 vesicouterine pouch
5. 阴道 vagina
6. 输尿管 ureter
7. 膀胱筋膜 vesical fascia
8. 膀胱 urinary bladder
9. 耻骨后间隙 retropubic space
10. 耻骨上支 superior ramus of pubis
11. 闭孔外肌 obturator externus
12. 肛提肌 levator ani
13. 膀胱阴道隔 veslcovaginal septum
14. 直肠后隙 retrorectal space
15. 直肠前隙 anterior rectal space
16. 直肠阴道隔 rectovaginal septum
17. 直肠壶腹 ampulla of rectum
18. 直肠筋膜 rectal fascia
19. 腹膜 peritoneum

图 284　男性盆腔的血管（侧面观）▶
Blood vessels of male pelvic cavity.Lateral view

1. 乙状结肠 sigmoid colon
2. 脐动脉 umbilical a.
3. 膀胱上动脉 superior vesical a.
4. 膀胱下动、静脉 inferior vesical a.and v.
5. 膀胱 urinary bladder
6. 前列腺 prostate
7. 盆膈下筋膜 inferior fascia of pelvic diaphragm
8. 前列腺支 prostatic branch
9. 直肠下动、静脉 inferior rectal a.and v.
10. 阴部神经 pudendal n.
11. 阴部内动、静脉 internal pudendal a.and v.
12. 坐骨神经 sciatic n.
13. 髂腰动脉 iliolumbar a.
14. 右髂总动脉 right common iliac a.

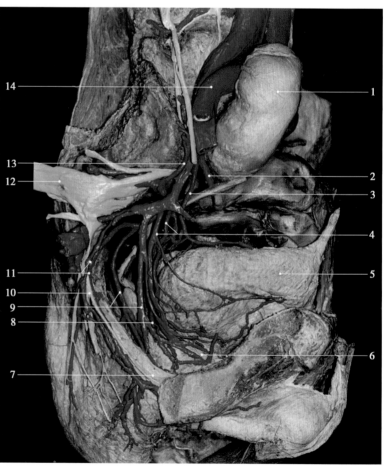

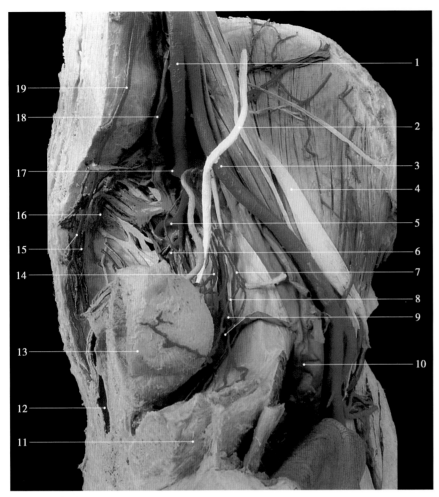

◀ 图285　男性盆腔的血管(内侧面观)
Blood vessels of male pelvic
cavity.Medial view

1. 髂内动脉 internal iliac a.
2. 输尿管 ureter
3. 髂外动脉 external iliac a.
4. 股神经 femoral n.
5. 臀下动脉 inferior gluteal a.
6. 阴部内动脉 internal pudendal a.
7. 脐动脉 umbilical a.
8. 膀胱上动脉 superior vesical a.
9. 闭孔动、静脉 obturator a.and v.
10. 股静脉 femoral v.
11. 耻骨 pubis
12. 直肠 rectum
13. 膀胱 urinary bladder
14. 膀胱下动脉 inferior vesical a.
15. 骶正中动、静脉 median sacral a.and v.
16. 骶外侧动脉 lateral sacral a.
17. 臀上动脉 superior gluteal a.
18. 髂内静脉 internal iliac v.
19. 骶正中动脉 median sacral a.

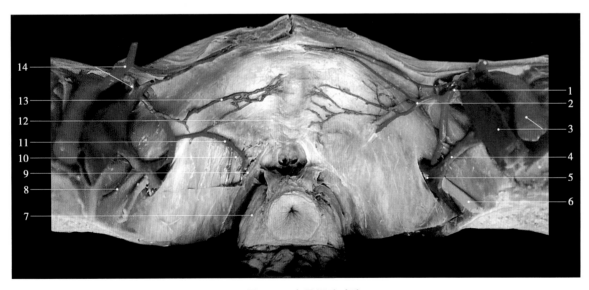

▲ 图 286　变异闭孔动脉
Variant obturator artery

1. 变异闭孔动脉 variant obturator a.
2. 闭孔动脉耻骨支 pubic branch of obturator a.
3. 髂外动、静脉 external iliac a.and v.
4. 耻静脉 pubic v.
5. 闭膜管 obturator canal
6. 闭孔神经 obturator n.
7. 前列腺 prostate
8. 闭孔静脉 obturator v.
9. 肛提肌 levator ani
10. 闭孔内肌 obturator internus
11. 闭孔内肌肌支 muscular branch of obturator internus
12. 耻骨联合后面 posterior surface of pubic symphysis
13. 腹壁下静脉耻骨支 pubic branch of inferior epigastric v.
14. 腹壁下动、静脉 inferior epigastric a.and v.

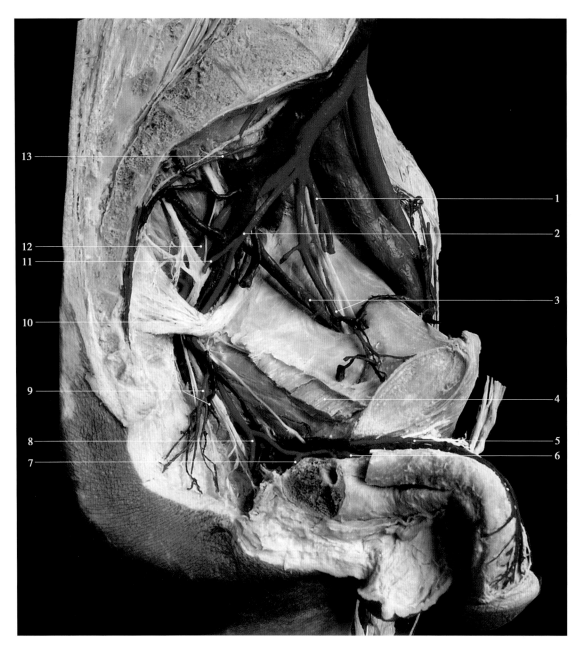

▲ 图 287　阴茎背动脉
Dorsal artery of penis

1. 脐动脉 umbilical a.
2. 阴部内动脉 internal pudendal a.
3. 闭孔动、静脉 obturator a.and v.
4. 肛提肌 levator ani
5. 阴茎背动脉 dorsal artery of penis
6. 阴茎深动脉 deep artery of penis
7. 尿道球动脉 urethral bulbar a.
8. 阴囊后动脉 posterior scrotal a.
9. 肛动、静脉 anal a.and v.
10. 坐骨棘 ischial spine
11. 直肠下动脉 inferior rectal a.
12. 臀下动脉 inferior gluteal a.
13. 骶外侧动脉 lateral sacral a.

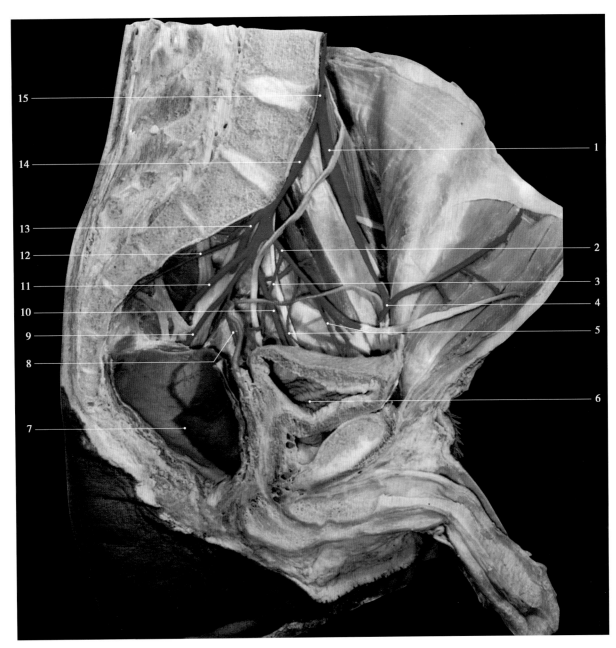

▲ 图 288　男性盆腔的动脉
Arteries of male pelvic cavity

1. 髂外动脉 external iliac a.
2. 脐动脉 umbilical a.
3. 膀胱下动脉 inferior vesical a.
4. 腹壁下动脉 inferior epigastric a.
5. 膀胱上动脉 superior vesical a.
6. 膀胱 urinary bladder
7. 直肠 rectum
8. 直肠下动脉 inferior rectal a.
9. 阴部内动脉 internal pudendal a.
10. 闭孔动脉 obturator a.
11. 臀下动脉 inferior gluteal a.
12. 骶外侧动脉 lateral sacral a.
13. 臀上动脉 superior gluteal a.
14. 髂内动脉 internal iliac a.
15. 髂总动脉 common iliac a.

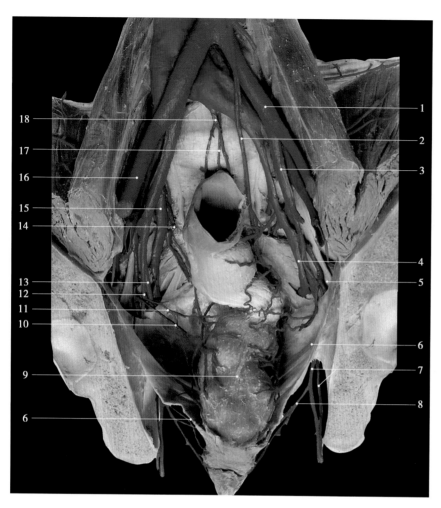

◀ 图 289　直肠和肛管的血管
Blood vessels of rectum and anal
canal.Anterior view

1. 髂总动脉 common iliac a.
2. 直肠上动脉 superior rectal a.
3. 髂内动脉 internal iliac a.
4. 臀下静脉 inferior gluteal v.
5. 坐骨神经 sciatic n.
6. 肛提肌 levator ani
7. 阴部内动、静脉 internal pudendal a.and v.
8. 肛动脉 anal a.
9. 直肠 rectum
10. 直肠下静脉 inferior rectal v.
11. 直肠下动脉 inferior rectal a.
12. 阴部内动脉 internal pudendal a.
13. 臀下动脉 inferior gluteal a.
14. 臀上静脉 superior gluteal v.
15. 髂内静脉 internal iliac v.
16. 髂外动脉 external iliac a.
17. 骶正中动脉 median sacral a.
18. 骶正中静脉 median sacral v.

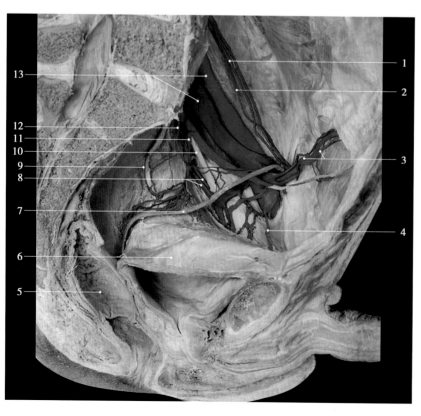

◀ 图 290　输精管的血管
Blood vessels of ductus deferens

1. 睾丸静脉 testicular v.
2. 睾丸动脉 testicular a.
3. 腹壁下动、静脉 inferior epigastric a.and v.
4. 膀胱上动脉 superior vesical a.
5. 直肠 rectum
6. 膀胱 urinary bladder
7. 输精管盆段 pelvic part of deferent duct
8. 闭孔动、静脉 obturator a.and v.
9. 输尿管动脉 ureteric a.
10. 闭孔神经 obturator n.
11. 膀胱下动脉 inferior vesical a.
12. 输精管动脉 deferential a.
13. 髂外动、静脉 external iliac a.and v.

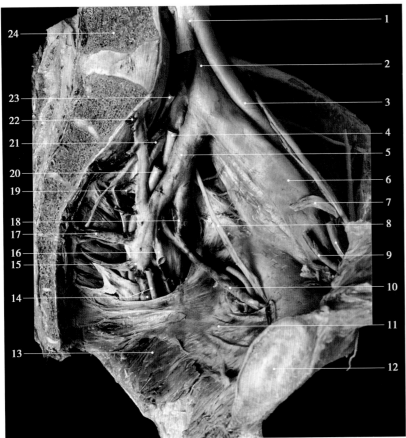

◀图 291　髂内静脉及其属支
Internal iliac vein and its tributaries

1. 髂总动脉 common iliac a.
2. 髂总静脉 common iliac v.
3. 髂外动脉 external iliac a.
4. 臀上动脉 superior gluteal a.
5. 髂内静脉 internal iliac v.
6. 髂外静脉 external iliac v.
7. 输精管 ductus deferens
8. 闭孔神经 obturator n.
9. 腹壁下动、静脉 inferior epigastric a.and v.
10. 闭孔静脉 obturator v.
11. 闭孔筋膜 obturator fascia
12. 耻骨联合面 symphysial surface
13. 肛提肌 levator ani
14. 阴部内动、静脉 internal pudendal a.and v.
15. 臀下静脉 inferior gluteal v.
16. 膀胱静脉 vesical v.
17. 骶静脉丛 sacral venous plexus
18. 臀上静脉 superior gluteal v.
19. 脊支 spinal branch
20. 臀下动脉 inferior gluteal a.
21. 骶外侧静脉 lateral sacral v.
22. 骶正中静脉 median sacral v.
23. 髂腰动脉 iliolumbar a.
24. 第 5 腰椎 the 5th lumbar vertebra

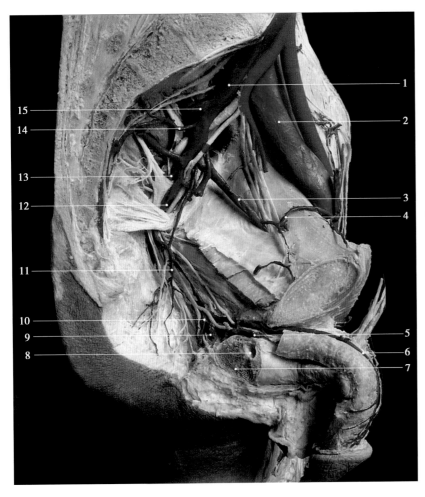

◀图 292　阴部内静脉
Internal pudendal vein

1. 髂内静脉 internal iliac v.
2. 髂外静脉 external iliac v.
3. 闭孔静脉 obturator v.
4. 耻静脉 pubic v.
5. 阴茎深静脉 deep vein of penis
6. 阴茎背深静脉 deep dorsal vein of penis
7. 尿道球 bulb of urethra
8. 尿道 urethra
9. 尿道球静脉 urethral bulbar v.
10. 阴囊后静脉 posterior scrotal v.
11. 肛静脉 anal v.
12. 阴部内静脉 interal pudendal v.
13. 臀下静脉 inferior gluteal v.
14. 骶外侧静脉 lateral sacral v.
15. 臀上静脉 superior gluteal v.

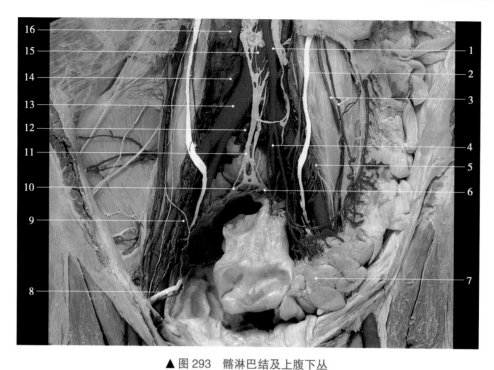

▲ 图 293　髂淋巴结及上腹下丛
Iliac lymph nodes and superior hypogastric plexus

1. 肠系膜下动脉 inferior mesenteric a.
2. 输尿管 ureter
3. 睾丸动、静脉 testicular a.and v.
4. 直肠上动脉 superior rectal a.
5. 髂外外侧淋巴结 lateral external iliac lymph nodes
6. 左腹下神经 left hypogastric n.
7. 乙状结肠 sigmoid colon
8. 输精管 ductus deferens
9. 髂内淋巴结 internal iliac lymph nodes
10. 右腹下神经 right hypogastric n.
11. 上腹下丛 superior hypogastric plexus
12. 主动脉下淋巴结 subaortic lymph nodes
13. 髂总动脉 common iliac a.
14. 下腔静脉 inferior vena cava
15. 腹主动脉 abdominal aorta
16. 腔静脉前淋巴结 precaval lymph nodes

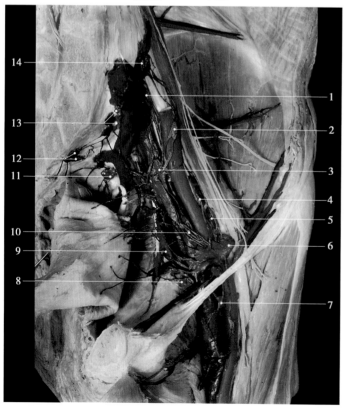

◀ 图 294　男性盆腔淋巴结
Lymph nodes of male pelvic cavity

1. 髂总内侧淋巴结 medial common iliac lymph nodes
2. 髂总外侧淋巴结 lateral common iliac lymph nodes
3. 髂外内侧淋巴结 medial external iliac lymph nodes
4. 髂外中间淋巴结 intermediate iliac lymph nodes
5. 髂外外侧淋巴结 lateral external iliac lymph nodes
6. 腔隙外侧淋巴结 lateral lacunar lymph node
7. 腹股沟深淋巴结 deep inguinal lymph nodes
8. 腔隙内侧淋巴结 medial lacunar lymph node
9. 闭孔淋巴结 obturator lymph nodes
10. 淋巴管 lymphatic vessel
11. 骶外侧淋巴结 latera sacral lymph nodes
12. 骶淋巴结 sacral lymph nodes
13. 主动脉下淋巴结 subaortic lymph nodes
14. 髂总淋巴结 common iliac lymph nodes

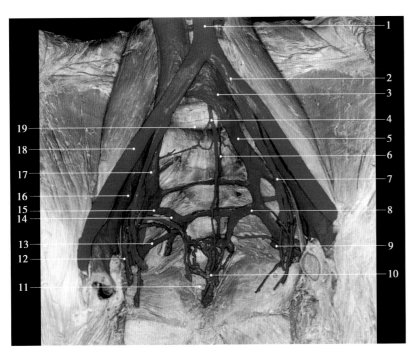

◀ 图 295　骶前部的血管
Blood vessels of anterior sacral region

1. 腹主动脉 abdominal aorta
2. 左髂总动脉 left common iliac a.
3. 左髂总静脉 left common iliac v.
4. 骶正中动脉 median sacral a.
5. 左髂内静脉 left internal iliac v.
6. 骶正中静脉 median sacral v.
7. 髂内动脉 internal iliac a.
8. 骶外侧静脉 lateral sacral v.
9. 臀下静脉 inferior gluteal v.
10. 骶静脉丛 sacral venous plexus
11. 尾骨 coccyx
12. 闭孔静脉 obturator v.
13. 骶外侧静脉下支 inferior branch of lateral sacral v.
14. 骶外侧静脉上支 superior branch of lateral sacral v.
15. 臀上静脉 superior gluteal v.
16. 右髂外静脉 right external iliac v.
17. 右髂内静脉 right internal iliac v.
18. 右髂外动脉 right external iliac a.
19. 岬 promontory

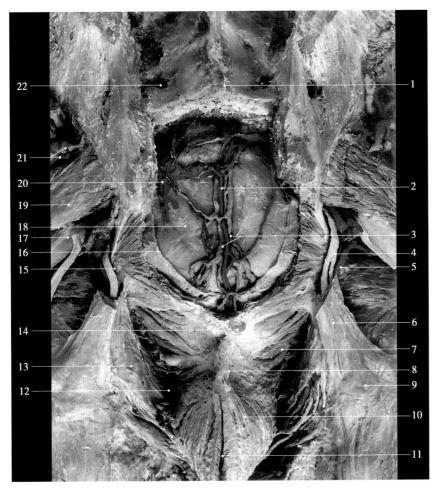

◀ 图 296　直肠后间隙局解（后面观 1 ）
Regional anatomy of retrorectal space. Posterior view (1)

1. 第 3 骶椎 the 3rd sacral vertebra
2. 骶正中动脉 median sacral a.
3. 骶正中静脉 median sacral v.
4. 阴部神经 pudendal n.
5. 阴部内动脉 internal pudendal a.
6. 骶结节韧带 sacrotuberous lig.
7. 肛提肌 levator ani
8. 肛尾韧带 anococcygeal lig.
9. 坐骨结节 ischial tuberosity
10. 肛门外括约肌 sphincter ani externus
11. 肛门 anus
12. 坐骨肛门窝 ischioanal fossa
13. 闭孔筋膜 obturator fascia
14. 尾骨 coccyx
15. 坐骨棘 ischial spine
16. 骶前筋膜 anterior sacral fascia
17. 坐骨神经 sciatic n.
18. 直肠筋膜 rectal fascia
19. 梨状肌 piriformis
20. 骶外侧动脉 lateral sacral a.
21. 臀上动、静脉 superior gluteal a.and v.
22. 骶后孔 posterior sacral foramina

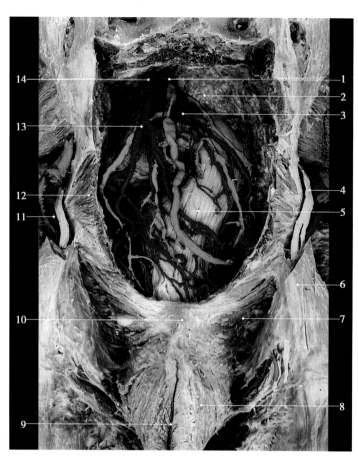

◀ 图 297　直肠后间隙局解（后面观 2 ）
Regional anatomy of retrorectal space.
Posterior view（2）

1. 直肠上静脉 superior rectal v.
2. 直肠周围脂肪 pararectal fat
3. 直肠上动脉右支 right branch of superior rectal a.
4. 阴部神经 pudendal n.
5. 直肠 rectum
6. 骶结节韧带 sacrotuberous lig.
7. 肛提肌 levator ani
8. 肛门外括约肌 sphincter ani externus
9. 肛门 anus
10. 肛尾韧带 anococcygeal lig.
11. 阴部内动脉 internal pudendal a.
12. 尾骨肌 coccygeus
13. 直肠上动脉左支 left branch of superior rectal a.
14. 直肠上动脉 superior rectal a.

图 298　直肠后间隙局解（后面观 3 ）▶
Regional anatomy of retrorectal space.Posterior view（3）

1. 乙状结肠直肠动脉 sigmoid rectus a.
2. 右腹下神经 right hypogastric n.
3. 直肠 rectum
4. 直肠上动脉右支 right branch of superior rectal a.
5. 输精管动脉 deferential a.
6. 输精管 ductus deferens
7. 直肠筋膜 fascia of rectum
8. 骶正中静脉 median sacral v.
9. 阴部内静脉 internal pudendal v.
10. 肛静脉 anal v.
11. 闭孔筋膜 obturator fascia
12. 阴囊后支 posterior scrotal branches
13. 肛门外括约肌 sphincter ani externus
14. 肛动脉 anal a.
15. 阴部神经 pudendal n.
16. 肛提肌 levator ani
17. 阴部内动脉 internal pudendal a.
18. 骶前筋膜 anterion sacral fascia
19. 直肠上动脉左支 left branch of superior rectal a.
20. 左腹下神经 left hypogastric n.
21. 直肠上动脉 superior rectal a.

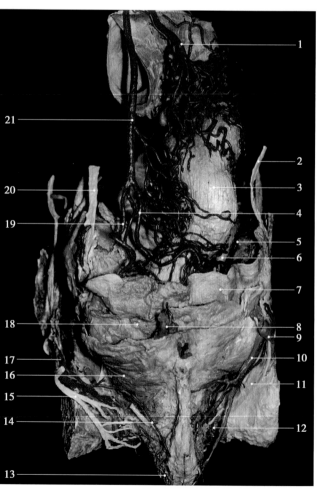

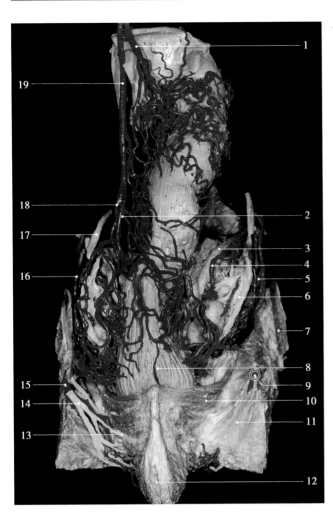

◀ 图 299 直肠后间隙局解（后面观 4）
Regional anatomy of retrorectal space.Posterior view（4）

1. 乙状结肠直肠动脉 sigmoid rectus a.
2. 直肠上动脉右支 right branch of superior rectal a.
3. 输精管 ductus deferens
4. 输精管动脉 deferential a.
5. 膀胱下动脉 inferior vesical a.
6. 下腹下丛 inferior hypogastric plexus
7. 耻骨 pubis
8. 直肠壶腹 ampulla of rectum
9. 阴部管 pudendal canal
10. 肛提肌 levator ani
11. 闭孔筋膜 obturator fascia
12. 肛门 anus
13. 肛神经 anal n.
14. 阴部神经 pudendal n.
15. 阴部内动脉 internal pudendal a.
16. 膀胱下静脉 inferior vesical v.
17. 输尿管 ureter
18. 直肠上动脉左支 left branch of superior rectal a.
19. 直肠上动脉 superior rectal a.

图 300 阴茎背神经 ▶
Dorsal nerve of penis

1. 腰骶干 lumbosacral trunk
2. 闭孔神经 obturator n.
3. 坐骨神经 sciatic n.
4. 肛提肌 levator ani
5. 阴茎背神经 dorsal nerve of penis
6. 阴茎 penis
7. 尿道 urethra
8. 会阴神经 perineal n.
9. 肛神经 anal n.
10. 骶棘韧带 sacrospinous lig.
11. 阴部神经 pudendal n.
12. 第 4 骶神经 the 4th sacral n.
13. 第 3 骶神经 the 3rd sacral n.
14. 第 1 骶神经 the 1st sacral n.

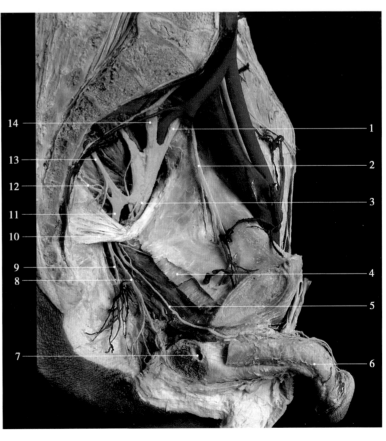

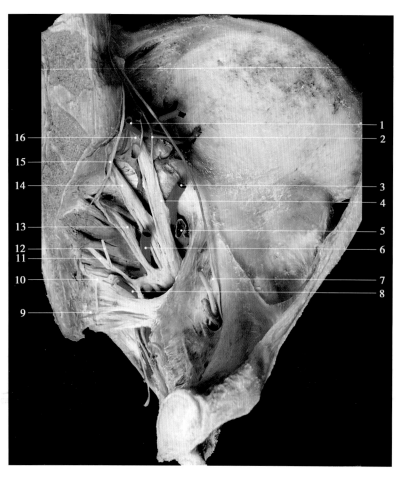

◀ 图 301　骶丛
Sacral plexus
1. 髂腰动脉 iliolumbar a.
2. 第 4 腰神经前支 anterior branch of the 4th lumbar n.
3. 臀上动脉 superior gluteal a.
4. 腰骶干 lumbosacral trunk
5. 臀上静脉 superior gluteal v.
6. 臀下动脉 inferior gluteal a.
7. 闭孔神经 obturator n.
8. 阴部内动脉 internal pudendal a.
9. 尾神经 coccygeal n.
10. 第 5 骶神经前支 anterior branch of the 5th sacral n.
11. 第 4 骶神经前支 anterior branch of the 4th sacral n.
12. 第 3 骶神经前支 anterior branch of the 3rd sacral n.
13. 第 2 骶神经前支 anterior branch of the 2nd sacral n.
14. 第 1 骶神经前支 anterior branch of the 1st sacral n.
15. 骶交感干 sacral sympathetic trunk
16. 第五腰神经前支 anterior branch of the 5th lumbar n.

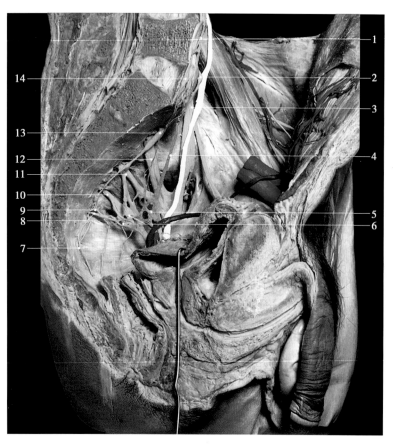

◀ 图 302　男性盆部内脏神经（内侧面观）
Splanchnic nerve of male pelvis Medial view
1. 上腹下丛 superior hypogastric plexus
2. 腰交感神经节 lumbar sympathetic ganglion
3. 腰骶干 lumbosacral trunk
4. 左腹下神经 left hypogastric n.
5. 下腹下丛 inferior hypogastric plexus
6. 盆内脏神经 pelvic splanchnic n.
7. 尾神经 coccygeal n.
8. 第 5 骶神经前支 anterior branch of the 5th sacral n.
9. 第 4 骶神经前支 anterior branch of the 4th sacral n.
10. 第 3 骶神经前支 anterior branch of the 3rd sacral n.
11. 第 2 骶神经前支 anterior branch of the 2nd sacral n.
12. 第 1 骶神经前支 anterior branch of the 1st sacral n.
13. 骶交感神经节 sacral sympathetic ganglion
14. 右腹下神经 right hypogastric n.

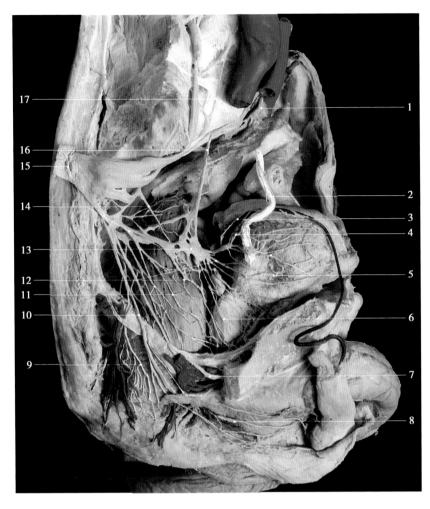

◀图 303 男性盆部内脏神经（侧面观）
Splanchnic nerve of male pelvis Lateral view

1. 左腹下神经 left hypogastric n.
2. 输尿管 ureter
3. 输精管丛 deferential plexus
4. 输尿管丛 ureteric plexus
5. 膀胱丛 vesical plexus
6. 前列腺丛 prostatic plexus
7. 阴茎背神经 dorsal nerve of penis
8. 阴囊后神经 posterior scrotal n.
9. 肛神经 anal n.
10. 阴部神经 pudendal n.
11. 直肠丛 rectal plexus
12. 下腹下丛 inferior hypogastric plexus
13. 盆神经节 pelvic ganglia
14. 盆内脏神经 pelvic splanchnic n.
15. 坐骨神经 sciatic n.
16. 右腹下神经 right hypogastric n.
17. 交感干 sympathetic trunk

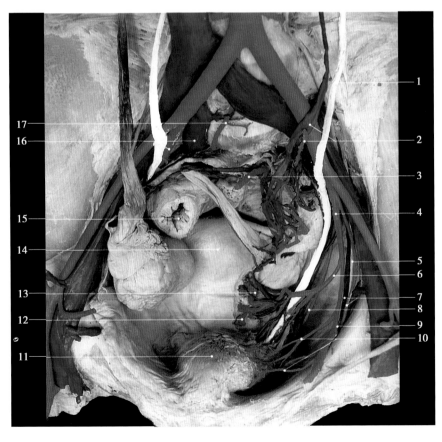

◀图 304 输尿管盆部与子宫动脉的关系
Relationship of pelvic part of ureter and uterine artery

1. 输尿管 ureter
2. 卵巢动、静脉 ovarian a.and v.
3. 直肠上动脉 superior rectal a.
4. 髂内动脉 internal iliac a.
5. 闭孔神经 obturator n.
6. 子宫动脉 uterine a.
7. 闭孔动、静脉 obturator a.and v.
8. 膀胱下动脉 inferior vesical a.
9. 脐动脉 umbilical a.
10. 膀胱上动脉 superior vesical a.
11. 膀胱 urinary bladder
12. 子宫动脉阴道支 vaginal branch of uterine a.
13. 子宫动脉螺旋支 spiral branch of uterine a.
14. 子宫 uterus
15. 直肠 rectum
16. 髂内动、静脉 internal iliac a.and v.
17. 骶正中动脉 median sacral a.

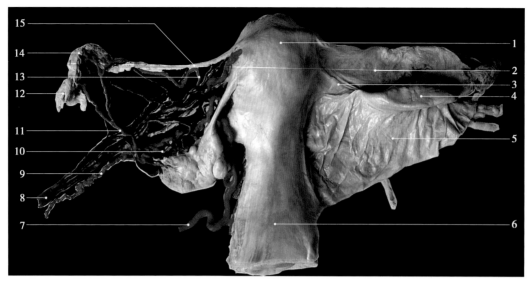

▲ 图 305　女性内生殖器的血管
Blood vessels of female internal genital organs

1. 子宫底 fundus of uterus
2. 输卵管系膜 mesosalpinx
3. 卵巢固有韧带 proper ligament of ovary
4. 卵巢 ovary
5. 子宫系膜 mesometrium
6. 阴道 vagina
7. 子宫动脉 uterine a.
8. 卵巢静脉 ovarian v.
9. 卵巢动脉 ovarian a.
10. 卵巢动脉卵巢支 ovarian branches of ovarian a.
11. 卵巢动脉输卵管支 tubal branches of ovarian a.
12. 输卵管伞 fimbriae of uterine tube
13. 子宫动脉输卵管支 tubal branch of uterine a.
14. 输卵管壶腹 ampulla of uterine tube
15. 输卵管 uterine tube

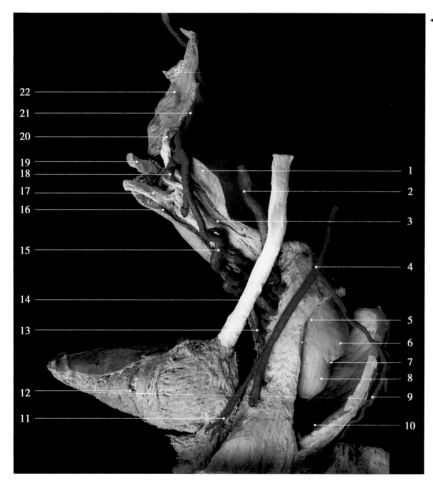

◀图 306　女性内生殖器的动脉（侧面观）
Arteries of female internal genital organs.Lateral view

1. 子宫阔韧带后叶 posterior layer of broad ligament of uterus
2. 子宫动脉 uterine a.
3. 子宫左缘 left margin of uterus
4. 阴道动脉 vaginal a.
5. 子宫颈阴道部 vaginal part of cervix
6. 后唇 posterior lip
7. 子宫口 orifice of uterus
8. 前唇 anterior lip
9. 直肠支 rectal branch
10. 阴道 vagina
11. 尿道支 urethral branch
12. 膀胱 urinary bladder
13. 子宫动脉阴道支 vaginal branch of uterine a.
14. 输尿管 ureter
15. 子宫动脉螺旋支 spiral branch of uterine a.
16. 子宫阔韧带前叶 anterior layer of broad ligament of uterus
17. 子宫圆韧带 round ligament of uterus
18. 子宫动脉宫底支 branch of fundus of uterine a.
19. 输卵管 uterine tube
20. 卵巢固有韧带 proper ligament of ovary
21. 卵巢动脉 ovarian a.
22. 卵巢 ovary

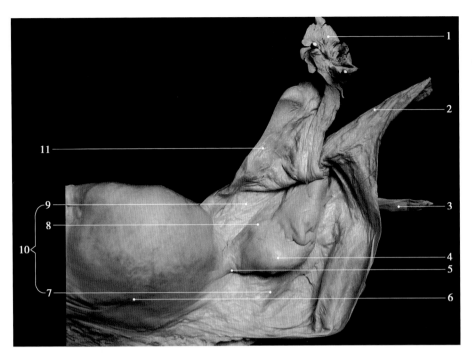

◀图 307　子宫阔韧带（后面观）
Broad ligament of uterus.
Posterior view

1. 输卵管伞 fimbriae of uterine tube
2. 卵巢悬韧带 suspensory ligament of ovary
3. 子宫圆韧带 round ligament of uterus
4. 卵巢 ovary
5. 卵巢固有韧带 proper ligament of ovary
6. 子宫 uterus
7. 子宫系膜 mesometrium
8. 卵巢系膜 mesovarium
9. 输卵管系膜 mesosalpinx
10. 子宫阔韧带 broad ligament of uterus
11. 输卵管 uterine tube

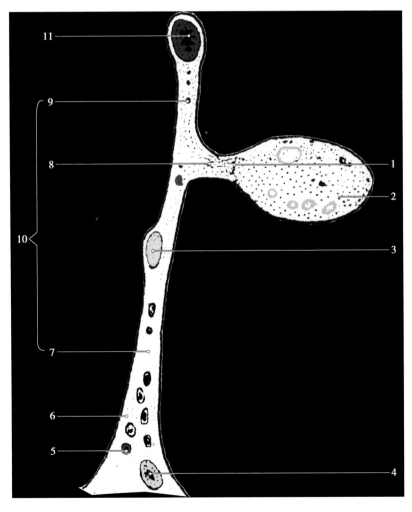

◀图 308　子宫阔韧带（矢状切面）
Broad ligament of uterus.Sagittal section

1. 卵巢门 hilum of ovary
2. 卵巢 ovary
3. 子宫圆韧带 round ligament of uterus
4. 输尿管 ureter
5. 子宫动脉 uterine a.
6. 子宫主韧带 cardinal ligament of uterus
7. 子宫系膜 mesometrium
8. 卵巢系膜 mesovarium
9. 输卵管系膜 mesosalpinx
10. 子宫阔韧带 broad ligament of uterus
11. 输卵管 uterine tube

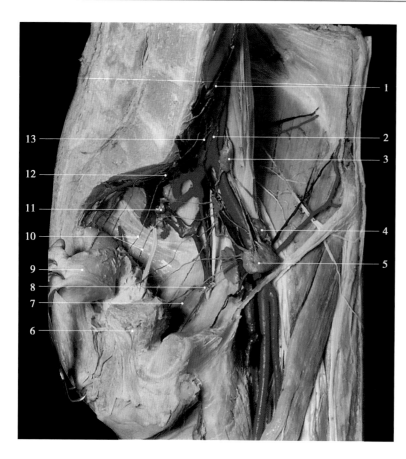

◀ 图 309　女性盆腔的淋巴结
Lymph nodes of female pelvic cavity

1. 主动脉下淋巴结 subaortic lymph nodes
2. 髂总动脉 common iliac a.
3. 髂总外侧淋巴结 lateral common iliac lymph nodes
4. 髂外外侧淋巴结 lateral external iliac lymph node
5. 腔隙外淋巴结 lateral lacunar lymph node
6. 膀胱 urinary bladder
7. 膀胱淋巴管 lymphatic vessel of urinary bladder
8. 闭孔淋巴结 obturator lymph node
9. 子宫 uterus
10. 子宫淋巴管 lymphatic vessel of uterus
11. 髂内淋巴结 medial iliac lymph nodes
12. 骶外侧淋巴结 lateral sacral lymph nodes
13. 髂总内侧淋巴结 medial common iliac lymph nodes

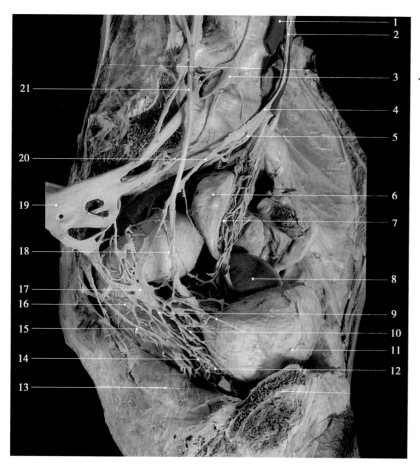

◀ 图 310　女性盆部内脏神经（侧面观）
Splanchnic plexus of female pelvis
Lateral view

1. 腹主动脉 abdorninal aorta
2. 腹主动脉丛 abdominal aortic plexus
3. 交感干神经节 ganglion of sympathetic trunk
4. 上腹下丛 superior hypogastric plexus
5. 右腹下神经 right hypogastric n.
6. 卵巢 ovary
7. 卵巢丛 ovarian plexus
8. 子宫 uterus
9. 左下腹下丛 left inferior hypogastric plexus
10. 膀胱丛 vesical plexus
11. 膀胱 urinary bladder
12. 阴道 vagina
13. 肛提肌 levator ani
14. 阴道神经 vaginal n.
15. 直肠丛 rectal plexus
16. 直肠 rectum
17. 盆神经节 pelvic ganglia
18. 输尿管丛 ureteric plexus
19. 坐骨神经 sciatic n.
20. 左腹下神经 left hypogastric n.
21. 输尿管 ureter

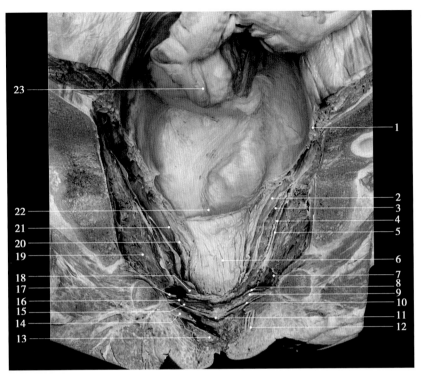

◀ 图 311　盆膈（冠状切面）
Pelvic diaphragm.Coronal section

1. 输尿管 ureter
2. 盆膈上筋膜 superior fascia of pelvic diaphragm
3. 肛提肌 levator ani
4. 盆膈下筋膜 inferior fascia of pelvic diaphragm
5. 闭孔筋膜 obturator fascia
6. 直肠 rectum
7. 阴部管 pudendal canal
8. 尿生殖膈上筋膜 superior fascia of urogenital diaphragm
9. 会阴深横肌 deep transverse muscle of perineum
10. 尿生殖膈下筋膜 inferior fascia of urogenital diaphragm
11. 会阴中心腱 perineal central tendon
12. 肛神经 anal n.
13. 肛门外括约肌 sphincter ani externus
14. 会阴浅横肌 superficial transverse muscle of perineum
15. 尿道球动脉 bulbourethral a.
16. 阴茎背动脉 dorsal artery of penis
17. 阴茎背神经 dorsal nerve of penis
18. 耻骨直肠肌 puborectalis
19. 闭孔内肌 obturator internus
20. 直肠筋膜 rectal fascia
21. 直肠周围间隙 pararectal space
22. 腹膜 peritoneum
23. 乙状结肠 sigmoid colon

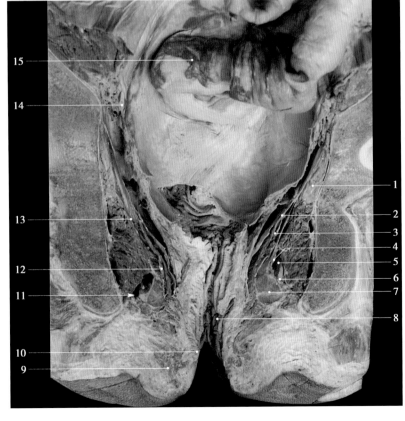

◀ 图 312　坐骨肛门窝（冠状切面）
Ischioanal fossa.Coronal section

1. 闭孔内肌 obturator internus
2. 盆膈上筋膜 superior fascia of pelvic diaphragm
3. 肛提肌 levator ani
4. 阴茎背神经 dorsal nerve of penis
5. 阴部内动脉 internal pudendal a.
6. 会阴神经 perineal n.
7. 坐骨肛门窝脂体 adipose body of ischioanal fossa
8. 肛管 anal canal
9. 肛门外括约肌 sphincter ani externus
10. 肛门内括约肌 sphincter ani internus
11. 阴部管 pudendal canal
12. 盆膈下筋膜 inferior fascia of pelvic diaphragm
13. 闭孔筋膜 obturator fascia
14. 输尿管 ureter
15. 乙状结肠 sigmoid colon

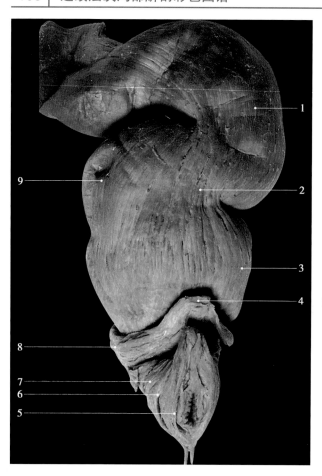

◀ 图 313　肛门外括约肌（后面观）
Sphincter ani externus.Posterior view

1. 直肠上方侧曲 flexura superior lateralis recti
2. 直肠纵肌层 longitudinal muscular layer of rectum
3. 直肠下方侧曲 flexura inferior lateralis recti
4. 尾骨直肠肌 rectococcygeal m.
5. 肛门外括约肌皮下部 subcutaneous part of sphincter ani externus
6. 肛门外括约肌浅部 superficial part of sphincter ani externus
7. 肛门外括约肌深部 deep part of sphincter ani externus
8. 肛提肌 levator ani
9. 直肠中间侧曲 flexura intermedia lateralis recti

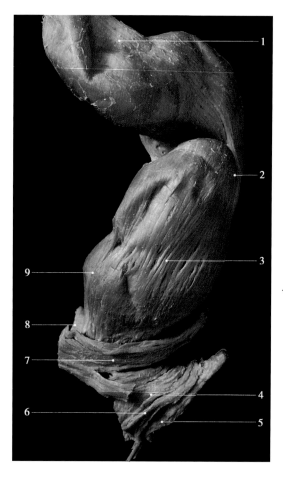

◀ 图 314　肛门外括约肌（侧面观）
Sphincter ani externus.Lateral view

1. 乙状结肠 sigmoid colon
2. 直肠骶曲 sacral flexure of rectum
3. 直肠纵肌层 longitudinal muscular layer of rectum
4. 肛门外括约肌深部 deep part of sphincter ani externus
5. 肛门外括约肌皮下部 subcutaneous part of sphincter ani externus
6. 肛门外括约肌浅部 superficial part of sphincter ani externus
7. 肛提肌 levator ani
8. 耻骨直肠肌 puborectalis
9. 会阴曲 perineal flexure

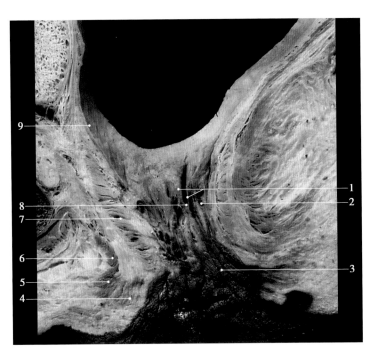

◀ 图 315　肛门矢状切面
Sagittal section of anus

1. 肛柱 anal column
2. 肛窦 anal sinuses
3. 肛门 anus
4. 肛门外括约肌皮下部 subcutaneous part of sphincter ani externus
5. 肛门外括约肌浅部 superficial part of sphincter ani externus
6. 肛门外括约肌深部 deep part of sphincter ani externus
7. 肛门内括约肌 sphincter ani internus
8. 肛瓣 anal valves
9. 直肠 rectum

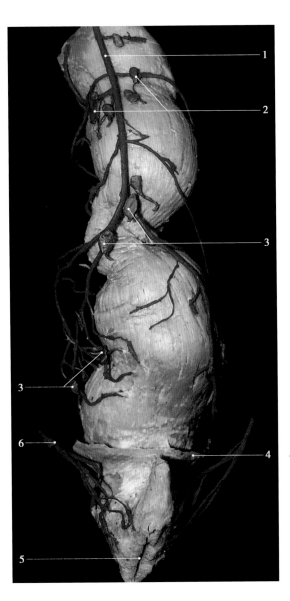

◀ 图 316　直肠的淋巴结（后面观）
Lymph nodes of rectum.Posterior view

1. 直肠上动脉 superior rectal a.
2. 直肠上淋巴结 superior rectal lymph nodes
3. 直肠旁淋巴结 pararectal lymph nodes
4. 肛提肌 levator ani
5. 肛门 anus
6. 肛动脉 anal a.

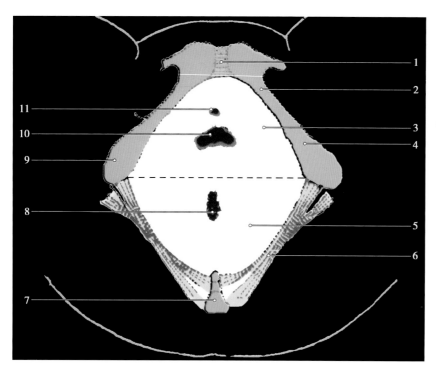

◀图 317　会阴的境界和分区（模式图）
Perineal boundary and zonation. Diagram

1. 耻骨联合 pubic symphysis
2. 耻骨下支 inferior ramus of pubis
3. 尿生殖区 urogenital region
4. 坐骨支 ramus of ischium
5. 肛区 anal region
6. 骶结节韧带 sacrotuberous lig.
7. 尾骨 coccyx
8. 肛门 anus
9. 坐骨结节 ischial tuberosity
10. 阴道口 vagina orifice
11. 尿道外口 external orifice of urethra

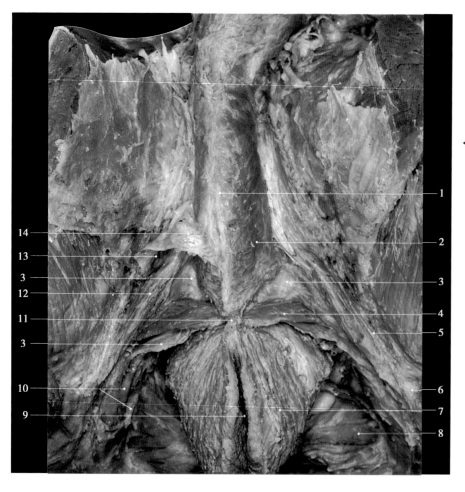

◀图 318　男性会阴浅隙（1）
Superficial perineal space of male（1）

1. 尿道球中隔 septum bulbi urethrae
2. 球海绵体肌 bulbocavernosus
3. 尿生殖膈下筋膜 inferior fascia of urogenital diaphragm
4. 会阴浅横肌 superficial transverse muscle of perineum
5. 坐骨支 ramus of ischium
6. 坐骨结节 ischial tuberosity
7. 肛门外括约肌 sphincter ani externus
8. 肛提肌 levator ani
9. 肛门 anus
10. 阴部内动、静脉 internal pudendal a.and v.
11. 会阴中心腱 perineal central tendon
12. 坐骨海绵体肌 ischiocavernosus
13. 会阴浅隙 superficial perineal space
14. 会阴浅筋膜 superficial fascia of perineum

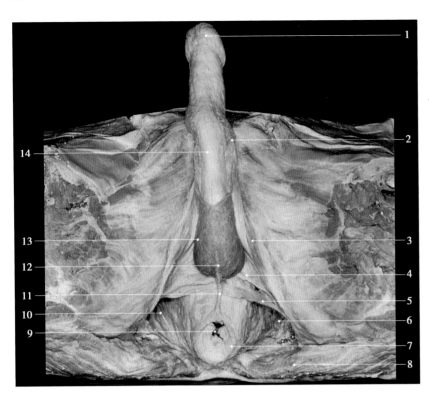

◀ 图 319 男性会阴浅隙（2）
Superficial perineal space of male(2)

1. 阴茎头 glans penis
2. 阴茎海绵体 cavernous body of penis
3. 坐骨海绵体肌 ischiocavernosus
4. 尿生殖膈下筋膜 inferior fascia of urogenital diaphragm
5. 会阴浅横肌 superficial transverse muscle of perineum
6. 坐骨肛门窝 ischioanal fossa
7. 肛门外括约肌 sphincter ani externus
8. 臀大肌 gluteus maximus
9. 肛门 anus
10. 肛提肌 levator ani
11. 会阴中心腱 perineal central tendon
12. 尿道球中隔 bulbourethral septum
13. 球海绵体肌 bulbocavernosus
14. 尿道海绵体 cavernous body of urethra

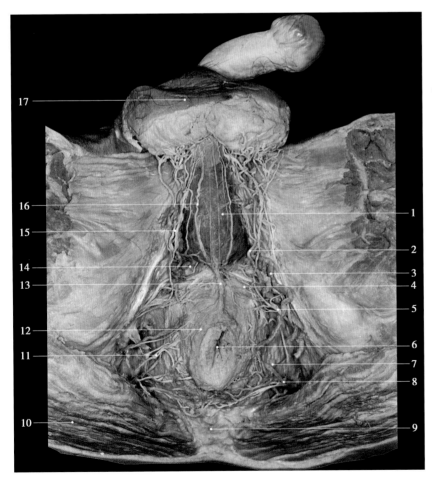

◀ 图 320 男性会阴浅隙及其结构
Structures in superficial perineal space of male

1. 球海绵体肌 bulbocavernosus
2. 阴囊后动脉 posterior scrotal a.
3. 阴囊后静脉 posterior scrotal v.
4. 会阴浅横肌 superficial transverse muscle of perineum
5. 会阴神经 perineal n.
6. 肛门 anus
7. 肛提肌 levator ani
8. 肛静脉 anal v.
9. 尾骨 coccyx
10. 臀大肌 gluteus maximus
11. 肛神经 anal n.
12. 肛门外括约肌 sphincter ani externus
13. 会阴中心腱 perineal central tendon
14. 尿生殖膈下筋膜 inferior fascia of urogenital diaphragm
15. 阴囊后神经外支 lateral branch of posterior scrotal n.
16. 阴囊后神经内支 medial branch of posterior scrotal n.
17. 阴囊 scrotum

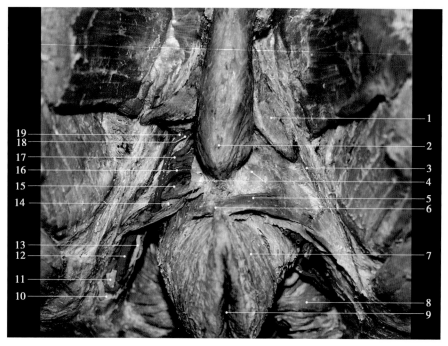

◀图 321　男性会阴深隙及其结构（1）
Structures in deep perineal space of male（1）

1. 阴茎脚 crus penis
2. 尿道球 bulb of urethra
3. 耻骨下支 inferior ramus pubis
4. 尿生殖膈下筋膜 inferior fascia of urogenital diaphragm
5. 会阴浅横肌 superficial transverse muscle of perineum
6. 会阴中心腱 perineal central tendon
7. 肛门外括约肌 sphincter ani externus
8. 肛提肌 levator ani
9. 肛门 anus
10. 阴部管 pudendal canal
11. 会阴神经 perineal n.
12. 阴部内动脉 internal pudendal a.
13. 阴茎背神经 dorsal nerve of penis
14. 尿生殖膈上筋膜 superior fascia of urogenital diaphragm
15. 会阴深横肌 deep transverse muscle of perineum
16. 尿道球动脉 urethral bulbar a.
17. 会阴深隙静脉丛 venous plexus of deep perineal space
18. 阴茎深动脉 deep artery of penis
19. 阴茎背动脉 dorsal artery of penis

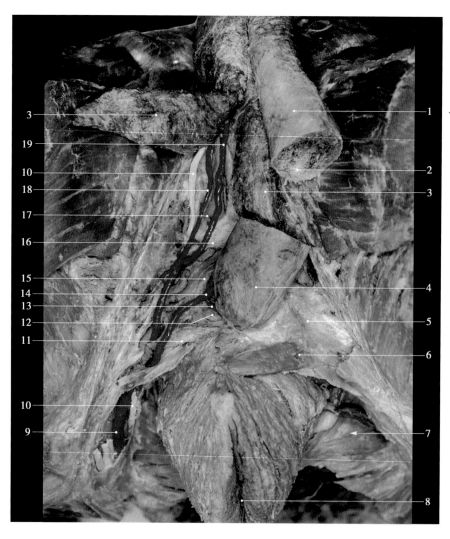

◀图 322　男性会阴深隙及其结构（2）
Structures in deep perineal space of male（2）

1. 尿道海绵体 cavernous body of urethra
2. 尿道 urethra
3. 阴茎脚 crus penis
4. 尿道球 bulb of urethra
5. 尿生殖膈下筋膜 inferior fascia of urogenital diaphragm
6. 会阴浅横肌 superficial transverse muscle of perineum
7. 坐骨肛门窝 ischioanal fossa
8. 肛门 anus
9. 阴部内动脉 internal pudendal a.
10. 阴茎背神经 dorsal nerve of penis
11. 会阴深横肌 deep transverse muscle of perineum
12. 尿道球腺 bulbourethral gland
13. 尿道球腺动脉 artery of bulbourethral gland
14. 尿道球动脉 urethral bulbar a.
15. 尿道括约肌 sphincter of urethra
16. 会阴横韧带 transverse ligament of perineum
17. 阴茎背深静脉 deep dorsal vein of penis
18. 阴茎背动脉 dorsal artery of penis
19. 阴茎深动脉 deep artery of penis

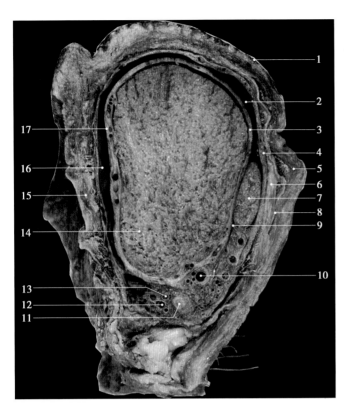

◀ 图 323 阴囊的层次结构（水平切面）
Different hierarchical structures of scrotum.Horizontal
section

1. 阴囊皮肤 skin of scrotum
2. 鞘膜腔 vaginal cavity
3. 白膜 tunica albuginea
4. 精索内筋膜 internal spermatic fascia
5. 肉膜 dartos coat
6. 提睾肌筋膜 cremasteric fascia
7. 附睾 epididymis
8. 精索外筋膜 external spermatic fascia
9. 附睾窦 sinus of epididymis
10. 蔓状静脉丛前组 anterior group of pampiniform plexus
11. 输精管 ductus deferens
12. 蔓状静脉丛后组 posterior group of pampiniform plexus
13. 睾丸动脉 testicular a.
14. 精曲小管 contorted seminiferous tubules
15. 阴囊隔 septum scrotum
16. 鞘膜壁层 parietal layer of tunica vaginalis
17. 鞘膜脏层 visceral layer of tunica vaginalis

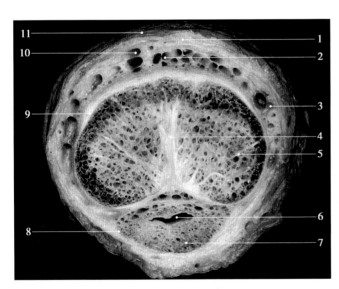

▲ 图 324 阴茎体横切面
Transverse section through body of penis

1. 阴茎浅筋膜 superficial fascia of penis
2. 阴茎背深静脉 deep dorsal vein of penis
3. 阴茎深筋膜 deep fascia of penis
4. 阴茎中隔 septum penis
5. 阴茎海绵体小梁 trabeculae of cavernous body of penis
6. 尿道 urethra
7. 尿道海绵体 cavernous body of urethra
8. 尿道海绵体白膜 albuginea of cavernous
   body of urethra
9. 阴茎海绵体白膜 albuginea of cavernous
   body of penis
10. 阴茎背浅静脉 superficial dorsal veins of penis
11. 皮肤 skin

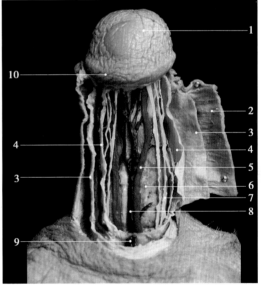

▲ 图 325 阴茎筋膜及血管、神经（背面观）
Blood vessels，nerves and fascia penis.
Dorsal view

1. 阴茎头 glans penis
2. 皮肤 skin
3. 阴茎浅筋膜 superficial fascia of penis
4. 阴茎深筋膜 deep fascia of penis
5. 阴茎背动脉 dorsal artery of penis
6. 阴茎海绵体 cavernous body of penis
7. 阴茎背神经 dorsal nerve of penis
8. 阴茎背深静脉 deep dorsal vein of penis
9. 阴茎背浅静脉 superficial dorsal vein of penis
10. 阴茎头冠 corona glandis

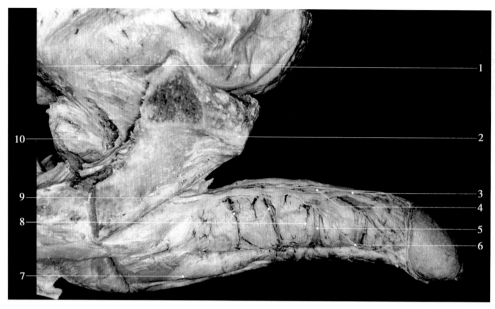

▲ 图 326　阴茎的血管、神经（侧面观）
Blood vessels and nerves of penis.Lateral view

1. 膀胱 urinary bladder
2. 耻骨 pubis
3. 阴茎背深静脉 deep dorsal vein of penis
4. 阴茎背动脉 dorsal artery of penis
5. 阴茎背动脉分支 branch of dorsal artery of penis
6. 阴茎背神经分支 branch of dorsal nerve of penis
7. 尿道海绵体 cavernous body of urethra
8. 阴茎背深静脉属支 branch of deep dorsal vein of penis
9. 阴茎背神经 dorsal nerve of penis
10. 前列腺 prostate

◀ 图 327　前列腺的血管（后面观）
Blood vessels of prostate.Posterior view

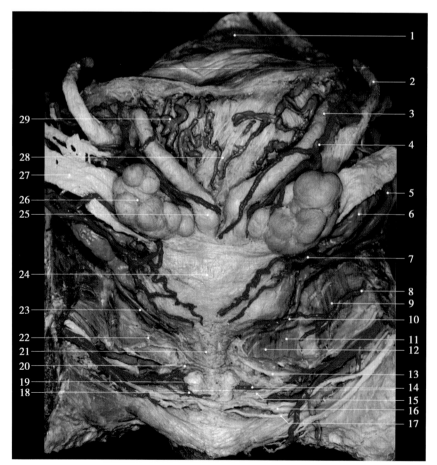

1. 膀胱尖 apex of bladder
2. 输尿管 ureter
3. 输精管 ductus deferens
4. 输精管动脉 deferential a.
5. 膀胱下动脉 inferior vesical a.
6. 膀胱静脉 vesical v.
7. 膀胱下动脉前列腺支 prostate branch of inferior vesical a.
8. 直肠下动脉 inferior rectal a.
9. 耻骨直肠肌 puborectalis
10. 直肠下动脉前列腺支 prostate branch of inferior rectal a.
11. 耻尾肌外侧部纤维 lateral fiber of pubococcygeus
12. 耻尾肌内侧部纤维 medial fiber of pubococcygeus
13. 盆膈下筋膜 inferior fascial of pelvic diaphragm
14. 尿道球动、静脉 urethral bulbar a.and v.
15. 会阴深横肌 deep transverse muscle of perineum
16. 尿生殖膈下筋膜 inferior fascial of urogenital diaphragm
17. 会阴神经深支 deep branch of perineal n.
18. 尿道动脉 urethral a.
19. 尿道球腺 bulbourethral gland
20. 尿生殖膈上筋膜 superior fascial of urogenital diaphragm
21. 尿道膜部 membranous part of urethra
22. 盆膈上筋膜 superior fascial of pelvic diaphragm
23. 前列腺静脉丛 prostatic venous plexus
24. 前列腺 prostate
25. 输精管壶腹 ampulla ductus deferentis
26. 精囊 seminal vesicle
27. 盆丛 pelvic plexus
28. 膀胱底 fundus of bladder
29. 膀胱静脉丛 vesical venous plexus

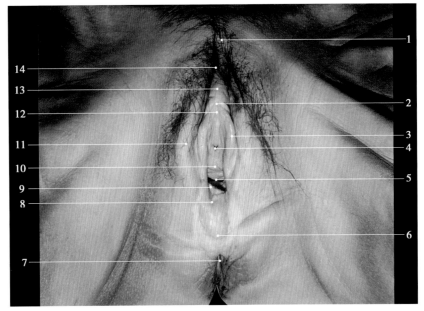

▲ 图 328　女性外生殖器
Female external genital organs

1. 阴阜 mons pubis
2. 阴蒂头 glans of clitoris
3. 小阴唇 lesser lip of pudendum
4. 尿道外口 external orifice of urethra
5. 阴道口 vaginal orifice
6. 唇后连合 posterior labial commissure
7. 肛门 anus
8. 阴唇系带 frenulum of pudendal labia
9. 处女膜 hymen
10. 阴道前庭 vaginal vestibule
11. 大阴唇 greater lip of pudendum
12. 阴蒂系带 frenulum of clitoris
13. 阴蒂包皮 prepuce of clitoris
14. 唇前连合 anterior labial commissure

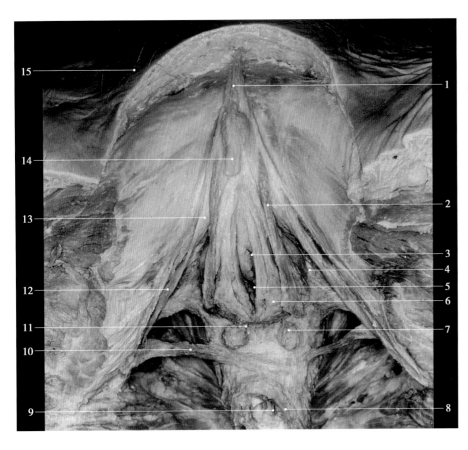

◀图 329　女性会阴浅隙（1）
Superficial perineal space of female（1）

1. 阴蒂悬韧带 suspensory ligament of clitoris
2. 球海绵体肌 bulbocavernosus
3. 尿道外口 external orifice of urethra
4. 尿生殖膈下筋膜 inferior fascia of urogenital diaphragm
5. 阴道口 vaginal orifice
6. 前庭球 bulb of vestibule
7. 前庭大腺 greater vestibular gland
8. 肛门外括约肌 sphincter ani externus
9. 肛门 anus
10. 会阴浅横肌 superficial transverse muscle of perineum
11. 前庭大腺小管 canaliculus of greater vestibular gland
12. 坐骨海绵体肌 ischiocavernosus
13. 阴蒂脚 crus of clitoris
14. 阴蒂头 glans of clitoris
15. 阴阜 mons pubis

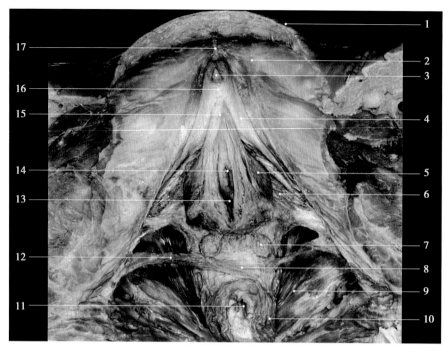

▲ 图 330　女性会阴浅隙（2）
Superficial perineal space of female（2）

1. 阴阜 mons pubis
2. 耻骨 pubis
3. 阴蒂头 glans of clitoris
4. 阴蒂脚 crus of clitoris
5. 前庭球外侧部 lateral part of vestibular bulbs
6. 尿生殖膈下筋膜 inferior fascia of urogenital diaphragm

7. 前庭大腺 greater vestibular gland
8. 会阴中心腱 perineal central tendon
9. 肛提肌 levator ani
10. 肛门外括约肌 sphincter ani externus
11. 肛门 anus
12. 会阴浅横肌 superficial transverse muscle of perineum

13. 阴道口 vaginal orifice
14. 尿道外口 external orifice of urethra
15. 前庭球中间部 intermediate part of bulbs
16. 阴蒂体 body of clitoris
17. 阴蒂悬韧带 suspensory ligament of clitoris

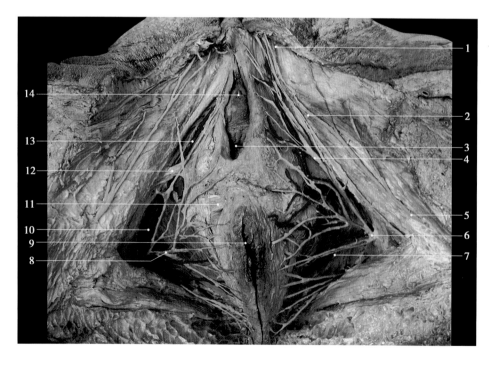

◀图 331　女性会阴浅隙及其结构 Structures in superficial perineal space of female

1. 耻骨 pubis
2. 耻骨下支 inferior ramus of pubis
3. 阴道口 vaginal orifice
4. 阴唇后神经 posterior labial n.
5. 会阴支 perineal branch
6. 会阴神经 perineal n.
7. 肛提肌 levator ani
8. 肛神经 anal n.
9. 肛门 anus
10. 阴部内动脉 internal pudendal a.
11. 会阴浅横肌 superficial transverse muscle of perineum
12. 尿生殖膈下筋膜 inferior fascia of urogenital diaphragm
13. 阴蒂背动脉 dorsal artery of clitoris
14. 尿道外口 external orifice of urethra

第六章

脊 柱 区

Chapter 6　Vertebral region

脊柱区又称背区，其范围是：上界自枕外隆凸和上项线，下至尾骨尖；两侧界是从斜方肌前缘、三角肌后缘上份、腋后襞与胸壁交界处、腋后线、髂嵴后份、髂后上棘至尾骨尖连线。脊柱区又分为项区、胸背区、腰区和骶尾区。

项区上界即脊柱区的上界，下界为第7颈椎棘突至两侧肩峰连线。

胸背区上界即项区下界，胸背区下界为第12胸椎棘突、第12肋下缘、第11肋前份连线。胸背区外上部为肩胛区。

腰区上界即胸背区下界，腰区下界为两髂嵴后份及两髂后上棘的连线。

骶尾区为两髂后上棘与尾骨尖三点间所围成的三角区。

菱形区范围是：左右髂后上棘与第5腰椎棘突和尾骨尖的连线构成。临床上腰椎或骶、尾椎骨折时，菱形区可变形。

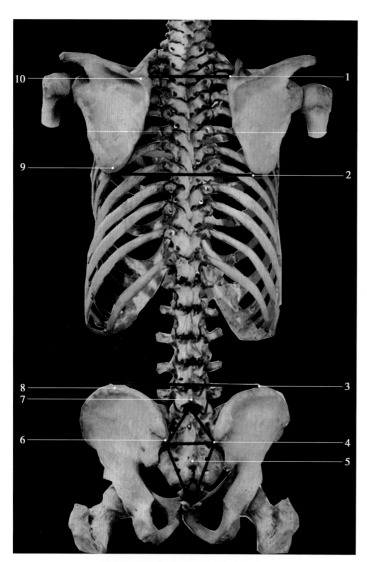

◀ 图 332 体表标志线及菱形区
Reference lines of body surface and rhomboid area

1. 两侧肩胛冈内侧端连线 connecting line between medial ends of scapular spines
2. 两侧肩胛骨下角连线 connecting line between inferior angles of scapulae
3. 两侧髂嵴最高点连线 connecting line between highest points of iliac crests
4. 两侧髂后上棘连线 connecting line between posterior superior iliac spines
5. 菱形区 rhomboid area
6. 髂后上棘 posterior superior iliac spine
7. 第 5 腰椎棘突 spinous process of the 5th lumbar uertebra
8. 髂嵴 iliac crest
9. 肩胛骨下角 inferior angles of scapulae
10. 肩胛冈 scapular spine

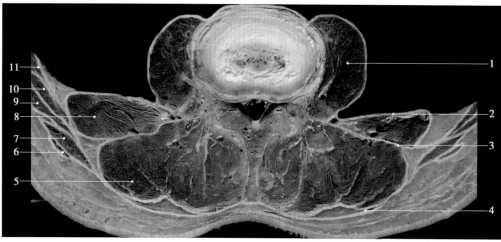

▲ 图 333 胸腰筋膜（水平切面）
Thoracolumbar fascia.Horizontal section

1. 腰大肌 psoas major
2. 胸腰筋膜深层 deep layer of thoracolumbar fascia
3. 胸腰筋膜中层 middle layer of thoracolumbar fascia
4. 胸腰筋膜浅层 superficial layer of thoracolumbar fascia
5. 竖脊肌 erector spinae
6. 背阔肌 latissimus dorsi
7. 下后锯肌 serratus posterior inferior
8. 腰方肌 quadratus lumborum
9. 腹外斜肌 obliquus externus abdominis
10. 腹内斜肌 obliquus internus abdominis
11. 腹横肌 transverses abdominis

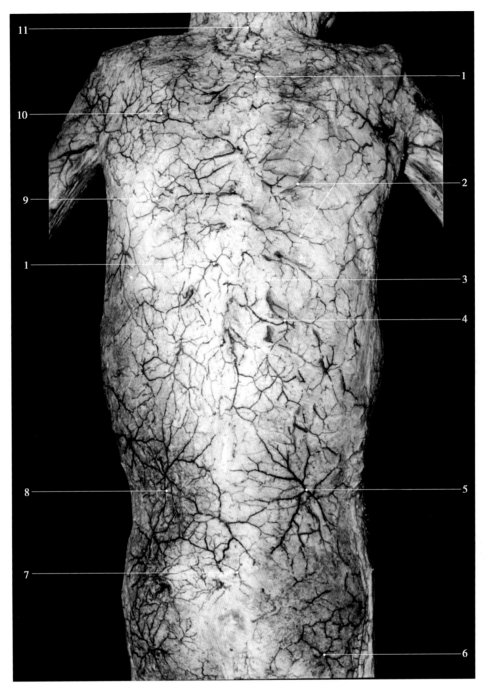

▲ 图 334　背部浅筋膜及浅血管
Superficial fascia and superficial blood vessels of back

1. 脊柱区动脉网 arterial rete of vertebral region
2. 肋间后动脉后支 posterior branch of posterior intercostal a.
3. 背部浅筋膜 superficial fascia of back
4. 背部静脉网 venous rete of back
5. 腰区静脉网 venous rete of lumbar region
6. 臀区静脉网 venous rete of gluteal region
7. 骶区动脉网 arterial rete of sacral region
8. 腰区动脉网 lumbar arterial rete
9. 肩胛下区动脉网 arterial rete of inferior scapular region
10. 肩胛区动脉网 arterial rete of scapular region
11. 项部动脉网 arterial rete of nuchae region

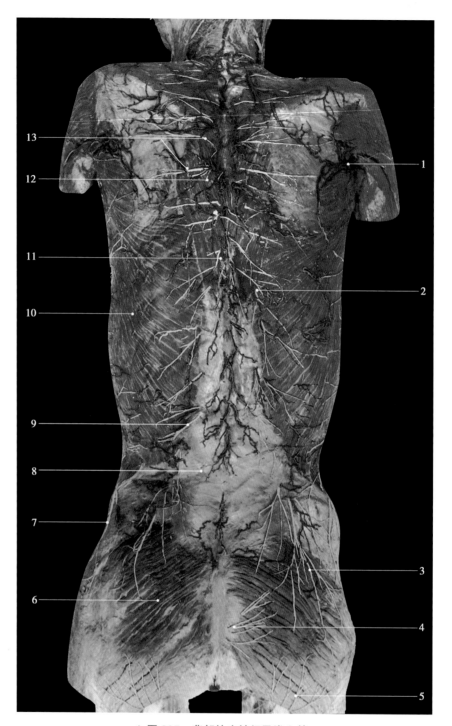

▲ 图 335　背部的皮神经及浅血管
Cutaneous nerves and superficial blood vessels of back

1. 旋肩胛动脉浅支 superficial branch of circumflex scapular a.
2. 肋间后动脉后支 posterior branch of posterior intercostal a.
3. 臀上皮神经 superior clunial n.
4. 臀内侧皮神经 medial clunial n.
5. 臀下皮神经 inferior clunial n.
6. 臀大肌 gluteus maximus
7. 髂腹下神经外侧皮支 lateral cutaneous branch of iliohypogastric n.
8. 胸腰筋膜浅层 superficial layer of thoracolumbar fascia

9. 腰神经后支外侧支 lateral branch of posterior branch of lumbar n.
10. 背阔肌 latissimus dorsi
11. 肋间后动脉背侧支 dorsal branch of posterior intercostal a.
12. 斜方肌 trapezius
13. 胸神经后支外侧支 lateral branch of posterior branch of thoracic n.

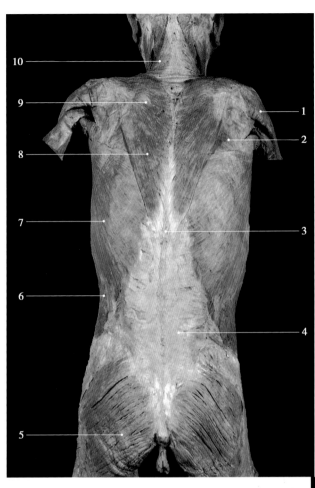

◀ 图 336 背部肌（1）
Muscles of back（1）

1. 三角肌 deltoid
2. 大菱形肌 rhomboideus major
3. 棘突 spinous process
4. 胸腰筋膜浅层 superficial layer of thoracolumbar fascia
5. 臀大肌 gluteus maximus
6. 腹外斜肌 obliquus externus abdominis
7. 背阔肌 latissimus dorsi
8. 斜方肌下部 inferior part of trapezius
9. 斜方肌中部 medial part of trapezius
10. 斜方肌上部 superior part of trapezius

图 337 背部肌（2）▶
Muscles of back（2）

1. 头半棘肌 semispinalis capitis
2. 头夹肌 splenius capitis
3. 上后锯肌 serratus posterior superior
4. 棘肌 spinalis
5. 胸最长肌 longissimus thoracis
6. 髂肋肌 iliocostalis
7. 腹外斜肌 obliquus externus abdominis
8. 腹内斜肌 obliquus internus abdominis
9. 臀大肌 gluteus maximus
10. 胸腰筋膜浅层 superficial layer of thoracolumbar fascia
11. 下后锯肌 serratus posterior inferior
12. 前锯肌 serratus anterior
13. 大菱形肌 rhomboideus major
14. 小菱形肌 rhomboideus minor
15. 肩胛提肌 levator scapulae

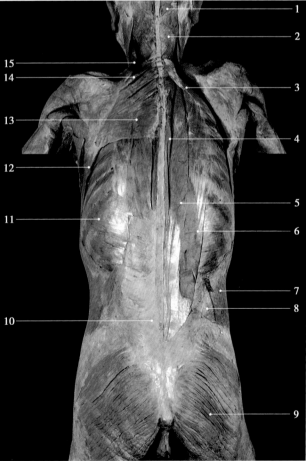

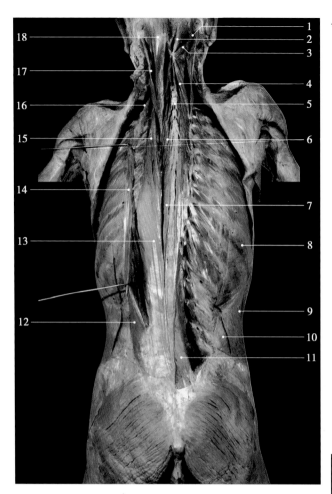

◀ 图 338 背部肌（3）
Muscles of back（3）

1. 头上斜肌 obliquus capitis superior
2. 头后大直肌 rectus capitis posterior major
3. 头下斜肌 obliquus capitis inferior
4. 颈半棘肌 semispinalis cervicis
5. 棘间肌 interspinales
6. 胸半棘肌 semispinalis thoracis
7. 胸棘肌 spinalis thoracis
8. 下后锯肌 serratus posterior inferior
9. 腹外斜肌 obliquus externus abdominis
10. 腹内斜肌 obliquus internus abdominis
11. 骶多裂肌 sacral multifidi
12. 腰髂肋肌 iliocostalis lumborum
13. 胸最长肌 longissimus thoracis
14. 胸髂肋肌 iliocostalis thoracis
15. 颈最长肌 longissimus cervicis
16. 颈髂肋肌 iliocostalis cervicis
17. 头最长肌 longissimus capitis
18. 头半棘肌 semispinalis capitis

图 339 背部肌（4）▶
Muscles of back（4）

1. 枢椎棘突 spinous process of axis
2. 第 7 颈椎棘突 spinous process of the 7th cervical vertebra
3. 棘间肌 interspinales
4. 肋提肌 levatores costarum
5. 胸横突间肌 intertransversarii thoracis
6. 胸腰筋膜中层 medial layer of thoracolumbar fascia
7. 腰横突间肌 intertransversarii lumborum
8. 骶多裂肌 sacral multifidi
9. 腰多裂肌 lumbar multifidi
10. 胸多裂肌 thoraco-multifidi
11. 胸回旋肌 rotatores thoracis
12. 颈棘间肌 interspinales cervicis
13. 头后小直肌 rectus capitis posterior minor

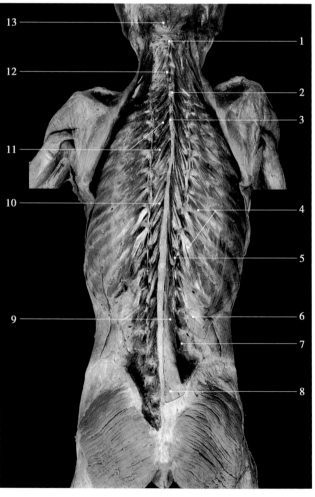

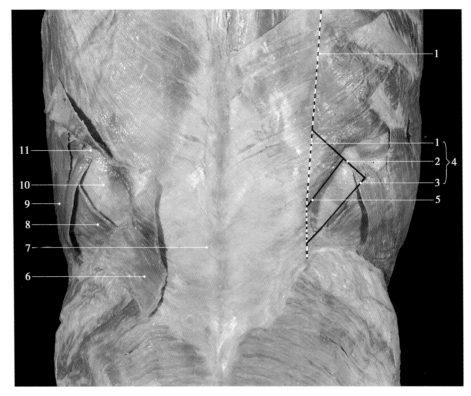

▲ 图 340　腰上三角
Superior lumbar triangle

1. 竖脊肌外缘 lateral border of erector spinae
2. 第 12 肋下缘 inferior border of the 12th rib
3. 腹内斜肌后缘 posterior border of obliquus internus abdominis
4. 腰上三角 superior lumbar triangle
5. 下后锯肌下缘 inferior border of serratus posterior inferior
6. 背阔肌 latissimus dorsi
7. 胸腰筋膜 thoracolumbar fascia
8. 腹内斜肌 obliquus internus abdominis
9. 腹外斜肌 obliquus externus abdominis
10. 腹横肌腱膜 aponeurosis of transverse abdominis
11. 第 12 肋 the 12th rib

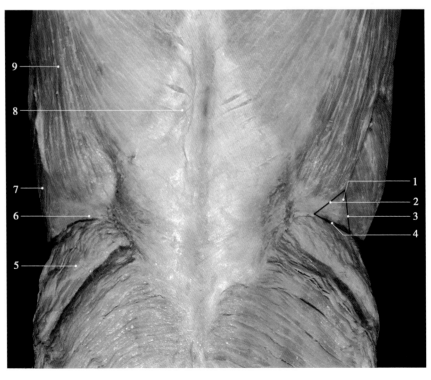

◀ 图 341　腰下三角
Inferior lumbar triangle

1. 腰下三角 inferior lumbar triangle
2. 背阔肌下缘 inferior border of latissimus dorsi
3. 腹外斜肌后缘 posterior border of obliquus externus abdominis
4. 髂嵴上缘 superior border of iliac crest
5. 臀中肌 gluteus medius
6. 髂嵴 iliac crest
7. 腹外斜肌 obliquus externus abdominis
8. 胸 腰 筋 膜 浅 层 superficial layer of thoracolumbar fascia
9. 背阔肌 latissimus dorsi

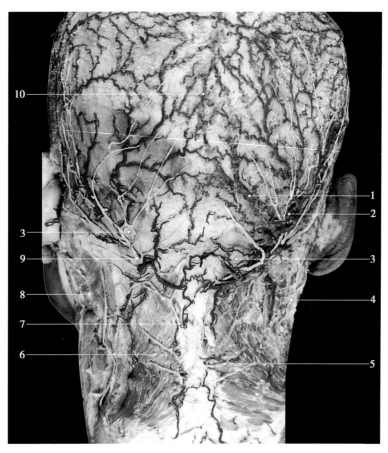

◀ 图 342　项部的血管、神经（1）
Blood vessels and nerves of nuchae（1）

1. 枕静脉 occipital v.
2. 枕动脉 occipital a.
3. 枕淋巴结 occipital lymph nodes
4. 枕小神经 lesser occipital n.
5. 第 4、第 5 颈神经后支的外侧支 lateral branch of posterior branches of the 4th，5th cervical n.
6. 斜方肌 trapezius
7. 第 3 枕神经 the 3rd occipital n.
8. 胸锁乳突肌 sternocleidomastoid
9. 枕大神经 greater occipital n.
10. 枕部动脉网 arterial rete of occipital region

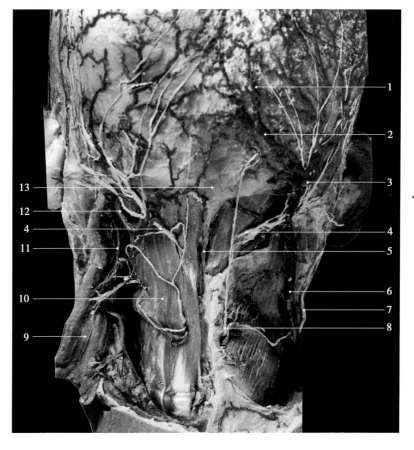

◀ 图 343　项部的血管、神经（2）
Blood vessels and nerves of nuchae（2）

1. 枕部动脉网 arterial rete of occipital region
2. 枕静脉 occipital v.
3. 枕动脉 occipital a.
4. 枕大神经 greater occipital n.
5. 项韧带 ligmentum nuchae
6. 颈后外静脉 posterior external jugular v.
7. 枕小神经 lesser occipital n.
8. 第 3 枕神经 the 3rd occipital n.
9. 头夹肌 splenius capitis
10. 头半棘肌 semispinalis capitis
11. 枕动脉降支 descending branch of occipital a.
12. 枕动脉枕支 occipital branch of occipital a.
13. 枕外隆凸 external occipital protuberance

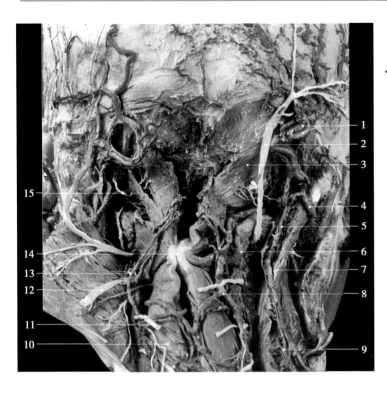

◀图 344 项部的血管、神经（3）
Blood vessels and nerves of nuchae （3）

1. 枕动、静脉枕支 occipital branch of occipital a.and v.
2. 枕大神经 greater occipital n.
3. 头后大直肌 rectus capitis posterior major
4. 枕动脉 occipital a.
5. 枕动脉降支 descending branch of occipital a.
6. 头下斜肌 obliquus capitis inferior
7. 头最长肌 longissimus capitis
8. 颈深静脉 deep cervical v.
9. 颈浅动脉升支 ascending branch of superficial cervical a.
10. 颈半棘肌 semipinalis cervicis
11. 第4颈神经后支 posterior branch of the 4th cervical n.
12. 第3颈神经后支 posterior branch of the 3rd cervical n.
13. 颈深动脉 deep cervical a.
14. 枢椎棘突 spinous process of axis
15. 枕下神经（第1颈神经后支）suboccipital n.

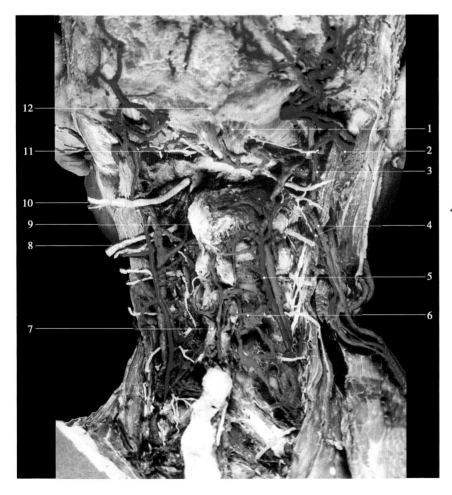

◀图 345 项部的血管、神经（4）
Blood vessels and nerves of nuchae （4）

1. 头后小直肌 rectus capitis posterior minor
2. 枕动脉 occipital a.
3. 枕动脉降支 descending branch of occipital a.
4. 颈浅动、静脉 superfical cervical a.and v.
5. 颈深动脉升支 ascending branch of deep cervical a.
6. 椎外后静脉丛 posterior external vertebral venous plexus
7. 颈棘间肌 interspinales cervicis
8. 第3颈神经 the 3rd cervical n.
9. 枢椎棘突 spinous process of axis
10. 枕大神经 greater occipital n.
11. 枕下神经 suboccipital n.
12. 枕外隆凸 external occipital protuberance

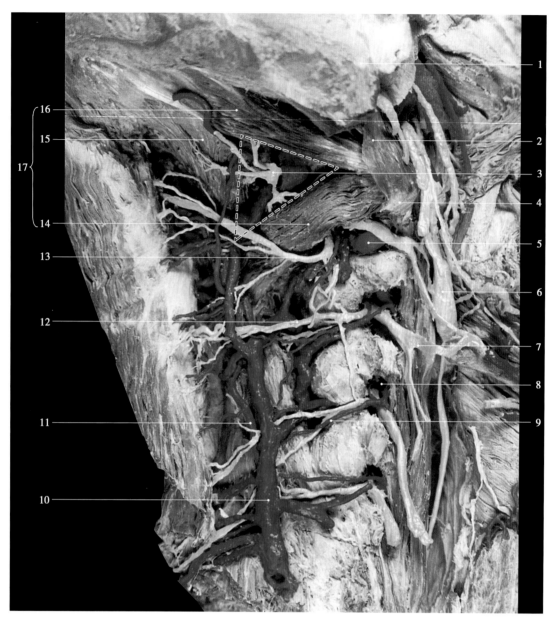

▲ 图 346 枕下三角
Suboccipital triangle

1. 乳突 mastoid process
2. 头外侧直肌 rectus capitis lateralis
3. 枕下神经 suboccipital n.
4. 寰椎横突 transverse process of atlas
5. 椎动脉 vertebral a.
6. 颈上神经节 superior cervical ganglion
7. 第 3 颈神经前支 anterior branch of the 3 rd cervical n.
8. 椎间孔 intervertebral foramen
9. 椎动脉肌支 muscular branches of vertebral a.

10. 颈深静脉 deep cervical v.
11. 颈深动脉 deep cervical a.
12. 第 3 枕神经 the 3rd occipital n.
13. 枕大神经 greater occipital n.
14. 头下斜肌 obliquus capitis inferior
15. 头后大直肌 rectus capitis posterior major
16. 头上斜肌 obliquus capitis superior
17. 枕下三角 suboccipital triangle

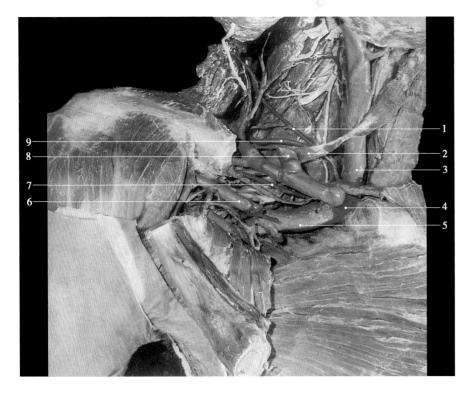

◀ 图 347　肩胛背血管（前面观 1）
Dorsal scapular blood vessels.
Anterior view（1）

1. 颈浅动脉 superficial cervical a.
2. 肩胛舌骨肌下腹 inferior belly of omohyoid
3. 颈内静脉 internal jugular v.
4. 右头臂静脉 right brachiocephalic v.
5. 锁骨下静脉 subclavian v.
6. 头静脉 cephalic v.
7. 肩胛上动脉 suprascapular a.
8. 颈外静脉 external jugular v.
9. 肩胛背动脉 dorsal scapular a.

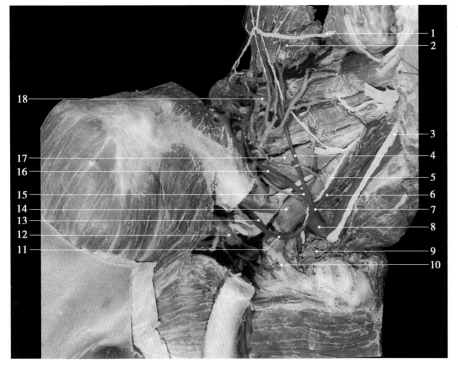

◀ 图 348　肩胛背血管（前面观 2）
Dorsal scapular blood vessels.
Anterior view（2）

1. 副神经 accessory n.
2. 斜方肌 trapezius
3. 迷走神经 vagus n.
4. 颈浅动脉 superficial cervical a.
5. 膈神经 phrenic n.
6. 甲状腺下动脉 inferior thyroid a.
7. 甲状颈干 thyrocervical trunk
8. 锁骨下动脉 subclavian a.
9. 右头臂静脉 right brachiocephalic v.
10. 第 1 肋 the 1st rib
11. 肩胛上动脉 suprascapular a.
12. 头静脉 cephalic v.
13. 臂丛 brachial plexus
14. 前斜角肌 scalenus anterior
15. 颈横动脉 transverse cervical a.
16. 肩胛背动脉 dorsal scapular a.
17. 中斜角肌 scalenus medius
18. 肩胛提肌 levator scapulae

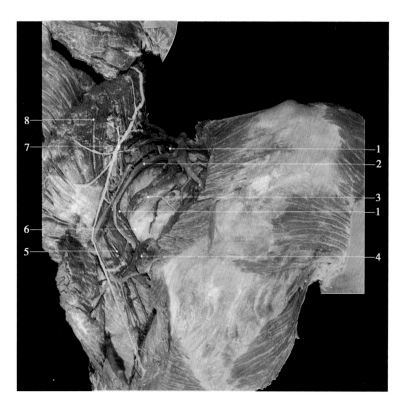

◀ 图 349　肩胛背血管和副神经（后面观 1）
Dorsal scapular blood vessels and accessory nerve.Posterior view（1）

1. 肩胛背动脉 dorsal scapular a.
2. 肩胛背静脉 dorsal scapular v.
3. 肩胛提肌（切断）levator scapulae
4. 小菱形肌 rhomboideus minor
5. 大菱形肌 rhomboideus major
6. 肩胛骨上角 superior angle of scapular
7. 副神经 accessory n.
8. 斜方肌 trapezius

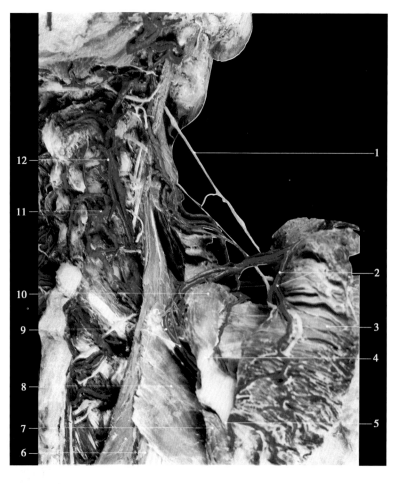

◀ 图 350　肩胛背血管和副神经（后面观 2）
Dorsal scapular blood vessels and accessory nerve. Posterior view（2）

1. 副神经 accessory n.
2. 颈浅动、静脉 superficial cervical a.and v.
3. 斜方肌 trapezius
4. 肩胛骨上角 superior angle of scapular
5. 肩胛骨内侧缘 medial border of scapular
6. 竖脊肌 erector spinae
7. 大菱形肌 rhomboideus major
8. 上后锯肌 serratus posterior superior
9. 肩胛背动、静脉 dorsal scapular a.and v.
10. 肩胛提肌 levator scapulae
11. 椎外后静脉丛 posterior external vertebral venous plexus
12. 颈深动脉深支 deep branch of deep cervical a.

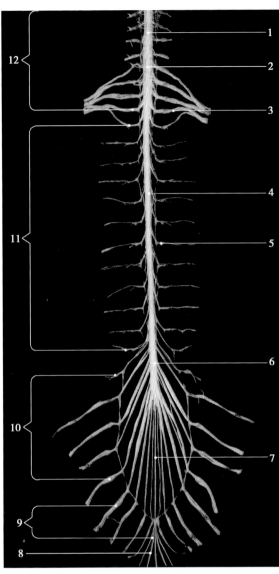

◀图 351　脊髓及脊神经全貌
General arrangement of spinal cord and spinal nerve

1. 颈段 cervical segments
2. 颈膨大 cervical enlargement
3. 脊神经 spinal n.
4. 胸段 thoracic segments
5. 脊神经节 spinal ganglia
6. 腰骶膨大 lumbosacral enlargement
7. 终丝 filum terminale
8. 尾神经 coccygeal n.
9. 骶神经 sacral n.
10. 腰神经 lumbar n.
11. 胸神经 thoracic n.
12. 颈神经 cervical n.

图 352　脊髓和脊神经与椎骨的关系▶
Relation of segment of spinal cord and spinal nerve with vertebrae

1. 第 1~8 颈神经 cervical n.（C_1~C_8）
2. 第 1~12 胸神经 thoracic n.（T_1~T_{12}）
3. 第 1~5 腰神经 lumbar n.（L_1~L_5）
4. 第 1~5 骶神经 sacral n.（S_1~S_5）
5. 尾神经 coccygeal n.
6. 尾骨 coccyx
7. 骶骨 sacrum
8. 第 5 腰椎 the 5th lumbar vertebra
9. 尾髓 tail core
10. 第 12 胸椎 the 12th thoracic vertebra
11. 第 1 骶段 the 1st sacral segment（S_1）
12. 第 1 腰段 the 1st lumbar segment（L_1）
13. 脊神经节 spinal ganglia
14. 第 1 胸段 the 1st thoracic segment（T_1）
15. 第 7 颈椎 the 7th cervical vertebra
16. 寰椎 atlas
17. 第 1 颈段 the 1st cervical segment（C_1）

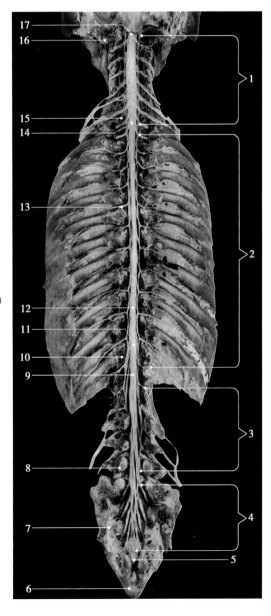

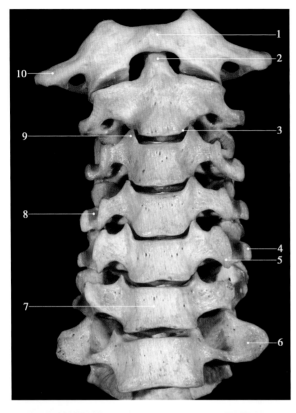

◀ 图 353　颈椎（前面观）
Cervical vertebrae.Anterior view

1.　寰椎前结节 anterior tubercle of atlas
2.　齿突 dens
3.　唇缘 border of lip
4.　横突后结节 posterior tubercle of transverse process
5.　横突前结节 anterior tubercle of transverse process
6.　第 7 颈椎横突 transverse process of the 7th cervical vertebrae
7.　椎体 vertebral body
8.　脊神经沟 sulcus for spinal n.
9.　椎体钩 uncus of vertebral body
10.　寰椎横突 transverse process of atlas

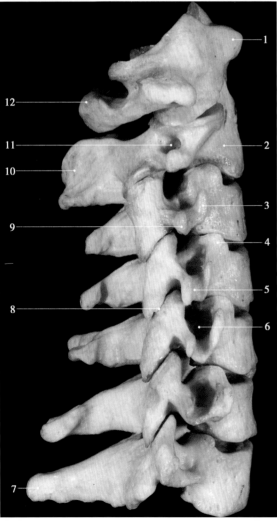

◀ 图 354　颈椎（侧面观）
Cervical vertebrae.Lateral view

1.　寰椎前结节 anterior tubercle of atlas
2.　枢椎体 vertebral body of axis
3.　横突前结节 anterior tubercle of transverse process
4.　椎体钩 uncus of vertebral body
5.　脊神经沟 sulcus for spinal n.
6.　椎间孔 intervertebral foramen
7.　隆椎棘突 spinous process of pprominent vertebra
8.　关节突关节 zygapophysial joint
9.　横突后结节 posterior tubercle of transverse process
10.　枢椎棘突 spinous process of axis
11.　横突孔 transverse foramen
12.　后弓 posterior arch

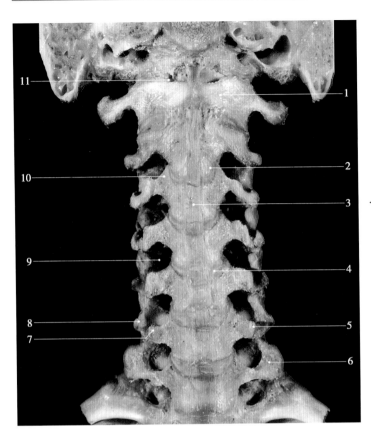

◀ 图 355 颈椎的连结及钩椎关节（1）
Connection of cervical vertebrae and Luschka
joints（1）

1. 寰椎 atlas
2. 唇缘 border of lip
3. 前纵韧带 anterior longitudinal lig.
4. 椎间盘 intervertebral disc
5. 横突 transverse process
6. 脊神经沟 sulcus for spinal n.
7. 前结节 anterior tubercle
8. 后结节 posterior tubercle
9. 椎间孔 intervertebral foramen
10. 椎体钩 uncus of vertebral body
11. 寰枕关节 atlantooccipital joint

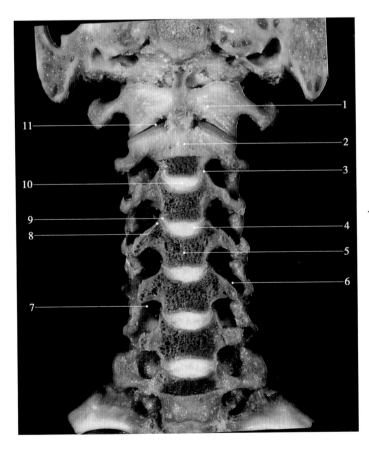

◀ 图 356 颈椎的连结及钩椎关节（2）
Connection of cervical vertebrae and Luschka
joints（2）

1. 寰椎 atlas
2. 枢椎体 vertebral body of axis
3. 钩椎关节（Luschka 关节）uncovertebral joint
4. 纤维环 anulus fibrosus
5. 椎体 vertebral body
6. 脊神经沟 sulcus for spinal n.
7. 椎间孔 intervertebral foramen
8. 椎体钩 uncus of vertebral body
9. 唇缘 border of lip
10. 髓核 nucleus pulposus
11. 寰枢外侧关节 lateral atlantoaxial joint

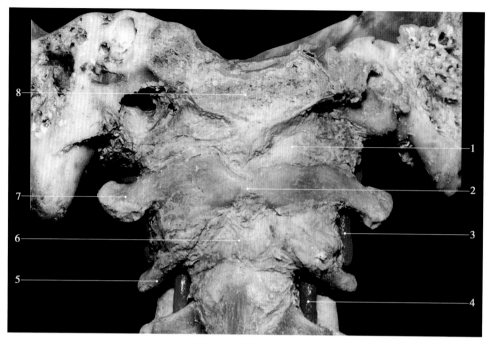

▲ 图 357　寰枕前膜
Anterior atlantooccipital membrane

1. 寰枕前膜 anterior atlantooccipital membrane
2. 寰椎前结节 anterior trbercle of atlas
3. 椎动脉 V3 段 V3 section of vartebral a.
4. 椎动脉 V1 段 V1 section of vartebral a.
5. 枢椎横突 transverse process of axis
6. 枢椎 axis
7. 寰椎横突 transverse process of atlas
8. 枕骨基底部 basilar part of occipital bone

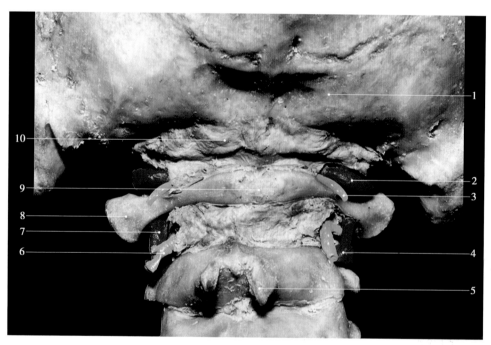

▲ 图 358　寰枕后膜
Posterior atlantooccipital membrane

1. 枕骨 occipital bone
2. 椎动脉 V4 段 V4 section of vertebral a.
3. 第 1 颈神经 the 1st cervical n.
4. 椎动脉 V2 段 V2 section of vertebral a.
5. 枢椎棘突 spinous process of axis
6. 第 2 颈神经 the 2nd cervical n.
7. 椎动脉 V3 段 V3 section of vertebral a.
8. 寰椎横突 transverse process of atlas
9. 寰椎后弓 posterior arch of atlas
10. 寰枕后膜 posterior atlantooccipital membrane

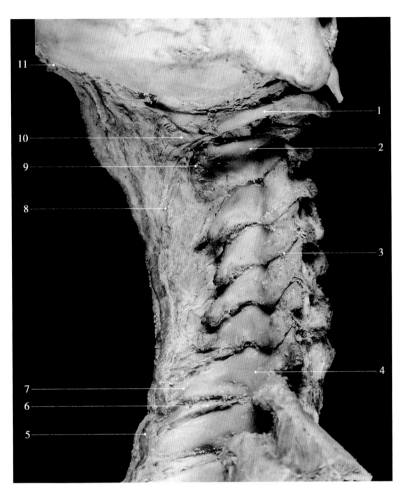

▶ 图 359　项韧带
Ligamentum nuchae

1. 寰椎 atlas
2. 枢椎 axis
3. 关节突关节 zygaophysial joint
4. 隆椎 prominent vertebra
5. 棘上韧带 supraspinal lig.
6. 棘间韧带 interspinal lig.
7. 隆椎棘突 spinous process of prominent vertebra
8. 项韧带 ligamentum nuchae
9. 枢椎棘突 spinous process of axis
10. 寰椎后弓 posterior arch of atlas
11. 枕外隆凸 external occipital protuberance

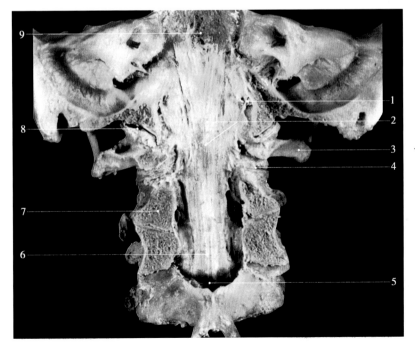

▶ 图 360　寰枕关节及覆膜（后面观）
Atlantooccipital joint and tectorial membrane.posterior view

1. 舌下神经管 hypoglossal canal
2. 覆膜 tectorial membrane
3. 寰椎横突 transverse process of atlas
4. 寰枢外侧关节 lateral atlantoaxial joint
5. 硬脊膜 spinal dura mater
6. 后纵韧带 posterior longitudinal lig.
7. 枢椎 axis
8. 寰枕关节 atlantooccipital joint
9. 斜坡 clivus

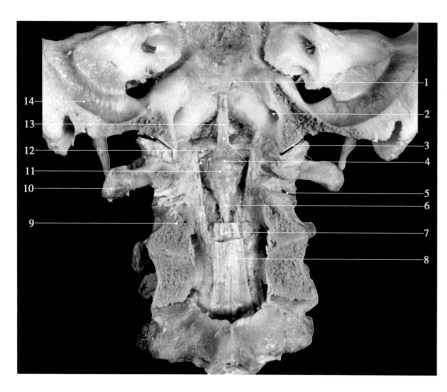

◀ 图 361 寰椎十字韧带和翼状韧带（1）

Cruciform ligament of atlas and alar ligament（1）

1. 斜坡 clivus
2. 舌下神经管 hypoglossal canal
3. 寰枕关节 atlantooccipital joint
4. 寰椎十字韧带 cruciform ligament of atlas
5. 寰枢外侧关节 lateral atlantoaxial joint
6. 下纵束 inferior longitudinal band
7. 覆膜 tectorial membrane
8. 后纵韧带 posterior longitudinal lig.
9. 枢椎 axis
10. 寰椎横突 transverse process of atlas
11. 寰椎横韧带 transverse ligament of atlas
12. 翼状韧带 alar lig.
13. 上纵束 superior longitudinal band
14. 乙状窦沟 sulcus for sigmoid sinus

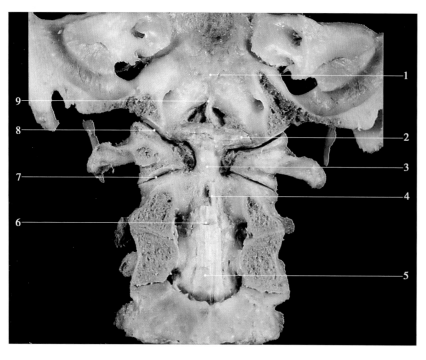

◀ 图 362 寰椎十字韧带和翼状韧带（2）

Cruciform ligament of atlas and alar ligament（2）

1. 斜坡 clivus
2. 翼状韧带 alar lig.
3. 齿突 dens
4. 下纵束 inferior longitudinal band
5. 后纵韧带 posterior longitudinal lig.
6. 覆膜 tectorial membrane
7. 寰枢外侧关节 lateral atlantoaxial joint
8. 寰枕关节 atlantooccipital joint
9. 齿突尖韧带 apical ligament of dens

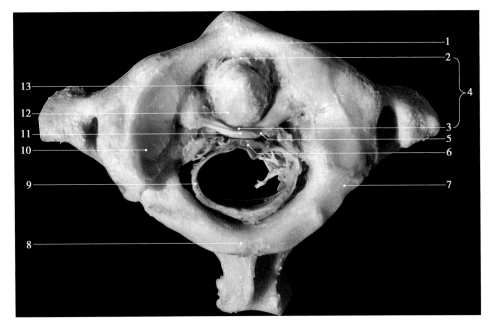

▲ 图 363 寰枢正中关节（上面观）
Median atlantoaxial joint.Superior view

1. 寰椎前弓 anterior arch of atlas
2. 寰齿前关节 anterior atlantodens joint
3. 寰齿后关节 posterior atlantodens joint
4. 寰枢正中关节 median atlantoaxial joint
5. 寰椎横韧带 transverse ligament of atlas

6. 覆膜 tectorial membrane
7. 椎动脉沟 groove for vertebral a.
8. 寰椎后弓 posterior arch of atlas
9. 硬脊膜 spinal dura mater

10. 上关节面 superior articular surface
11. 上纵束 suferior longitudinal band
12. 齿突 dens
13. 齿突尖韧带 apical ligament of dens

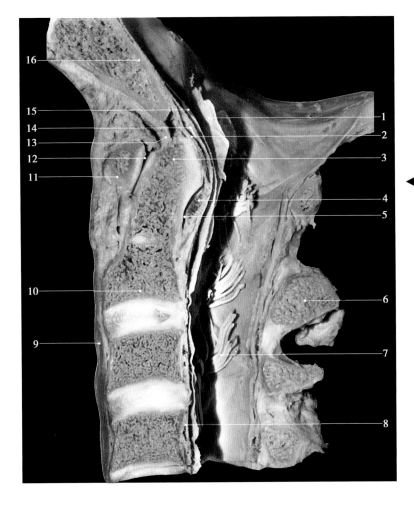

◄ 图 364 寰枕寰枢关节（矢状断面）
Atlantooccipital joint and atlantoaxial.Sagittal section

1. 蛛网膜 arachnoid mater
2. 上纵束 superior longitudinal band
3. 齿突 dens
4. 寰椎横韧带 transverse ligament of atlas
5. 寰齿后关节 posterior atlantodens joint
6. 枢椎棘突 spinous process of axis
7. 脊神经根丝 rootlets of spinal n.
8. 后纵韧带 posterior longitudinal Lig.
9. 前纵韧带 anterior longitudinal Lig.
10. 枢椎 axis
11. 寰椎前弓 anterior arch of atlas
12. 寰齿前关节 anterior atlantodens joint
13. 齿突尖韧带 apical ligament of dens
14. 覆膜 tectorial membrane
15. 硬脑膜 cerebral dura mater
16. 斜坡 clivus

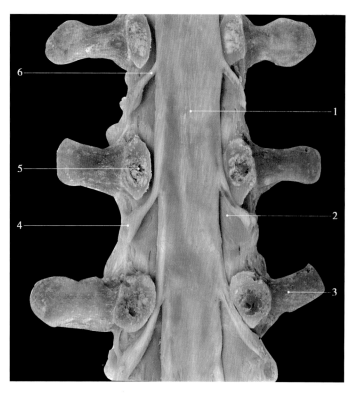

◀ 图 365　脊髓被膜（1）
Coverings of spinal cord（1）

1. 硬脊膜 spinal dura mater
2. 黄韧带 ligamenta flava
3. 腰椎横突 transverse process of lumbar vertebrae
4. 腰神经节 lumbar ganglia
5. 椎弓根 pedicle of vertebral arch
6. 脊神经根 root of spinal n.

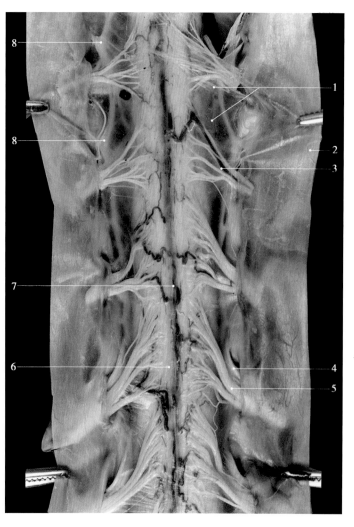

◀ 图 366　脊髓被膜（2）
Coverings of spinal cord（2）

1. 脊髓蛛网膜 spinal arachnoid mater
2. 硬脊膜 spinal dura mater
3. 前根静脉 anterior radicular v.
4. 后根 posterior root
5. 前根 anterior root
6. 脊髓 spinal cord
7. 脊髓前静脉 anterior spinal v.
8. 齿状韧带 denticulate lig.

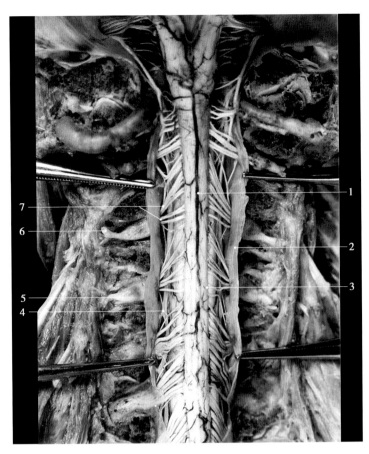

◀ 图 367 齿状韧带（后面观）
Denticulate ligament.posterior view

1. 脊髓后静脉 posterior spinal v.
2. 硬脊膜 spinal dura mater
3. 软脊膜及脊髓 spinal pia mater and spinal cord
4. 齿状韧带 denticulate lig.
5. 脊神经节 spinal ganglia
6. 脊神经后支 posterior branch of spinal n.
7. 脊神经后根 posterior root of spinal n.

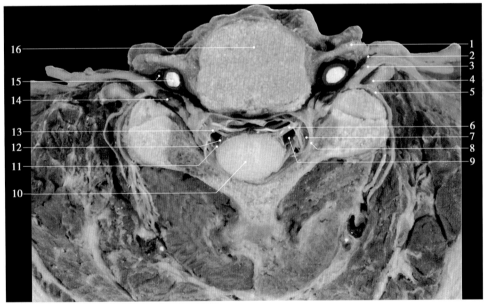

▲ 图 368 脊膜腔及脊神经的分支（上面观）
Branches of spinal nerve and cavity of spinal meninges.superior view

1. 横突前结节 anterior tubercle of transverse process
2. 脊神经沟 sulcus for spinal n.
3. 脊神经前支 anterior branch of spinal n.
4. 横突后结节 posterior tubercle of transverse process
5. 脊神经后支 posterior branch of spinal n.
6. 脊神经前根 anterior root of spinal n.
7. 硬膜下隙 subdural space
8. 硬脊膜 spinal dura mater
9. 蛛网膜下隙 subarachnoid space
10. 脊髓 spinal cord
11. 后根 posterior root of spinal n.
12. 软脊膜 spinal pia mater
13. 脊髓蛛网膜 spinal arachnoid mater
14. 脊神经节 spinal ganglia
15. 椎动、静脉 vertebral a.and v.
16. 椎体 vertebral body

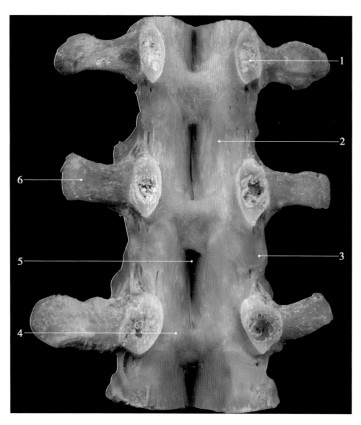

◀ 图 369　黄韧带
Ligamenta flava

1. 椎弓根 pedicle of vertebral arch
2. 黄韧带 ligamenta flava
3. 与关节突关节囊混合部 mixed part of ligamenta flava with articular capsule of zygapophysial joint
4. 椎弓板 lamina of vertebral arch
5. 黄韧带间隙 interspace of ligamenta flava
6. 横突 transverse process

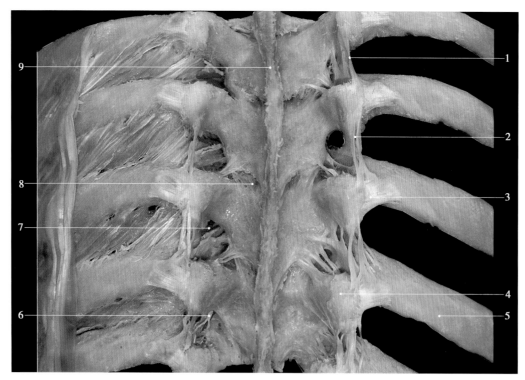

▲ 图 370　椎骨间的连结
Intervertebral joints

1. 横突间韧带 intertransverse lig.
2. 肋横突上韧带 superior costotransverse lig.
3. 肋横突外侧韧带 lateral costotransverse lig.
4. 横突 transverse process
5. 肋骨 cost bone

6. 胸神经后支 posterior branch of thoracic n.
7. 肋间后动脉背侧支 dorsal branch of posterior intercostal a.
8. 黄韧带 ligamenta flava
9. 棘上韧带 supraspinal lig.

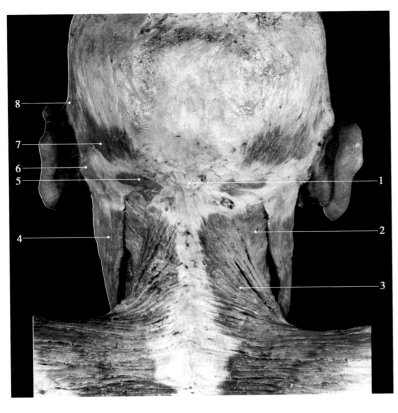

◀ 图 371 项部肌（1）
Nuchal muscles（1）

1. 枕外隆凸 external occipital protuberance
2. 头夹肌 splenius capitis
3. 斜方肌 trapezius
4. 胸锁乳突肌 sternocleidomastoid
5. 项横肌 transversus nuchae
6. 耳后肌 auricularis posterior
7. 枕额肌枕腹 occipital belly of occipitofrontalis
8. 耳上肌 auricularis superior

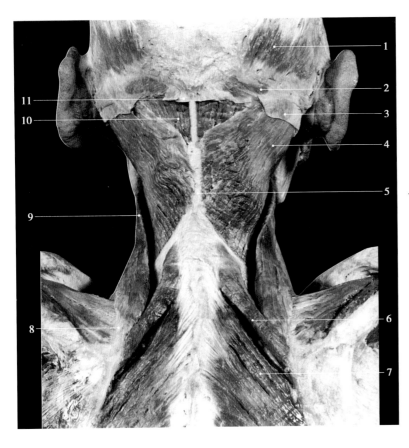

◀ 图 372 项部肌（2）
Nuchal muscles（2）

1. 枕额肌枕腹 occipital belly of occipitofrontalis
2. 项横肌 transversus nuchae
3. 胸锁乳突肌腱 tendon of sternocleidomastoid
4. 头夹肌 splenius capitis
5. 项韧带 ligamentum nuchae
6. 小菱形肌 rhomboideus minor
7. 大菱形肌 rhomboideus major
8. 肩胛骨上角 superior angle of scapula
9. 肩胛提肌 levator scapulae
10. 头半棘肌 semispinalis capitis
11. 斜方肌腱 tendon of trapezius

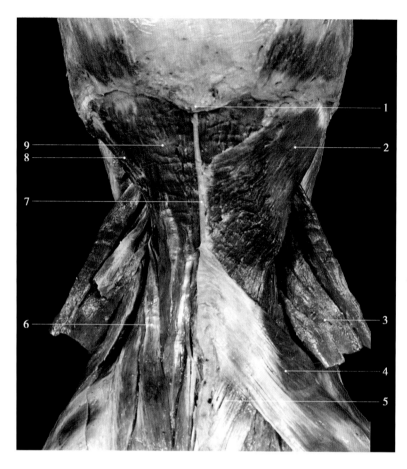

◀ 图 373　项部肌（3）
Nuchal muscles（3）

1. 枕外隆凸 external occipital protuberance
2. 头夹肌 splenius capitis
3. 肩胛提肌 levator scapulae
4. 上后锯肌 serratus posterior superior
5. 颈夹肌 splenius cervicis
6. 颈最长肌 longissimus cervicis
7. 项韧带 ligamentum nuchae
8. 头最长肌 longissimus capitis
9. 头半棘肌 semispinalis capitis

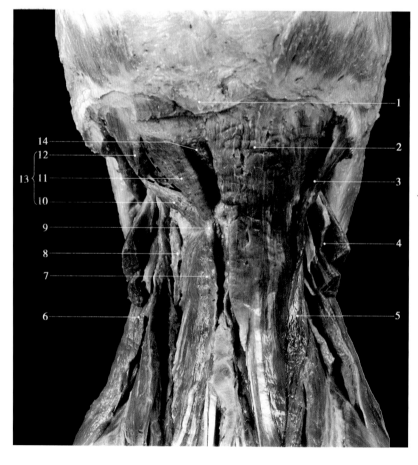

◀ 图 374　项部肌（4）
Nuchal muscles（4）

1. 枕外隆凸 external occipital protuberance
2. 头半棘肌 semispinalis capitis
3. 头最长肌 longissimus capitis
4. 肩胛提肌 levator scapulae
5. 颈最长肌 longissimus cervicis
6. 后斜角肌 scalenus posterior
7. 颈半棘肌 semispinalis cervicis
8. 颈夹肌 splenius cervicis
9. 枢椎棘突 spinous process of axis
10. 头下斜肌 obliquus capitis inferior
11. 头后大直肌 rectus capitis posterior major
12. 头上斜肌 obliquus capitis superior
13. 枕下三角 suboccipital triangle
14. 头后小直肌 rectus capitis posterior minor

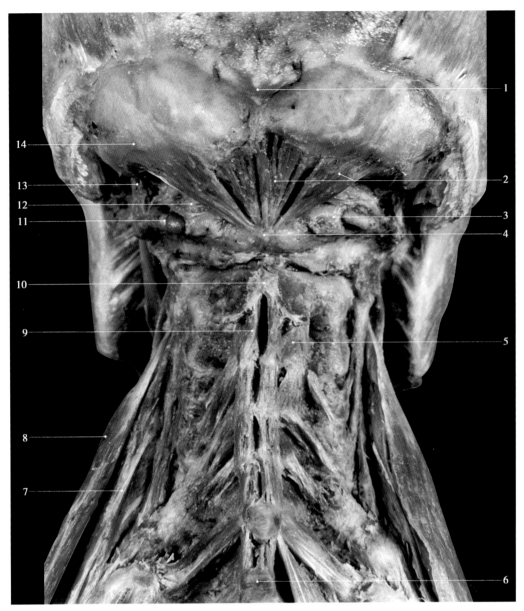

▲ 图 375　项部肌（5）
Nuchal muscles（5）

1. 枕外隆凸 external occipital protuberance
2. 头后小直肌 rectus capitis posterior minor
3. 内侧硬膜环 medial dural ring
4. 寰椎后结节 posterior tubercle of atlas
5. 颈回旋肌 rotatores cervicis
6. 隆椎棘突 spinous process of prominent vertebra
7. 中斜角肌 scalenus medius
8. 后斜角肌 scalenus posterior
9. 颈棘间肌 interspinales cervicis
10. 枢椎棘突 spinous process of axis
11. 椎动脉 vertebral a.
12. 寰枕后膜 posterior atlantooccipital membrane
13. 头外侧直肌 rectus capitis lateralis
14. 下项线 inferior nuchal line

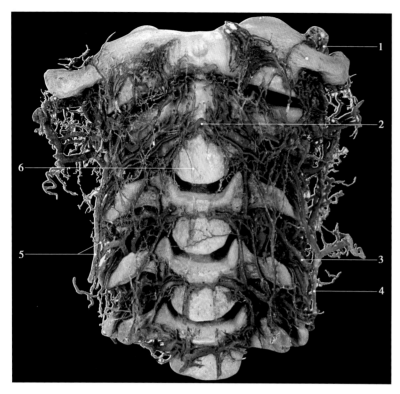

◀ 图 376　椎外前静脉丛（前面观）
Anterior external vertebral venous
plexus.Anterior view

1. 椎静脉 vertebral v.
2. 椎外前静脉丛 anterior external vertebral
   venous plexus
3. 椎间静脉 intervertebral v.
4. 颈深静脉 deep cervical v.
5. 颈升动、静脉 ascending cervical a.and v.
6. 椎体 vertebral body

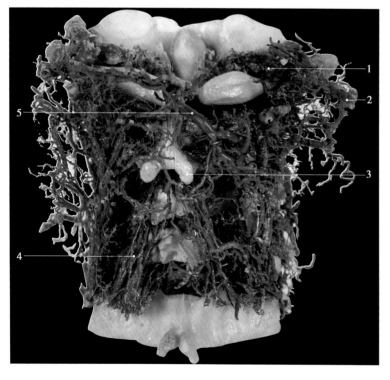

◀ 图 377　椎外后静脉丛（后面观）
Posterior external vertebral venous
plexus.Posterior view

1. 椎动脉旁静脉丛 venous plexus around vertebral a.
2. 枕静脉 occipital v.
3. 棘突 spinous process
4. 椎外后静脉丛 posterior external vertebral
   venous plexus
5. 枕下静脉丛 suboccipital venous plexus

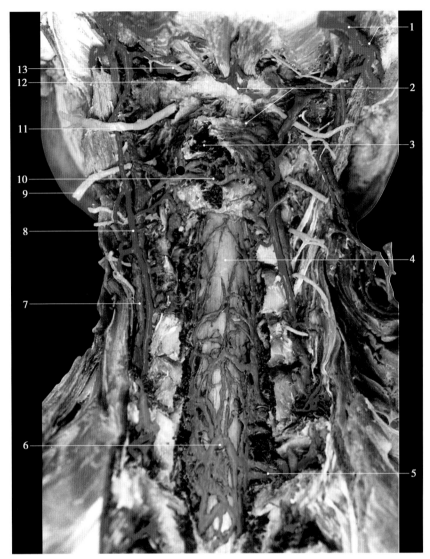

▲ 图 378　椎内后静脉丛（后面观）
Posterior internal vertebral venous plexus.Posterior view

1. 枕动、静脉 occipital a.and v.
2. 枕下静脉丛 suboccipital venous plexus
3. 枢椎（棘突切掉）atlas
4. 硬脊膜 spinal dura mater
5. 椎间静脉 intervertebral v.
6. 椎内后静脉丛 posterior internal vertebral venous plexus
7. 颈深静脉 deep cervical v.
8. 颈深动脉 deep cervical a.
9. 第3颈神经（第3枕神经）the 3rd cervical n.
10. 椎外后静脉丛 posterior external vertebral venous plexus
11. 第2颈神经（枕大神经）the 2nd cervical n.
12. 寰椎后弓 posterior arch of atlas
13. 第1颈神经（枕下神经）the 1st cervical n.

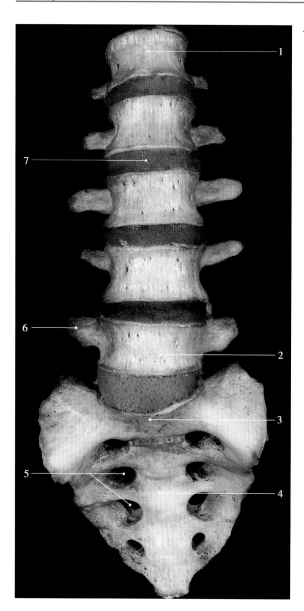

◀ 图 379　腰椎和骶骨（前面观）
Lumbar vertebra and sacrum.Anterior view

1. 第 1 腰椎体 body of the 1st lumbar vertebra
2. 第 5 腰椎体 body of the 5th lumbar vertebra
3. 岬 promontory
4. 盆面 pelvic surface
5. 骶前孔 anterior sacral foramina
6. 第 5 腰椎横突 transverse process of the 5th lumbar vertebra
7. 椎间盘 intervertebral disc

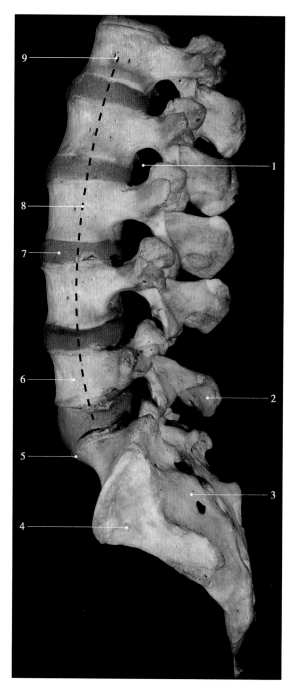

图 380　腰椎和骶骨（侧面观）▶
Lumbar vertebra and sacrum.Lateral view

1. 椎间孔 intervertebral foramina
2. 第 5 腰椎棘突 spinous process of 5th lumbar vertebra
3. 骶骨 sacrum
4. 耳状面 auricular surface
5. 岬 promontory
6. 第 5 腰椎体 body of the 5th lumbar vertebra
7. 椎间盘 intervertebral disc
8. 腰曲 lumbar curve
9. 第 1 腰椎体 body of the 1st lumbar vertebra

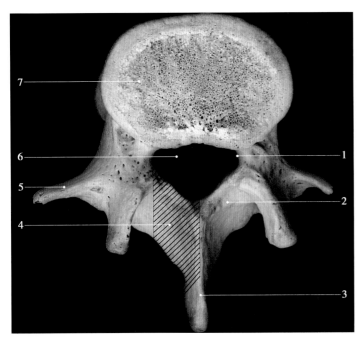

▲ 图 381　腰椎管的侧隐窝（1）
Laterorecessus of lumbar spinal canal（1）

1. 侧隐窝 laterorecessus
2. 椎弓板 lamina of vertebral arch
3. 棘突 spinous process
4. 手术减压区 reduced pressure zone of operation
5. 横突 transverse process
6. 椎孔 vertebral foramen
7. 腰椎体 body of lumbar vertebra

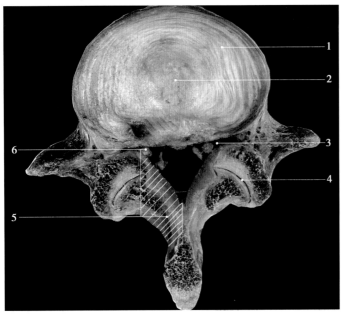

▲ 图 382　腰椎管的侧隐窝（2）
Laterorecessus of lumbar spinal canal（2）

1. 纤维环 anulus fibrosus
2. 髓核 nucleus pulposus
3. 侧隐窝 laterorecessus
4. 关节突关节 zygaophysial joint
5. 手术减压区 reduced pressure zone of operation
6. 腰神经根 root of lumbar n.

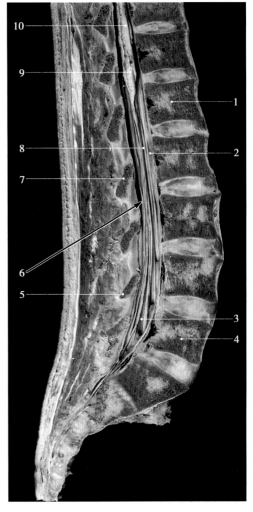

▲ 图 383　骶管及硬脊膜囊
Sacral canal and dural sac

1. 第 1 腰椎 the1st lumbar vertebra
2. 硬脊膜 spinal dura mater
3. 蛛网膜下隙 subarachnoid space
4. 第 5 腰椎 the 5th lumbar vertebra
5. 第 4 腰椎棘突 spinous process of the 4th lumbar vertebra
6. 硬膜外隙进针 needle entering epidural space
7. 第 2 腰椎棘突 spinous process of the 2nd lumbar vertebra
8. 马尾 cauda equina
9. 脊髓圆锥 conus medullaris
10. 脊髓 spinal cord

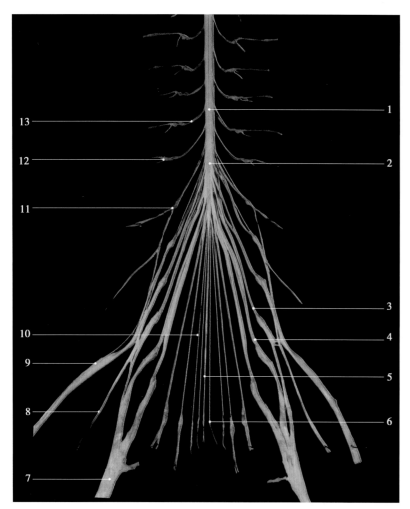

◀图 384　马尾与终丝
Cauda equina and filum terminale

1. 脊髓 spinal cord
2. 脊髓圆锥 conus medullaris
3. 第 5 腰神经 the 5th lumbar n.
4. 第 1 骶神经 the 1st sacral n.
5. 终丝 filum terminale
6. 尾神经 coccygeal n.
7. 坐骨神经 sciatic n.
8. 闭孔神经 obturator n.
9. 股神经 femoral n.
10. 第 5 骶神经 the 5th sacral n.
11. 第 2 腰神经 the 2nd lumbar n.
12. 第 1 腰神经 the 1st lumbar n.
13. 第 12 胸神经 the 12th thoracic n.

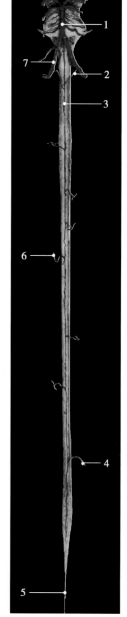

图 385　脊髓动脉（前面观）▶
Spinal arteries.Anterior view

1. 基底动脉 basilar a.
2. 椎动脉脊支 spinal branches of vertebral a.
3. 脊髓前动脉 anterior spinal a.
4. 腰动脉的根动脉 radicular artery of lumbar a.
5. 终丝 filum terminale
6. 肋间后动脉的根动脉 radicular artery of posterior intercostal a.
7. 椎动脉颅内段 intracranial part of vertebral a.

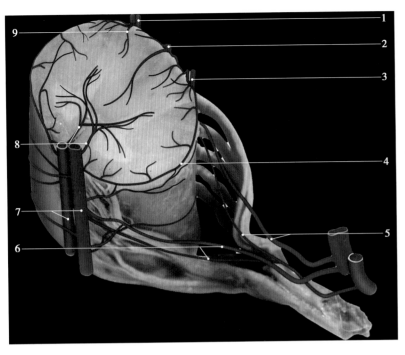

▶ 图 386　脊髓内部的血管分布
Distribution of blood vessels in spinal cord

1. 右脊髓后动脉 right posterior spinal a.
2. 脊髓后静脉 posterior spinal v.
3. 左脊髓后外侧静脉 left spinal external posterior v.
4. 动脉冠 vasocorona
5. 后根动、静脉 posterior radicular a.and v.
6. 前根动、静脉 anterior radicular a.and v.
7. 脊髓前动、静脉 anterior spinal a.and v.
8. 沟动、静脉 sulcus a.and v.
9. 周围支 peripheral branches

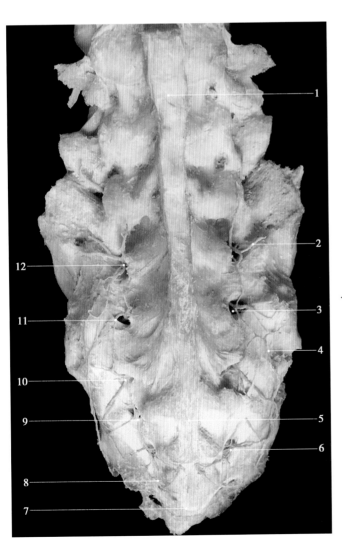

▶ 图 387　骶尾神经后支
Posterior branches of sacral and coccygeal nerves

1. 棘上韧带 supraspinal lig.
2. 第 1 骶神经后支外侧支 lateral branch of posterior branch of the 1st sacral n.
3. 骶后孔 posterio sacral foramina
4. 骶神经后支神经襻 nerve loop of posterior branch of sacral n.
5. 骶尾后浅韧带 superficial posterior sacrococcygeal lig.
6. 第 5 骶神经后支 posterior branch of the 5th sacral n.
7. 尾骨 coccyx
8. 尾神经后支 posterior branch of coccygeal n.
9. 第 4 骶神经后支 posterior branch of the 4th sacral n.
10. 第 3 骶神经后支 posterior branch of the 3rd sacral n.
11. 第 2 骶神经后支 posterior branch of the 2nd sacral n.
12. 第 1 骶神经后支 posterior branch of the 1st sacral n.

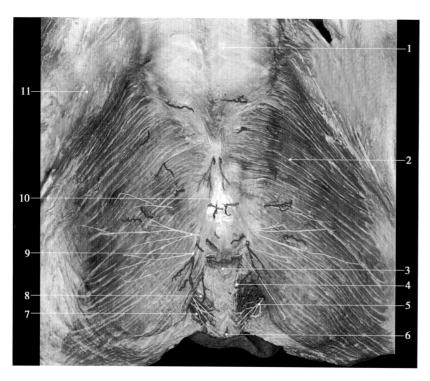

◀ 图 388　骶后区局解（1）
Regional anatomy of posterior sacral region（1）

1. 胸腰筋膜浅层 superficial layer of thoracolumbar fascia
2. 臀大肌 gluteus maximus
3. 尾骨 coccyx
4. 尾神经后支 posterior branch of coccygeal n.
5. 肛神经 anal n.
6. 肛门 anus
7. 肛动脉 anal a.
8. 肛静脉 anal v.
9. 臀内侧皮神经 medial clunial n.
10. 骶骨 sacrum
11. 臀中肌筋膜 fascia of gluteus medius

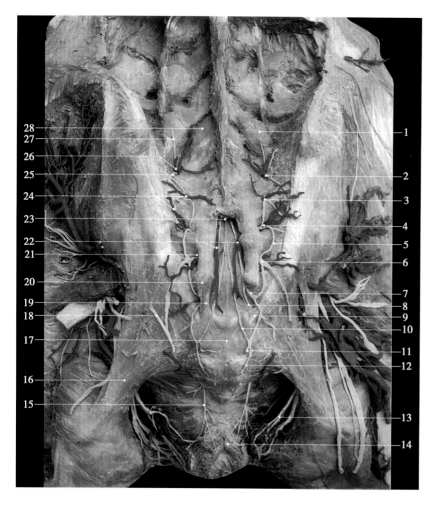

◀ 图 389　骶后区局解（2）
Regional anatomy of posterior sacral region（2）

1. 关节突关节 zygapophysial joint
2. 第 1 骶神经后支 posterior branch of the 1st sacral n.
3. 第 2 骶神经后支 posterior branch of the 2nd sacral n.
4. 第 3 骶神经后支 posterior branch of the 3th sacral n.
5. 骶神经后支神经襻 nerve loop of posterior branch of sacral n.
6. 第 4 骶神经后支 posterior branch of the 4th sacral n.
7. 第 5 骶神经后支 posterior branch of the 5th sacral n.
8. 第 5 骶神经前支 anterior branch of the 5th sacral n.
9. 骶尾外侧韧带 lateral sacrococcygeal lig.
10. 尾神经 coccygeal n.
11. 尾神经前支 anterior branch of coccygeal n.
12. 尾神经后支 posterior branch of coccygeal n.
13. 肛神经 anal n.
14. 肛门外括约肌 sphincter ani externa
15. 肛门外括约肌神经 nerve to sphincter ani externa
16. 骶结节韧带 sacrotuberous lig.
17. 外终丝 filum terminale externa
18. 肛尾神经 anococcygeal n.
19. 骶尾关节韧带 ligament of sacrococcygeal joint
20. 骶角 sacral cornu
21. 骶后孔 posterior sacral foramina
22. 椎内后静脉丛 posterior internal vertebral venous plexus
23. 骶管裂孔 sacral hiatus
24. 骶外侧动脉下支肌支 muscular branch of inferior branch of lateral sacral a.
25. 第 1 骶神经后支外侧支 lateral branch of posterior branch of the 1st sacral n.
26. 骶外侧动脉上支末支 terminal superior branch of lateral sacral a.
27. 第 1 骶神经后支内侧支 medial branch of posterior branch of the1st sacral n.
28. 黄韧带 ligamenta flava

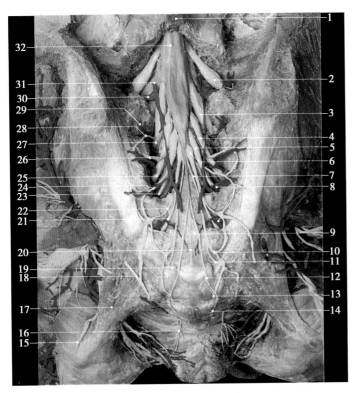

▲ 图 390　骶后区局解（3）
Regional anatomy of posterior sacral region（3）

1. 棘突 spinous process
2. 第 5 腰神经节 the 5th lumbar ganglion
3. 第 1 骶神经节 the 1st sacral ganglion
4. 第 2 骶神经节 the 2nd sacral ganglion
5. 第 3 骶神经节 the 3rd sacral ganglion
6. 第 4 骶神经节 the 4th sacral ganglion
7. 第 5 骶神经 the 5th sacral n.
8. 骶外侧动脉脊支 spinal branch of lateral sacral a.
9. 后纵韧带 posterior longitudinal lig.
10. 第 5 骶神经后支 posterior branch of the the 5th sacral n.
11. 第 5 骶神经前支 anterior branch of the the 5th sacral n.
12. 尾神经 coccygeal n.
13. 尾神经前支 anterior branch of coccygeal n.
14. 尾神经后支 posterior branch of coccygeal n.
15. 穿皮神经 perforating cutaneous n.
16. 肛门外括约肌神经 nerve to sphincter ani externus
17. 骶结节韧带 sacrotuberous lig.
18. 肛尾神经 anococcygeal n.
19. 尾骨角 coccygeal cornu
20. 外终丝 filum terminale externa
21. 第 4 骶神经前支 anterior branch of the 4th sacral n.
22. 第 4 骶神经后支 posterior branch of the 4th sacral n.
23. 第 3 骶神经前支 anterior branch of the3rd sacral n.
24. 第 3 骶神经后支 posterior branch of the 3rd sacral n.
25. 第 2 骶神经前支 anterior branch of the 2nd sacral n.
26. 第 2 骶神经后支 posterior branch of the 2nd sacral n.
27. 第 1 骶神经前支 anterior branch of the 1st sacral n.
28. 第 1 骶神经后支 posterior branch of the 1st sacral n.
29. 骶外侧动脉上支 superior branch of lateral sacral a.
30. 椎间静脉 intervertebral v.
31. 椎内后静脉丛 posterior internal vertebral venous plexus
32. 硬脊膜 spinal dura mater

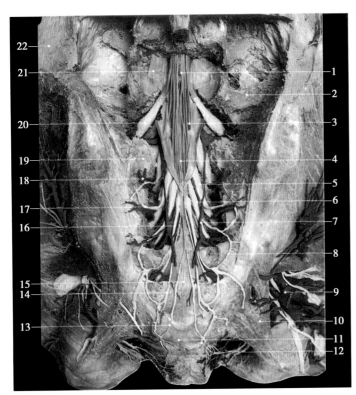

▲ 图 391　骶后区局解（4）
Regional anatomy of posterior sacral region（4）

1. 马尾 cauda equina
2. 第 5 腰椎横突 transverse process of the 5th lumbar vertebra
3. 第 1 骶神经后根 posterior root of the 1st sacral n.
4. 内终丝 filum terminal internum
5. 第 2 骶神经节 the 2nd sacral ganglia
6. 第 3 骶神经节 the 3rd sacral ganglia
7. 椎内后静脉丛 posterior internal vertebral venous plexus
8. 骶神经后支神经襻 nerve loop of posterior branch of sacral n.
9. 臀下静脉 inferior gluteal v.
10. 骶结节韧带 sacrotuberous lig.
11. 尾骨 coccyx
12. 尾神经前支 anterior branch of coccygeal n.
13. 尾神经 coccygeal n.
14. 第 5 骶神经后支 posterior branch of the 5th sacral n.
15. 外终丝 filum terminale externa
16. 第 4 骶神经 the 4th sacral n.
17. 第 2 骶神经后支 posterior branch of the 2nd sacral n.
18. 骶外侧动脉上支肌支 muscular branch of superior branch of lateral sacral a.
19. 骶骨 sacrum
20. 第 5 腰神经节 the 5th lumbar ganglia
21. 硬脊膜 spinal dura mater
22. 髂后上棘 posterior superior iliac spine

连续层次局部解剖

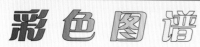

第七章

上 肢

Chapter 7　Upper limb

上肢借肩、腋区与颈、胸和背区相连。境界以锁骨上缘外 1/3 段及肩峰至第 7 颈椎棘突连线的外 1/3 段与颈部为界；以三角肌前、后缘上份与腋前、后襞下缘中点的连线与胸、背区为界。

上肢可分为肩、臂、肘、前臂和手部。各部又分为若干区。

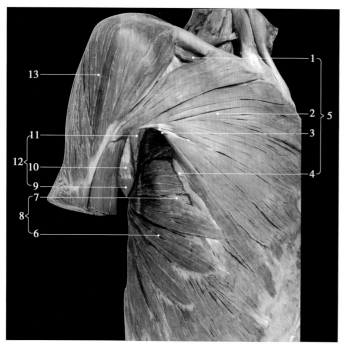

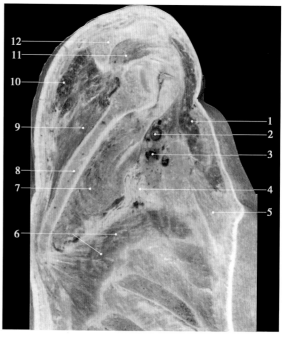

▲ 图 392　腋窝的界限
Boundaries of axillary fossa

1. 锁骨下肌 subclavius
2. 胸大肌 pectoralis major
3. 胸大肌下缘 inferior border of pectoralis major
4. 胸小肌 pectoralis minor
5. 腋窝前壁 anterior wall of axillary forssa
6. 前锯肌 serratus anterior
7. 第 1 至第 4 肋骨 the 1st~4th costal bone
8. 腋窝内侧壁 inner wall of axillary fossa
9. 大圆肌 teres major
10. 背阔肌 latissimus dorsi
11. 肩胛下肌 subscapularis
12. 腋窝后壁 posterior wall of axillary fossa
13. 三角肌 deltoid

▲ 图 393　腋窝的界限（矢状切面）
Boundaries of axillary fossa.Sagittal section

1. 胸大肌 pectoralis major
2. 腋动脉 axillary a.
3. 腋静脉 axillary v.
4. 臂丛 brachial plexus
5. 胸小肌 pectoralis minor
6. 前锯肌 serratus anterior
7. 肩胛下肌 subscapularis
8. 肩胛骨 scapular
9. 冈下肌 infraspinatus
10. 斜方肌 trapezius
11. 冈上肌 supraspinatus
12. 肩峰 acromion

◀ 图 394　腋窝的界限（水平切面）
Boundaries of axillary fossa.
Horizontal section

1. 胸大肌 pectoralis major
2. 胸小肌 pectoralis minor
3. 腋窝前壁 anterior wall of axillary fossa
4. 臂丛 brachial plexus
5. 腋动、静脉 axillary a.and v.
6. 肋骨 costal bone
7. 前锯肌 serratus anterior
8. 腋窝内侧壁 inner wall of axillary fossa
9. 冈下肌 infraspinatus
10. 肩胛下肌 subscapularis
11. 小圆肌 teres minor
12. 大圆肌 teres major
13. 背阔肌 latissimus dorsi
14. 腋窝后壁 posterior wall of axillary fossa
15. 三角肌 deltoid
16. 肱三头肌长头 long head of triceps brachii
17. 肱二头肌长头 long head of biceps brachii
18. 喙肱肌 coracobrachialis
19. 肱二头肌短头 short head of biceps brachii
20. 外侧壁 lateral wall

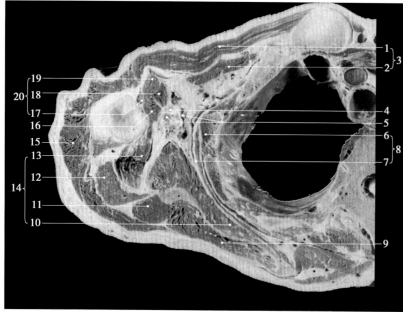

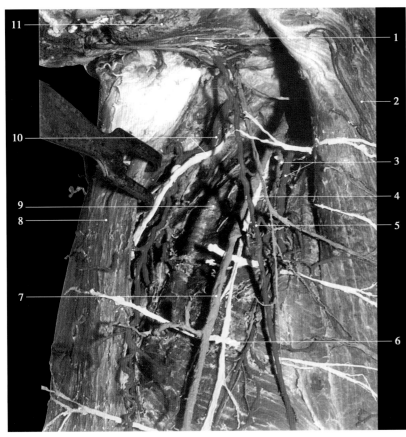

◀ 图 395 腋窝的内容（侧面观）
Contents of axillary fossa.Lateral view

1. 喙肱肌 coracobrachialis
2. 胸大肌 pectoralis major
3. 胸外侧动、静脉 lateral thoracic a.and v.
4. 胸长神经 long thoracic n.
5. 肱胸皮动脉 brachiithoracic cutaneous a.
6. 肋间神经外侧皮支 lateral cutaneous branch of intercostal n.
7. 胸腹壁静脉 thoracoepigastric v.
8. 背阔肌 latissimus dorsi
9. 前锯肌 serratus anterior
10. 胸背动脉、神经 thoracodorsal a.and n.
11. 肱二头肌 biceps brachii

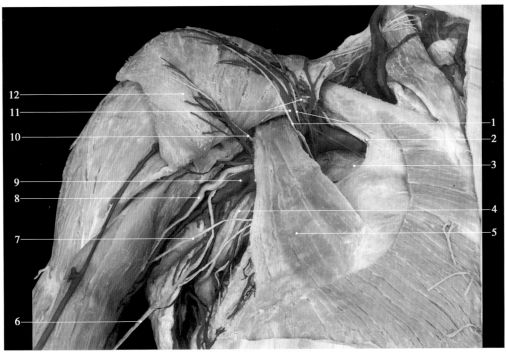

▲ 图 396 腋窝的内容（前面观 1 ）
Contents of axillary fossa.Anterior view（1）

1. 胸外侧神经 lateral pectoral n.
2. 锁骨下肌 subclavius
3. 第 1 肋骨 the 1st rib
4. 胸背神经 thoracodorsal n.
5. 胸小肌 pectoralis minor
6. 前臂内侧皮神经 medial antebrachial cutaneous n.
7. 肋间臂神经 intercostobrachial n.
8. 正中神经 median n.
9. 腋静脉 axillary v.
10. 胸内侧神经 medial pectoral n.
11. 胸肩峰动、静脉 thoracoacromial a.and v.
12. 胸大肌 pectoralis major

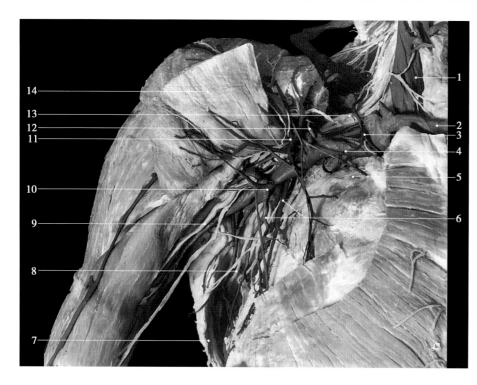

◀图397 腋窝的内容(前面观2)
Contents of axillary fossa.
Anterior view (2)

1. 颈内静脉 internal jugular v.
2. 颈静脉弓 jugular venous arch
3. 右淋巴导管 right lymphatic duct
4. 锁骨下静脉 subclavian v.
5. 第 1 肋 the 1st rib
6. 胸外侧动、静脉 lateral thoracic a.and v.
7. 背阔肌 latissimus dorsi
8. 胸背神经 thoracodorsal n.
9. 正中神经 median n.
10. 腋静脉 axillary v.
11. 胸肩峰动脉 thoracoacromial a.
12. 头静脉 cephalic v.
13. 臂丛 brachial plexus
14. 胸小肌 pectoralis minor

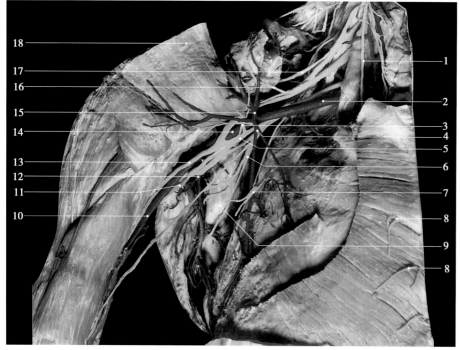

1. 膈神经 phrenic n.
2. 锁骨下动脉 subclavian a.
3. 胸内侧神经 medial pectoral n.
4. 胸外侧动脉 lateral thoracic a.
5. 内侧束 medial cord
6. 胸背神经 thoracodorsal n.
7. 肋间臂神经 intercostobrachial n.
8. 肋间神经前皮支 anterior cutaneous branch of intercostal n.
9. 肩胛下肌 subscapularis
10. 肱动脉 brachial a.
11. 尺神经 ulnar n.
12. 肩胛下动脉 subscapular a.
13. 正中神经 median n.
14. 腋动脉 axillary a.
15. 胸肩峰动脉 thoracoacromial a.
16. 胸外侧神经 lateral pectoral n.
17. 肩胛上神经 suprascapular n.
18. 胸小肌 pectoralis minor

▲ 图 398　腋窝的内容 （前面观 3 ）
Contents of axillary fossa.Anterior view (3)

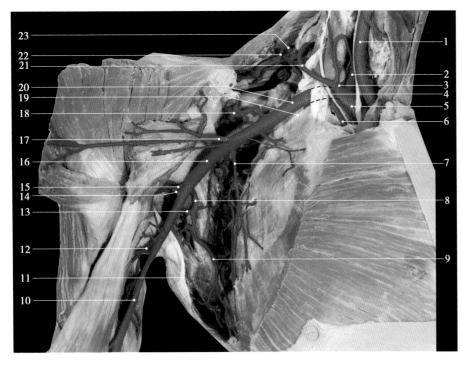

1. 颈总动脉 common carotid a.
2. 椎动脉 vertebral a.
3. 甲状颈干 thyrocervical trunk
4. 锁骨下动脉第 2 段 the 2nd segment of subclavian a.
5. 锁骨下动脉第 1 段 the 1st segment of subclavian a.
6. 胸廓内动脉 internal thoracic a.
7. 胸外侧动脉 lateral thoracic a.
8. 肩胛下动脉 subscapular a.
9. 胸背动脉 thoracodorsal a.
10. 肱动脉 brachial a.
11. 背阔肌下缘 inferior border of latissimus dorsi
12. 肱深动脉 deep brachial a.
13. 旋肩胛动脉 circumflex scapular a.
14. 旋肱前动脉 anterior humeral circumflex a.
15. 旋肱后动脉 posterior humeral circumflex a.
16. 腋动脉 axillary a.
17. 胸肩峰动脉 thoracoacromial a.
18. 肩胛上动脉 suprascapular a.
19. 第 1 肋 the 1 st rib
20. 锁骨下动脉第 3 段 the 3rd segment of subclavian a.
21. 颈横动脉 transverse cervical a.
22. 颈浅动脉 superficial cervical a.
23. 肩胛背动脉 dorsal scapular a.

▲ 图 399　锁骨下动脉和腋动脉
Subclavian artery and axillary artery

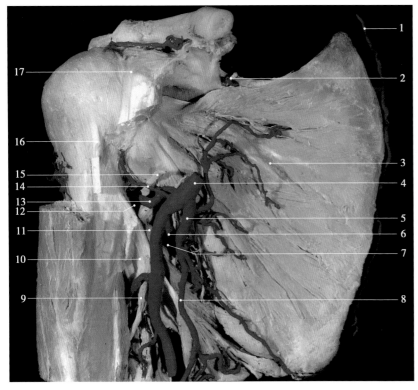

1. 肩胛背动脉 dorsal scapular a.
2. 肩胛上动脉 suprascapular a.
3. 肩胛下肌 subscapularis
4. 腋动脉 axillary a.
5. 肩胛下动脉 subscapular a.
6. 旋肩胛动脉 circumflex scapular a.
7. 三边孔 trilateral foramen
8. 胸背动脉 thoracodorsal a.
9. 桡神经 radial n.
10. 背阔肌 latissimus dorsi
11. 大圆肌 teres major
12. 四边孔 quadrilateral foramen
13. 旋肱后动脉 posterior humeral circumflex a.
14. 旋肱前动脉 anterior humeral circumflex a.
15. 腋神经 axillary n.
16. 肱二头肌长头 long head of biceps brachii
17. 喙突 coracoid process

▲ 图 400　三边孔与四边孔（前面观）
Trilateral foramen and quadrilateral foramen.Anterior view

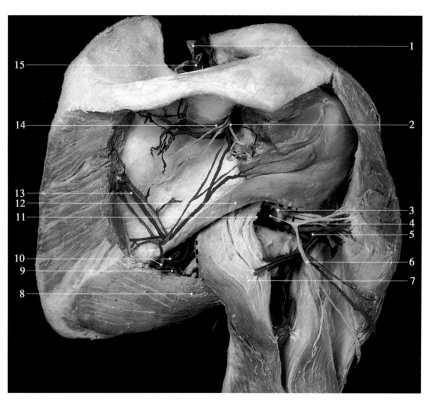

1. 肩胛上神经 suprascapular n.
2. 冈下肌神经 infraspinatus n.
3. 小圆肌支 muscular branch of teres minor
4. 腋神经 axillary n.
5. 旋肱后动脉 posterior humeral circumflex a.
6. 臂外侧上皮神经 superior lateral brachial cutaneous n.
7. 肱三头肌长头 long head of triceps brachii
8. 大圆肌 teres major
9. 三边孔 trilateral foramen
10. 旋肩胛动、静脉浅支 superficial branch of circumflex scapular a.and v.
11. 四边孔 quadrilateral foramen
12. 小圆肌 teres minor
13. 肩胛动脉网 arterial rete of scapular region
14. 冈下肌支 muscular branch of infraspinatus
15. 肩胛上动脉 suprascapular a.

▲ 图 401　三边孔与四边孔（后面观）
Trilateral foramen and quadrilateral foramen.Posterior view

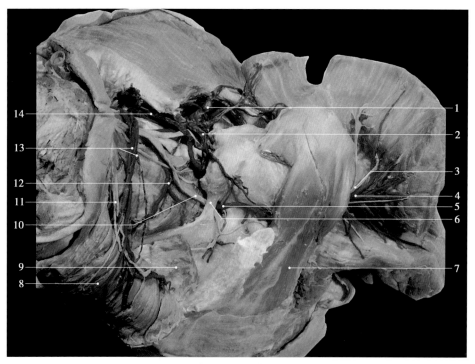

▲ 图 402　肩胛上区结构（上面观）
Structures of superior scapular region.Superior view

1. 头静脉 cephalic v.
2. 肩胛上静脉 suprascapular v.
3. 腋神经 axillary n.
4. 旋肱后动脉 posterior humeral circumflex a.
5. 肩胛上动脉 suprascapular a.
6. 肩胛上横韧带 superior transverse scapular lig.
7. 冈下肌 infraspinatus
8. 斜方肌 trapezius
9. 冈上肌 supraspinatus
10. 肩胛上神经 suprascapular n.
11. 副神经 accessory n.
12. 肩胛背动脉 dorsal scapular a.
13. 颈浅动、静脉 superficial cervical a.and v.
14. 锁骨下静脉 subclavian v.

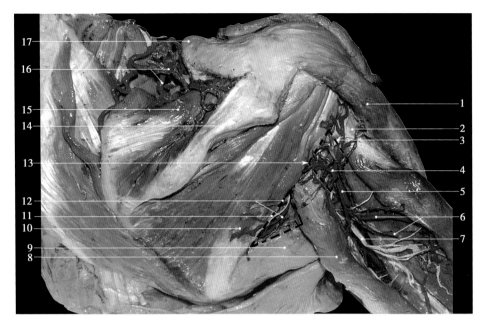

▲ 图 403　三角肌区及肩胛区结构（后面观）
Structures of deltoid and scapular regions.Posterior view

1. 三角肌 deltoid
2. 肱骨 humerus
3. 腋神经 axillary n.
4. 旋肱后动脉 posterior humeral circumflex a.
5. 肱深动脉返支 recurrent branch of deep brachial a.
6. 肱深动、静脉 deep brachial a.and v.
7. 桡神经 radial n.
8. 肱三头肌长头 long head of triceps brachii
9. 大圆肌 teres major

10. 小圆肌 teres minor
11. 三边孔 trilateral foramen
12. 旋肩胛动、静脉浅支 superficial branch of circumflex scapular a.and v.
13. 四边孔 quadrilateral foramen
14. 肩胛冈 spine of scapula
15. 冈上肌 supraspinatus
16. 肩胛上动、静脉 suprascapular a.and v.
17. 锁骨 clavicle

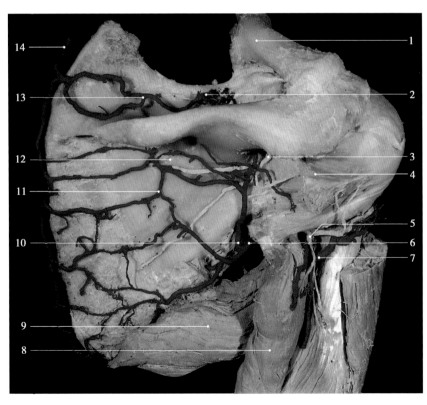

◀图 404　肩胛骨周围的动脉吻合（后面观）
Arterial anastomoses around scapula.
Posterior view

1. 锁骨 clavicle
2. 肩胛上动脉 suprascapular a.
3. 冈下肌肌支 muscular branch of infraspinatus
4. 冈下肌 infraspinatus
5. 腋神经 axillary n.
6. 肩胛下动脉 subscapular a.
7. 旋肱后动脉 posterior humeral circumflex a.
8. 肱三头肌长头 long head of triceps brachii
9. 大圆肌 teres major
10. 旋肩胛动脉 circumflex scapular a.
11. 肩胛动脉网 arterial rete of scapular region
12. 冈下窝 infraspinous fossa
13. 冈上肌肌支 muscular branch of supraspinatus
14. 肩胛背动脉 dorsal scapular a.

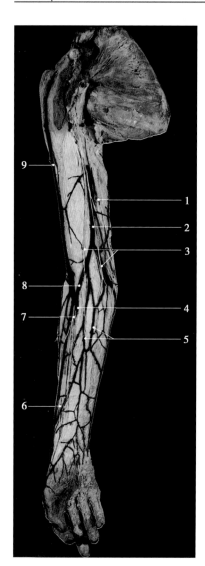

◀ 图 405　上肢皮神经及浅静脉
Cutaneous nerves and superficial veins of upper limb

1. 臂内侧皮神经 medial brachial cutaneous n.
2. 贵要静脉 basilic v.
3. 前臂内侧皮神经 medial antebrachial cutaneous n.
4. 深静脉交通支 communicating branch with deep veins
5. 前臂正中静脉 median antebrachial v.
6. 桡神经浅支 superficial branch of radial n.
7. 前臂外侧皮神经 lateral antebrachial cutaneous n.
8. 肘正中静脉 median v.
9. 头静脉 cephalic v.

图 406　臂丛的分支 ▶
Branches of brachial plexus

1. 第 5 颈神经 the 5th cervical n.
2. 第 8 颈神经 the 8th cervical n.
3. 第 1 胸神经 the 1st thoracic n.
4. 膈神经 phrenic n.
5. 胸长神经 long thoracic n.
6. 臂内侧皮神经 medial brachial cutaneous n.
7. 前臂内侧皮神经 medial antebrachial cutaneous n.
8. 桡神经深支 deep branch of radial n.
9. 骨间后神经 posterior interosseous n.
10. 尺神经 ulnar n.
11. 交通支 communicating branch
12. 指掌侧固有神经 proper palmar digital n.
13. 正中神经 median n.
14. 桡神经浅支 superficial branch of radial n.
15. 桡神经 radial n.
16. 前臂后侧皮神经 posterior antebrachial cutaneous n.
17. 臂外侧下皮神经 inferior lateral brachial cutaneous n.
18. 肌皮神经 musculocutaneous n.
19. 腋神经 axillary n.
20. 肩胛上神经 suprascapular n.
21. 肩胛背神经 dorsal scapular n.

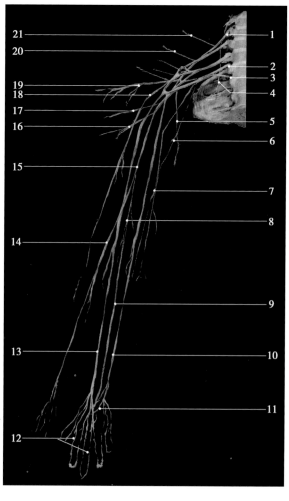

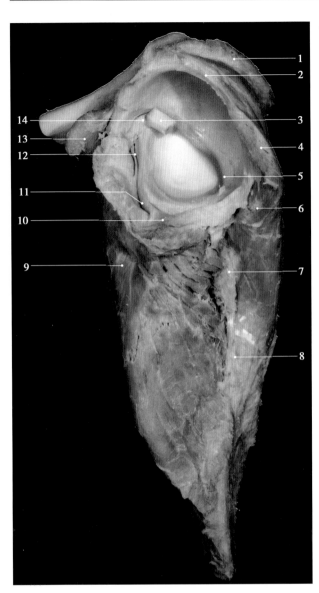

1. 肩峰 acromion
2. 冈上肌腱 tendon of supraspinatus
3. 肱二头肌腱（长头）biceps brachii tendon（long head）
4. 冈下肌腱 tendon of infraspinatus
5. 关节盂唇 glenoid labrum
6. 小圆肌 teres minor
7. 肱三头肌长头 long head of triceps brachii
8. 肩胛骨外侧缘 lateral border of scapular
9. 肩胛下肌 subscapularis
10. 腋隐窝 axillary recess
11. 盂肱下韧带 inferior glenohumeral lig.
12. 盂肱中韧带 middle glenohumeral lig.
13. 喙突 coracoid process
14. 盂肱上韧带 superior glenohumeral lig.

图 408 盂肱韧带 ▶
Glenohumeral ligament

1. 肩峰下囊 subacromial bursa
2. 冈上肌 supraspinatus
3. 肩峰 acromion
4. 肱二头肌腱（长头）biceps brachii tendon（long head）
5. 冈下肌 infraspinatus
6. 关节盂 glenoid cavity
7. 小圆肌 teres minor
8. 肱三头肌长头 long head of triceps brachii
9. 盂肱下韧带 inferior glenohumeral lig.
10. 肩胛下肌 subscapularis
11. 肩胛下肌腱下囊 subtendinous bursa of subscapularis
12. 盂肱中韧带 middle glenohumeral lig.
13. 喙突 coracoid process
14. 盂肱上韧带 superior glenohumeral lig.
15. 喙肩韧带 coracoacromial lig.

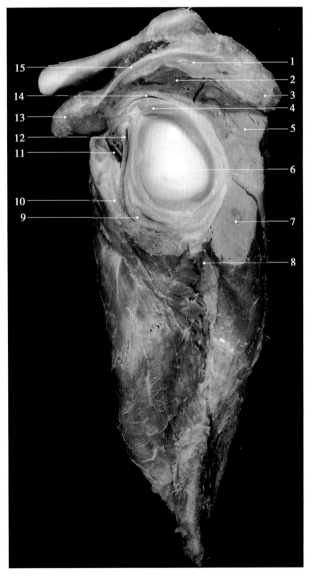

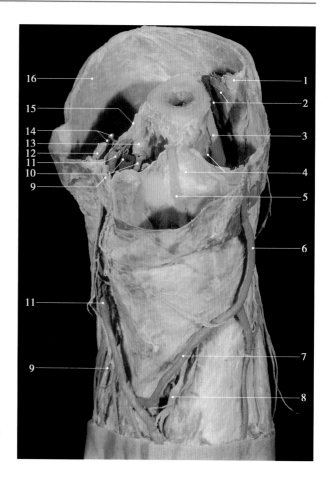

图 409 臂部骨筋膜鞘 ▶
Osseofascial sheaths of arm

1. 臂外侧肌间隔 lateral brachial intermuscular septum
2. 桡侧副动、静脉 radial collateral a.and v.
3. 桡神经 radial n.
4. 前骨筋膜鞘 anterior osseofascial sheath
5. 肌皮神经 musculocutaneous n.
6. 头静脉 cephalic v.
7. 肘正中静脉 median cubital v.
8. 前臂外侧皮神经 lateral antebrachial cutaneous n.
9. 前臂内侧皮神经 medial antebrachial cutaneous n.
10. 肱动、静脉 brachial a.and v.
11. 贵要静脉 basilic v.
12. 尺神经 ulnar n.
13. 正中神经 median n.
14. 尺侧上副动、静脉 superior ulnar collateral a.and v.
15. 臂内侧肌间隔 medial brachial intermuscular septum
16. 后骨筋膜鞘 posterior osseofascial sheath

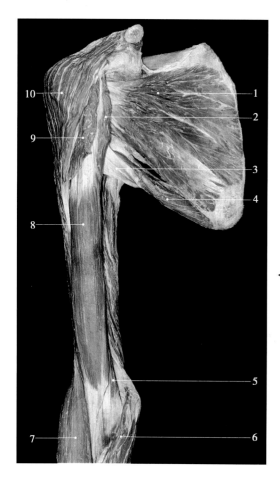

◀图 410 肩臂部肌（前面观 1）
Muscles of shoulder and upper arm.Anterior view（1）

1. 肩胛下肌 subscapularis
2. 喙肱肌 coracobrachialis
3. 背阔肌腱 tendon of latissimus dorsi
4. 大圆肌 teres major
5. 肱肌 brachialis
6. 旋前圆肌 pronator teres
7. 肱桡肌 brachioradialis
8. 肱二头肌 biceps brachii
9. 胸大肌 pectoralis major
10. 三角肌 deltoid

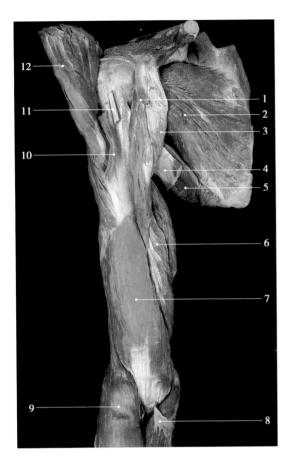

◀ 图 411　肩臂部肌（前面观 2）
Muscles of shoulder and upper arm.Anterior view（2）

1. 肱二头肌短头 short head of biceps brachii
2. 肩胛下肌 subscapularis
3. 喙肱肌 coracobrachialis
4. 背阔肌腱 tendon of latissimus dorsi
5. 大圆肌 teres major
6. 肱三头肌内侧头 medial head of triceps brachii
7. 肱肌 brachialis
8. 肱二头肌腱膜 bicipital aponeurosis
9. 肱桡肌 brachioradialis
10. 胸大肌腱 tendon of pectoralis major
11. 肱二头肌长头 long head of biceps brachii
12. 三角肌 deltoid

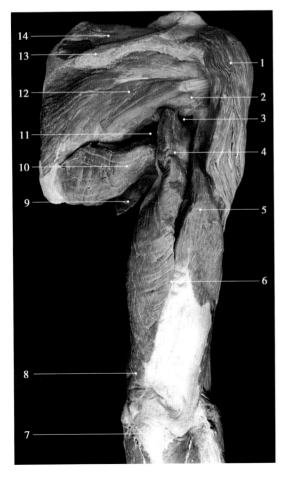

◀ 图 412　肩臂部肌（后面观）
Muscles of shoulder and upper arm.Posterior view

1. 三角肌 deltoid
2. 小圆肌 teres minor
3. 四边孔 quadrilateral foramen
4. 肱三头肌长头 long head of triceps brachii
5. 肱三头肌外侧头 lateral head of triceps brachii
6. 肱三头肌 triceps brachii
7. 鹰嘴 olecranon
8. 肱三头肌内侧头 medial head of triceps brachii
9. 背阔肌 latissimus dorsi
10. 大圆肌 teres major
11. 三边孔 trilateral foramen
12. 冈下肌 infraspinatus
13. 肩胛冈 spine of scapula
14. 冈上肌 supraspinatus

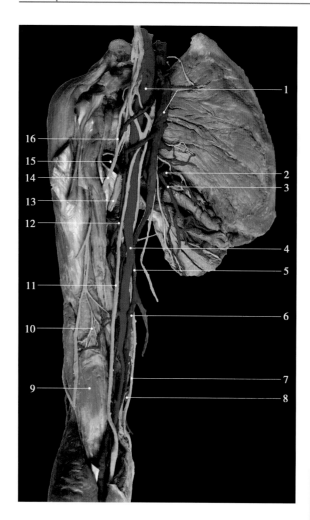

◀ 图 413　臂前区的结构（1）
Structures of anterior brachial region（1）

1. 腋动、静脉 axillary a.and v.
2. 旋肩胛动脉 circumflex scapular a.
3. 胸背动脉 thoracodorsal a.
4. 肱动脉 brachial a.
5. 尺侧上副动脉 superior ulnar collateral a.
6. 肱静脉 brachial v.
7. 尺神经 ulnar n.
8. 尺侧下副动脉 inferior ulnar collateral a.
9. 肱肌 brachialis
10. 肌支 muscular branches
11. 正中神经 median n.
12. 肱深动脉 deep brachial a.
13. 桡神经 radial n.
14. 肌皮神经 musculocutaneous n.
15. 旋肱后动脉 posterior humeral circumflex a.
16. 腋神经 axillary n.

图 414　臂前区的结构（2）▶
Structures of anterior brachial region（2）

1. 膈神经 phrenic n.
2. 前斜角肌 scalenus anterior
3. 锁骨下动脉 subclavian a.
4. 胸肩峰动脉 thoracoacromial a.
5. 后束 posterior cord
6. 内侧束 medial cord
7. 肩胛下动脉 subscapular a.
8. 胸背神经 thoracodorsal n.
9. 胸背动脉 thoracodorsal a.
10. 臂内侧皮神经 medial brachial cutaneous n.
11. 尺神经 ulnar n.
12. 前臂内侧皮神经 medial antebrachial cutaneous n.
13. 尺动脉（高位分支）ulnar a.
14. 桡动脉（高位分支）radial a.
15. 肱动脉 brachial a.
16. 肱深动脉 deep brachial a.
17. 正中神经 median n.
18. 旋肱后动脉 posterior humeral circumflex a.
19. 旋肱前动脉 anterior humeral circumflex a.
20. 腋神经 axillary n.
21. 肌皮神经 musculocutaneous n.
22. 外侧束 lateral cord
23. 肩胛背神经 dorsal scapular n.

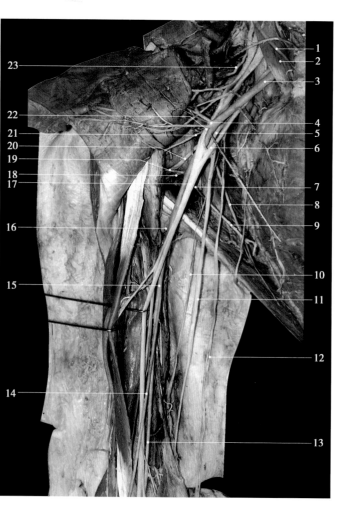

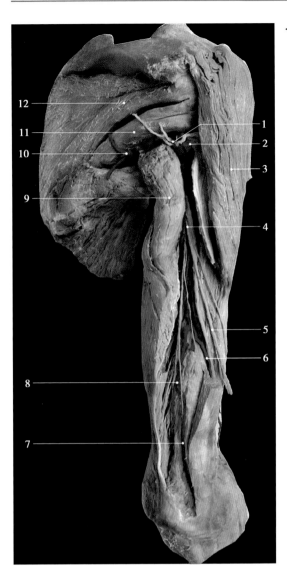

1. 腋神经 axillary n.
2. 旋肱后动脉 posterior humeral circumflex a.
3. 三角肌 deltoid
4. 桡神经 radial n.
5. 前臂后皮神经 posterior antebrachial cutaneous n.
6. 桡侧副动脉 radial collateral a.
7. 肘肌支 anconeus branch
8. 中副动脉 middle collateral a.
9. 肱三头肌长头 long head of triceps brachii
10. 旋肩胛动脉浅支 superficial branch of circumflex scapular a.
11. 小圆肌 teres minor
12. 冈下肌 infraspinatus

图 416　肘前区的浅层结构 ▶
Superficial structures of anterior cubital region

1. 贵要静脉 basilic v.
2. 臂内侧皮神经 medial brachial cutaneous n.
3. 前臂内侧皮神经 medial antebrachial cutaneous n.
4. 肘正中静脉 median cubital v.
5. 前臂正中静脉 median antebrachial v.
6. 前臂外侧皮神经 lateral antebrachial cutaneous n.
7. 深、浅静脉交通支 communicating branch between superficial and deep v.
8. 头静脉 cephalic v.
9. 臂筋膜 brachial fascia

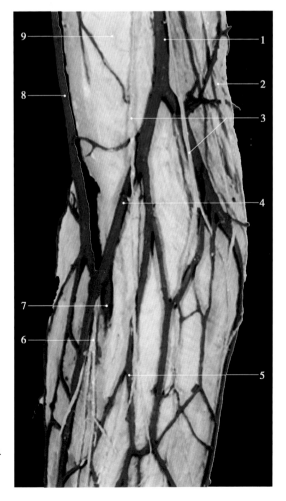

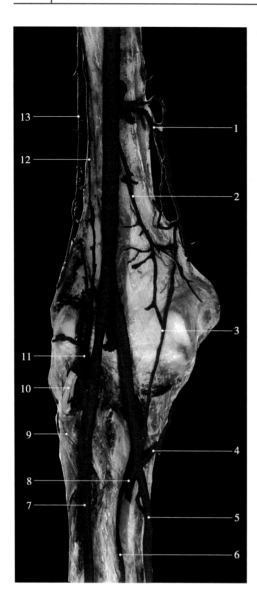

◀ **图 417　肘关节动脉网（前面观）**
Arterial rete of elbow joint.Anterior view

1. 尺侧上副动脉 superior ulnar collateral a.
2. 尺侧下副动脉 inferior ulnar collateral a.
3. 前支 anterior branch
4. 尺侧返动脉 ulnar recurrent a.
5. 尺动脉 ulnar a.
6. 骨间前动脉 anterior interosseous a.
7. 桡动脉 radial a.
8. 骨间总动脉 common interosseous a.
9. 旋后肌 supinator
10. 桡神经深支 deep branch of radial n.
11. 桡侧返动脉 radial recurrent a.
12. 桡侧副动脉 radial collateral a.
13. 中副动脉 middle collateral a.

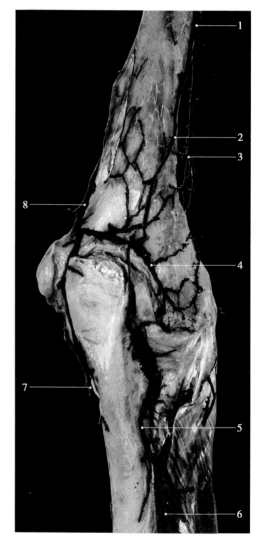

图 418　肘关节动脉网（后面观）▶
Arterial rete of elbow joint.Posterior view

1. 肱深动脉 deep brachial a.
2. 中副动脉 middle collateral a.
3. 桡侧副动脉 radial collateral a.
4. 肘关节动脉网 arterial rete of elbow joint
5. 骨间返动脉 recurrent interosseous a.
6. 骨间后动脉 posterior interosseous a.
7. 尺侧返动脉 ulnar recurrent a.
8. 尺侧下副动脉 inferior ulnar collateral a.

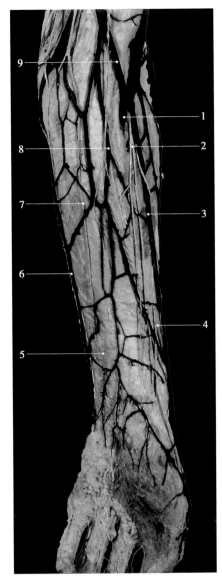

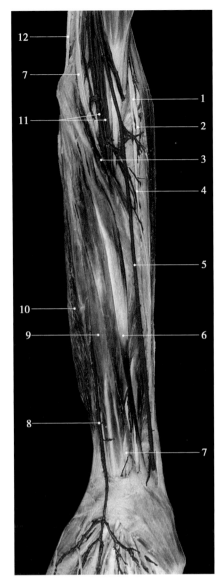

▲ 图 419 前臂前区浅层结构
Superficial structures of anterior region of forearm

1. 深、浅静脉交通支 communicating branch between superficial and deep v.
2. 前臂外侧皮神经 lateral antebrachial cutaneous n.
3. 头静脉 cephalic v.
4. 桡神经浅支 superficial branch of radial n.
5. 深筋膜 deep fascia
6. 贵要静脉 basilic v.
7. 前臂内侧皮神经 medial antebrachial cutaneous n.
8. 前臂正中静脉 median antebrachial v.
9. 肘正中静脉 median cubital v.

▲ 图 420 前臂前区深层结构（1）
Deep structures of anterior region of forearm（1）

1. 桡神经 radial n.
2. 桡神经深支 deep branch of radial n.
3. 旋前圆肌 pronator teres
4. 桡神经浅支 superficial branch of radial n.
5. 桡动脉（高位分支）radial a.
6. 桡侧腕屈肌 flexor carpi radialis
7. 正中神经 median n.
8. 尺动脉 ulnar a.
9. 指浅屈肌 flexor digitorum superficialis
10. 尺侧腕屈肌 flexor carpi ulnaris
11. 尺动、静脉 ulnar a.and v.
12. 尺神经 ulnar n.

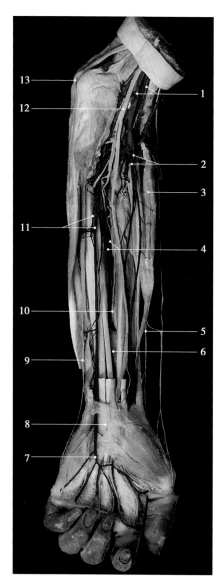

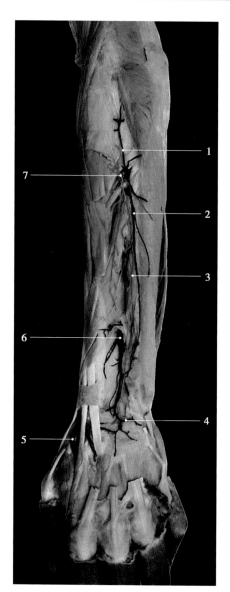

▲ 图 421　前臂前区深层结构（2）
Deep structures of anterior region of
forearm（2）

1. 肱动、静脉 brachial a.and v.
2. 桡动、静脉 radial a.and v.
3. 肱桡肌 brachioradialis
4. 骨间前动、静脉 anterior interosseous a.and v.
5. 桡神经浅支 superficial branch of radial n.
6. 旋前方肌 pronator quadratus
7. 掌浅弓 superficial palmar arch
8. 屈肌支持带 flexor retinaculum
9. 尺神经手背支 dorsal branch of ulnar n.
10. 骨间前神经 anterior interosseous n.
11. 尺动、静脉 ulnar a.and v.
12. 正中神经 median n.
13. 尺神经 ulnar n.

▲ 图 422　前臂后区深层结构
Deep structures of posterior region of forearm

1. 骨间返动脉 recurrent interosseous a.
2. 骨间后动脉 posterior interosseous a.
3. 骨间后神经 posterior interosseous n.
4. 腕背网 dorsal carpal rete
5. 桡动脉 radial a.
6. 骨间前动、静脉背侧支 dorsal branch of anterior interosseous a.and v.
7. 桡神经深支 deep branch of radial n.

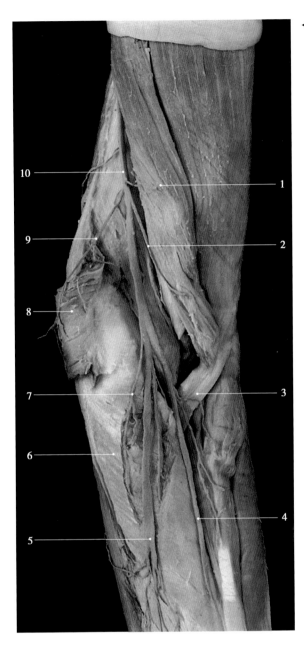

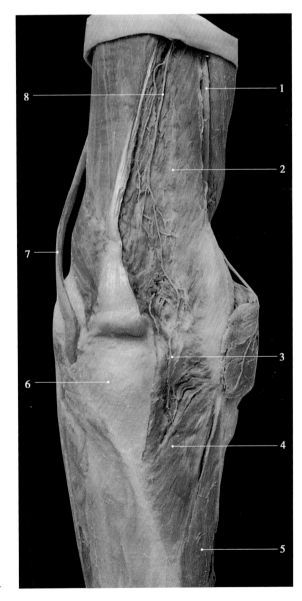

◀ 图 423 桡神经深支
Deep branch of radial nerve

1. 肱桡肌 brachioradialis
2. 肱桡肌肌支 muscular branches of brachioradialis
3. 肱二头肌腱 tendon of biceps brachii
4. 桡神经浅支 superficial branch of radial n.
5. 桡神经深支 deep branch of radial n.
6. 旋后肌 supinator
7. 旋后肌肌支 muscular branch of supinator
8. 桡侧腕短伸肌 extensor carpi radialis brevis
9. 桡侧腕短伸肌支 muscular branches of extensor carpi radialis brevis
10. 桡神经 radial n.

图 424 肘肌的神经 ▶
Nerve of anconeus

1. 桡神经 radial n.
2. 肱三头肌 triceps brachii
3. 肘肌支 muscular branches of anconeus
4. 肘肌 anconeus
5. 尺侧腕伸肌 extensor carpi ulnaris
6. 鹰嘴 olecranon
7. 尺神经 ulnar n.
8. 桡神经肌支 muscular branches of radial n.

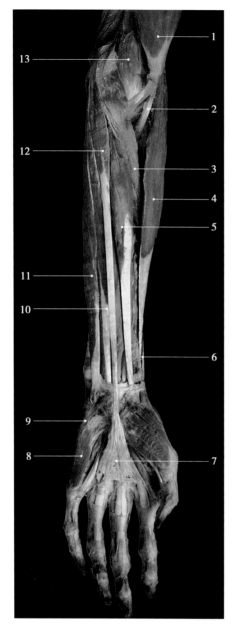

▲ 图 425　前臂肌（前面观 1）
Muscles of forearm.Anterior view（1）

1. 肱二头肌 biceps brachii
2. 肱二头肌腱 tendon of biceps brachii
3. 旋前圆肌 pronator teres
4. 肱桡肌 brachioradialis
5. 桡侧腕屈肌 flexor carpi radialis
6. 拇长展肌 abductor pollicis longus
7. 掌腱膜 palmar aponeurosis
8. 小指短屈肌 flexor digiti minimi brevis
9. 小指展肌 abductor digiti minimi
10. 指浅屈肌 flexor digitorum superficialis
11. 尺侧腕屈肌 flexor carpi ulnaris
12. 掌长肌 palmaris longus
13. 肱肌 brachialis

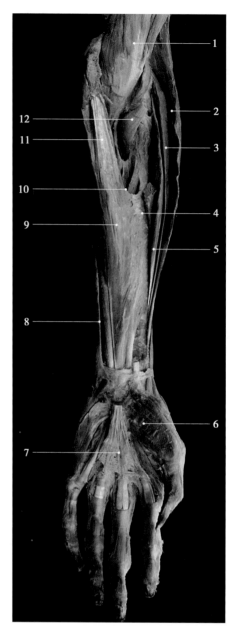

▲ 图 426　前臂肌（前面观 2）
Muscles of forearm.Anterior view（2）

1. 肱肌 brachialis
2. 肱桡肌 brachioradialis
3. 桡侧腕长伸肌 extensor carpi radialis longus
4. 指浅屈肌桡头 radial head of flexor digitorum superficialis
5. 桡侧腕短伸肌 extensor carpi radialis brevis
6. 鱼际肌 muscle of thenar
7. 掌腱膜 palmar aponeurosis
8. 尺侧腕屈肌 flexor carpi ulnaris
9. 指浅屈肌 flexor digitorum superficialis
10. 腱弓 arcus tendineus
11. 指浅屈肌肱尺头 humeroulnar head of flexor digitorum superficialis
12. 肱二头肌腱 tendon of biceps brachii

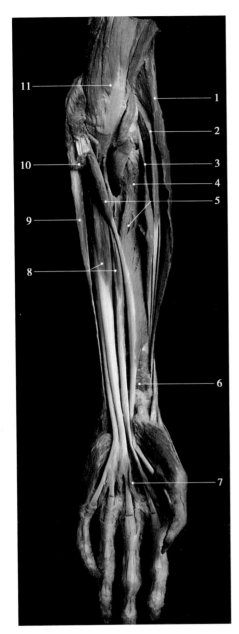

1. 肱桡肌 brachioradialis
2. 桡侧腕长伸肌 extensor carpi radialis longus
3. 桡侧腕短伸肌 extensor carpi radialis brevis
4. 旋后肌 supinator
5. 拇长屈肌 flexor pollicis longus
6. 旋前方肌 pronator quadratus
7. 蚓状肌 lumbricales
8. 指深屈肌 flexor digitorum profundus
9. 尺侧腕屈肌 flexor carpi ulnaris
10. 指浅屈肌肱尺头 humeroulnar head of flexor digitorum superficialis
11. 肱肌 brachialis

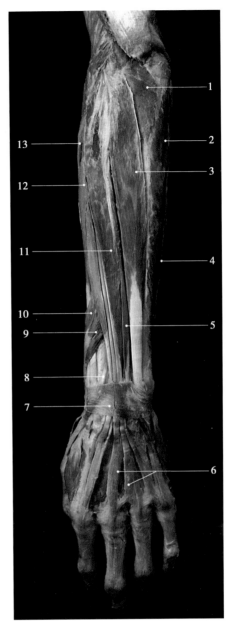

▲ 图 428　前臂肌（后面观 1）
Muscles of forearm.Posterior view（1）

1. 肘肌 anconeus
2. 指深屈肌 flexor digitorum profundus
3. 尺侧腕伸肌 extensor carpi ulnaris
4. 尺侧腕屈肌 flexor carpi ulnaris
5. 小指伸肌 extensor digiti minimi
6. 指伸肌腱 tendon of extensor digitorum
7. 伸肌支持带 extensor retinaculum
8. 拇长伸肌 extensor pollicis longus
9. 拇短伸肌 extensor pollicis brevis
10. 拇长展肌 abductor pollicis longus
11. 指伸肌 extensor digitorum
12. 桡侧腕短伸肌 extensor carpi radialis brevis
13. 桡侧腕长伸肌 extensor carpi radialis longus

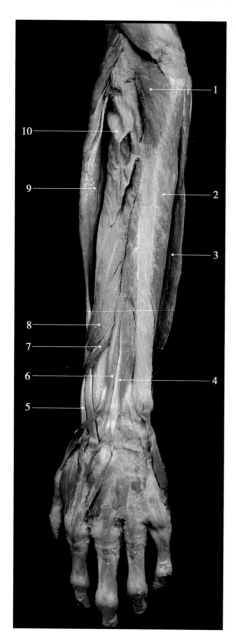

◀ 图 429　前臂肌（后面观 2 ）
Muscles of forearm.Posterior view（ 2 ）

1. 肘肌 anconeus
2. 指深屈肌 flexor digitorum profundus
3. 尺侧腕屈肌 flexor carpi ulnaris
4. 示指伸肌 extensor indicis
5. 桡侧腕长伸肌腱 tendon of extensor carpi radialis longus
6. 拇长伸肌 extensor pollicis longus
7. 拇短伸肌 extensor pollicis brevis
8. 拇长展肌 abductor pollicis longus
9. 桡侧腕短伸肌 extensor carpi radialis brevis
10. 旋后肌 supinator

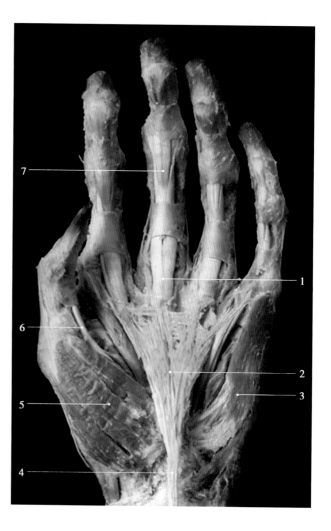

图 430　手肌（前面观 1 ）▶
Muscles of hand.Anterior view（ 1 ）

1. 指浅屈肌腱 tendon of flexor digitorum superficialis
2. 掌腱膜 palmar aponeurosis
3. 小鱼际肌 muscle of hypothenar
4. 掌长肌腱 tendon of palmaris longus
5. 鱼际肌 muscle of thenar
6. 拇长屈肌腱 tendon of flexor pollicis longus
7. 指深屈肌腱 tendon of flexor digitorum profundus

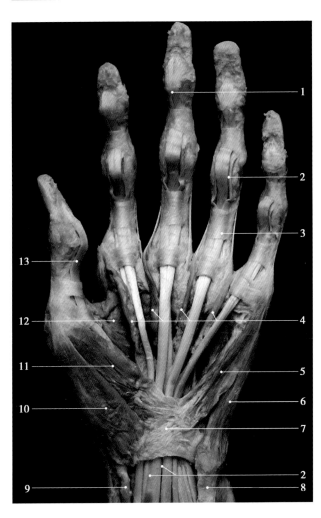

◀ 图 431　手肌（前面观 2 ）
Muscles of hand.Anterior view（2）

1. 指深屈肌腱 tendon of flexor digitorum profundus
2. 指浅屈肌腱 tendon of flexor digitorum superficialis
3. 指纤维鞘 digital fibrous sheath
4. 蚓状肌 lumbricales
5. 小指短屈肌 flexor digiti minimi brevis
6. 小指展肌 abductor digiti minimi
7. 屈肌支持带 flexor retinaculum
8. 尺侧腕屈肌腱 tendon of flexor carpi ulnaris
9. 桡侧腕屈肌腱 tendon of flexor carpi radialis
10. 拇短展肌 abductor pollicis brevis
11. 拇短屈肌 flexor pollicis brevis
12. 拇收肌 adductor pollicis
13. 拇长屈肌腱 tendon of flexor pollicis longus

图 432　手肌（前面观 3 ） ▶
Muscles of hand.Anterior view（3）

1. 指深屈肌腱 tendon of flexor digitorum profundus
2. 指浅屈肌腱 tendon of flexor digitorum superficialis
3. 指纤维鞘 digital fibrous sheath
4. 骨间背侧肌 dorsal interossei
5. 骨间掌侧肌 palmar interossei
6. 小指短屈肌 flexor digiti minimi brevis
7. 小指对掌肌 opponens digiti minimi
8. 腕管 carpal canal
9. 桡侧腕屈肌腱 tendon of flexor carpi radialis
10. 拇对掌肌 opponens pollicis
11. 拇收肌斜头 oblique head of adductor pollicis
12. 拇收肌横头 transverse head of adductor pollicis
13. 拇长屈肌腱 tendon of flexor pollicis longus

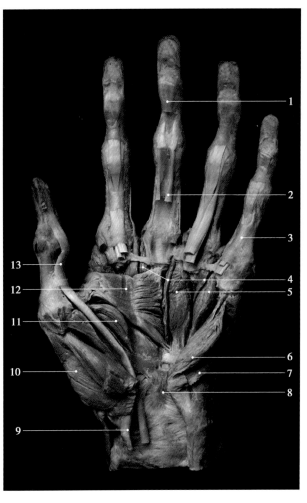

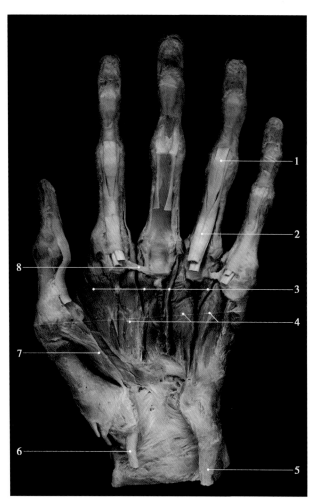

◀ 图 433　手肌（前面观 4）
Muscles of hand.Anterior view（4）

1. 指深屈肌腱 tendon of flexor digitorum profundus
2. 指浅屈肌腱 tendon of flexor digitorum superficialis
3. 骨间背侧肌 dorsal interossei
4. 骨间掌侧肌 palmar interossei
5. 尺侧腕屈肌腱 tendon of flexor carpi ulnaris
6. 桡侧腕屈肌腱 tendon of flexor carpi radialis
7. 拇短屈肌深头 deep head of flexor pollicis brevis
8. 掌深横韧带 deep transverse metacarpal lig.

图 434　骨间掌侧肌（前面观）▶
Palmar interossei.Anterior view

1. 掌板 volar plates
2. 骨间掌侧肌 palmar interossei
3. 拇长屈肌腱 tendon of flexor pollicis longus
4. 指浅屈肌腱 tendon of flexor digitorum superficialis
5. 指深屈肌腱 tendon of flexor digitorum profundus

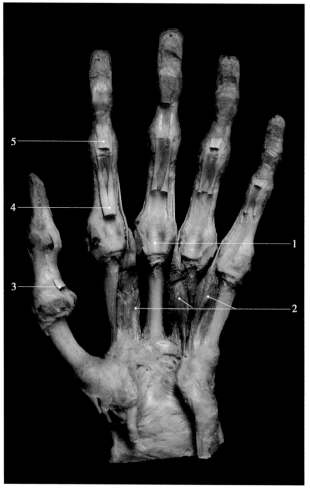

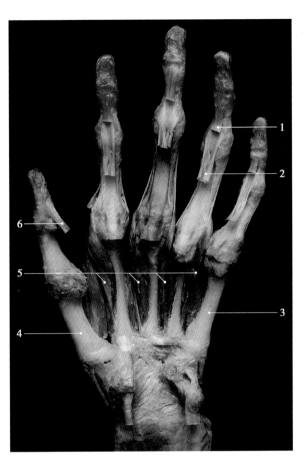

◀ 图 435　骨间背侧肌（前面观）
Dorsal interossei.Anterior view

1. 指深屈肌腱 tendon of flexor digitorum profundus
2. 指浅屈肌腱 tendon of flexor digitorum superficialis
3. 第 5 掌骨 the 5th metacarpal bone
4. 第 1 掌骨 the 1st metacarpal bone
5. 骨间背侧肌 dorsal interossei
6. 拇长屈肌腱 tendon of flexor pollicis longus

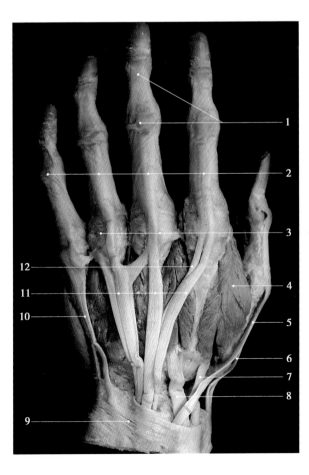

◀ 图 436　手肌（后面观 1）
Muscles of hand.Posterior view（1）

1. 指骨间关节 interphalangeal joints of hand
2. 指背腱膜 dorsal aponeurosis of fingers
3. 掌指关节 metacarpophalangeal joint
4. 第 1 骨间背侧肌 the 1st dorsal interossei
5. 拇长伸肌腱 tendon of extensor pollicis longus
6. 拇短伸肌腱 tendon of extensor pollicis brevis
7. 桡侧腕长伸肌腱 tendon of extensor carpi radialis longus
8. 桡侧腕短伸肌腱 tendon of extensor carpi radialis brevis
9. 伸肌支持带 extensor retinaculum
10. 小指伸肌腱 tendon of extensor digiti minimi
11. 指伸肌腱 tendon of extensor digitorum
12. 示指伸肌腱 tendon of extensor indicis

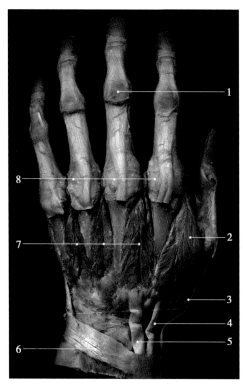

▲ 图 437　手肌（后面观 2）
Muscles of hand.Posterior view（2）

1. 指骨间关节 interphalangeal joints of hand
2. 第 1 骨间背侧肌 the 1st dorsal interossei
3. 拇短伸肌腱 tendon of extensor pollicis brevis
4. 桡侧腕长伸肌腱 tendon of extensor carpi radialis longus
5. 桡侧腕短伸肌腱 tendon of extensor carpi radialis brevis
6. 伸肌支持带 extensor retinaculum
7. 骨间背侧肌 dorsal interossei
8. 掌指关节 metacarpophalangeal joints

▲ 图 438　手指屈肌腱及腱纽
Flexor tendons and vincula tendinum of hand

1. 腱帽 tendon hood
2. 指伸肌腱 tendon of extensor digitorum
3. 骨间肌 interosseus
4. 长纽 long vincula
5. 蚓状肌 lumbricales
6. 指深屈肌腱 tendon of flexor digitorum profundus
7. 指浅屈肌腱 tendon of flexor digitorum superficialis
8. 短纽 short vincula
9. 外侧腱 lateral extensor tendon

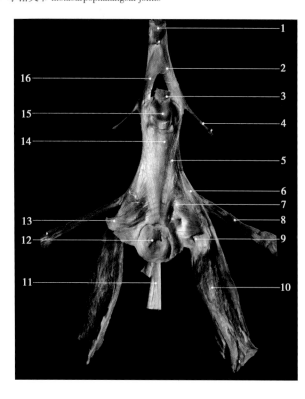

◀ 图 439　指背腱膜
Dorsal aponeurosis of fingers

1. 终腱 terminal extensor tendon
2. 三角韧带 deltoid lig.
3. 中间腱于手中节指骨的抵止 insertion of intermediate tendon
4. 支持韧带（斜束）retinacular lig.（oblique band）
5. 外侧束 lateral extensor band
6. 蚓状肌腱 tendon of lumbricales
7. 腱帽 tendon hood
8. 蚓状肌 lumbricales
9. 骨间肌于近节指骨抵止 insertion of interosseous
10. 骨间肌 interosseus
11. 指伸肌腱 tendon of extensor digitorum
12. 纤维软骨下方囊 capsule beneath fibrous cartilage
13. 矢状束 sagittal band
14. 中间束 intermediate extensor band
15. 纤维软骨 fibrous cartilage
16. 外侧腱 lateral extensor tendon

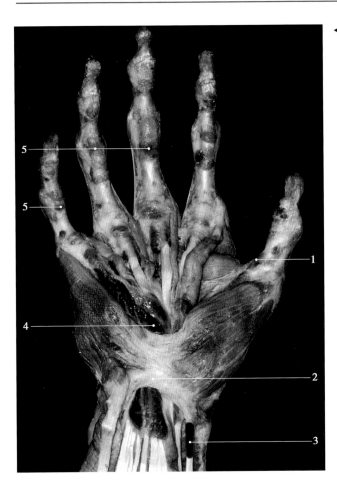

◀图 440　手腱鞘（前面观）
Tendinous sheaths of hand.Anterior view

1. 拇长屈肌腱鞘 tendinous sheath of flexor pollicis longus
2. 屈肌支持带 flexor retinaculum
3. 桡侧腕屈肌腱鞘 tendinous sheath of flexor carpi radialis
4. 屈肌总腱鞘 common flexor sheath
5. 指腱鞘 tendinous sheaths of fingers

图 441　手腱鞘（后面观）▶
Tendinous sheaths of hand.Posterior view

1. 小指伸肌腱鞘 tendinous sheath of extensor digitorum minimi
2. 指伸肌和示指伸肌腱鞘 tendinous sheath of extensor digitorum and extensor indicis
3. 桡侧腕短伸肌腱鞘 tendinous sheath of extensor carpi radialis brevis
4. 伸肌支持带 extensor retinaculum
5. 尺侧腕伸肌腱鞘 tendinous sheath of extensor carpi ulnaris
6. 拇长展肌和拇短伸肌腱鞘 tendinous sheath of abductor longus and extensor pollicis brevis
7. 桡侧腕长伸肌腱鞘 tendinous sheath of extensor carpi radialis longus
8. 拇长伸肌腱鞘 tendinous sheath of extensor pollicis longus

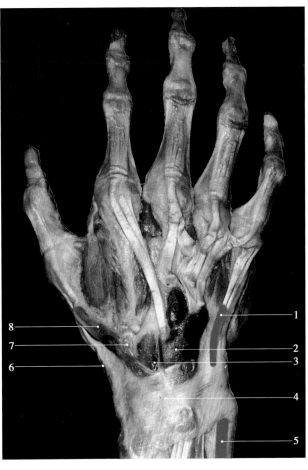

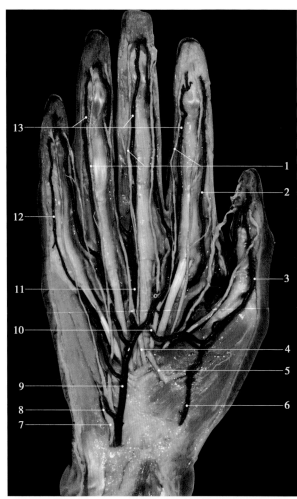

◀ **图 442　掌浅弓及正中神经的分支**
Branches of superficial palmar arch and median nerve

1. 指掌侧固有神经 proper palmar digital n.
2. 示指桡侧动脉 radial artery to index finger
3. 拇指桡掌侧动脉 radial palmar pollicis a.
4. 指掌侧总神经 common palmar digital n.
5. 正中神经返支 recurrent branch of median n.
6. 掌浅支 superficial palmar branch
7. 尺神经 ulnar n.
8. 尺神经深支 deep branch of ulnar n.
9. 尺动脉 ulnar a .
10. 掌浅弓 superficial palmar arch
11. 指掌侧总动脉 common palmar digital a.
12. 小指尺掌侧动脉 ulnar palmar artery of little finger
13. 指掌侧固有动脉 proper palmar digital a.

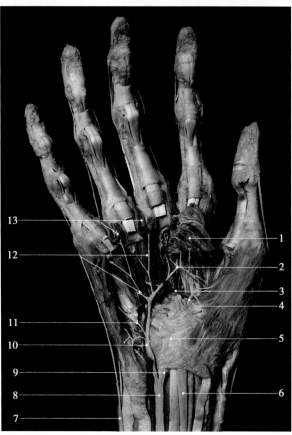

◀ **图 443　掌深弓及尺神经深支的分支**
Branches of deep palmar arch and deep branch of ulnar nerve

1. 拇收肌斜头 oblique head of adductor pollicis
2. 拇收肌神经 nerve of adductor pollicis
3. 掌深弓 deep palmar arch
4. 正中神经返支 recurrent branch of median n.
5. 屈肌支持带 flexor retinaculum
6. 正中神经 median n.
7. 尺神经手背支 dorsal branch of ulnar n.
8. 尺神经 ulnar n.
9. 尺神经浅支 superficial branch of ulnar n.
10. 尺神经深支 deep branch of ulnar n.
11. 小鱼际神经 nerves of hypothenar
12. 第 3、4 蚓状肌神经 nerves of the 3rd and 4th lumbricales
13. 蚓状肌 lumbricales

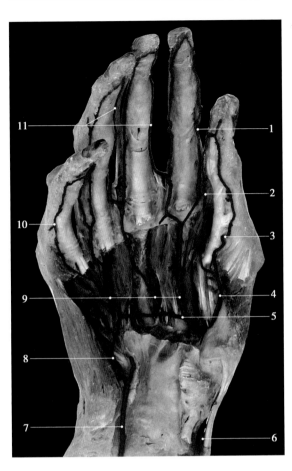

◀ 图 444　掌深弓及其分支
Branches of deep palmar arch

1. 示指桡侧动脉 radial artery to index finger
2. 拇指尺掌侧动脉 ulnar palmar pollicis a.
3. 拇指桡掌侧动脉 radial palmar pollicis a.
4. 拇主要动脉 principal artery of thumb
5. 掌深弓 deep palmar arch
6. 桡动脉 radial a.
7. 尺动脉 ulnar a.
8. 掌深支 deep palmar branch
9. 掌心动脉 palmar metacarpal a.
10. 小指尺掌侧动脉 ulnar palmar artery of little finger
11. 指掌侧固有动脉 proper palmar digital a.

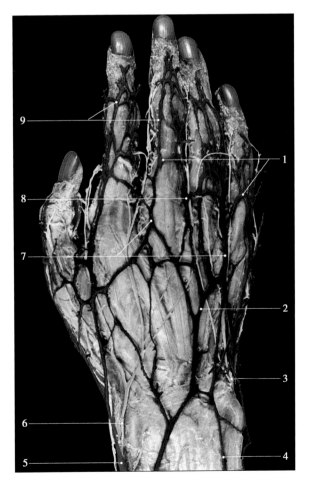

图 445　手背皮神经及浅静脉 ▶
Cutaneous nerves and superficial veins on dorsum of hand

1. 指静脉弓 digital venous arch
2. 手背静脉网 dorsal venous rete of hand
3. 尺神经手背支 dorsal branch of ulnar n.
4. 贵要静脉 basilic v.
5. 头静脉 cephalic v.
6. 桡神经浅支 superficial branch of radial n.
7. 掌背静脉 dorsal metacarpal v.
8. 掌骨头间静脉 intercapital v.
9. 指背静脉 dorsal digital v.

连续层次局部解剖

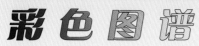 彩色图谱

第八章

下　肢

Chapter 8　Lower limb

下肢上界：前方以腹股沟与腹部分界，外侧和后方以髂嵴与腰、骶尾部分界，内侧与会阴相连。

下肢可分为臀、股、膝、小腿、踝和足等部。除臀部外，其余各部又可分为若干区。

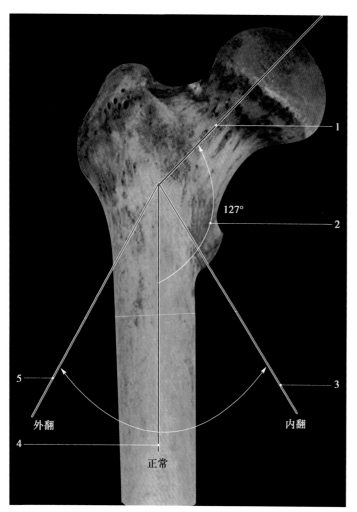

◀ 图 446　股骨颈干角
Angle of neck and body of femur
1. 股骨颈轴 axis of neck of femur
2. 颈干角 angle of neck and body
3. 髋内翻 coxa vara
4. 股骨干轴 axis of body of femur
5. 髋外翻 coxa valga

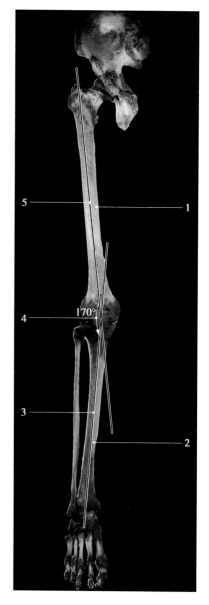

图 447　膝外翻角 ▶
Valgus angle of knee
1. 股骨干 body of femur
2. 胫骨干 body of tibia
3. 胫骨干轴 axis of body of tibia
4. 外翻角 genu valgum angle
5. 股骨干轴 axis of body of femur

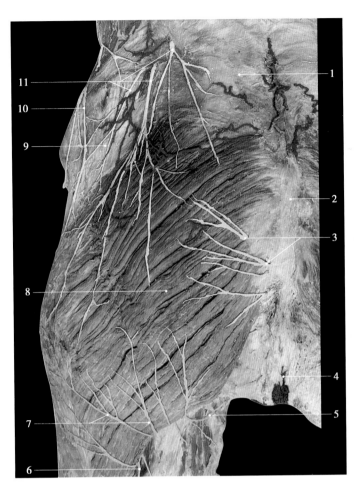

◀图 448　臀部血管、神经（1）
Blood vessels and nerves of gluteal region（1）

1. 胸腰筋膜浅层 superficial layer of thoracolumbar fascia
2. 骶骨 sacrum
3. 臀内侧皮神经 medial clunial n.
4. 肛门 anus
5. 股后皮神经会阴支 perineal branch of posterior femoral cutaneous n.
6. 股后皮神经 posterior femoral cutaneous n.
7. 臀下皮神经 inferior clunial n.
8. 臀大肌 gluteus maximus
9. 臀中肌筋膜 fascia of gluteus medius
10. 髂腹下神经外侧皮支 lateral cutaneous branch of iliohypogastric n.
11. 臀上皮神经 superior clunial n.

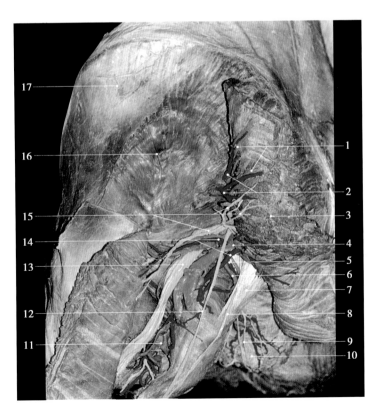

◀图 449　臀部血管、神经（2）
Blood vessels and nerves of gluteal region（2）

1. 臀上静脉 superior gluteal v.
2. 臀上动脉 superior gluteal a.
3. 臀大肌 gluteus maximus
4. 臀下静脉 inferior gluteal v.
5. 阴部内动脉 internal pudendal a.
6. 阴部内静脉 internal pudendal v.
7. 骶结节韧带 sacrotuberous lig.
8. 穿皮神经 perforating cutaneous n.
9. 肛神经 anal n.
10. 肛提肌 levator ani
11. 股方肌 quadratus femoris
12. 股后皮神经 posterior femoral cutaneous n.
13. 坐骨神经 sciatic n.
14. 臀下动脉 inferior gluteal a.
15. 臀下神经 inferior gluteal n.
16. 臀中肌 gluteus medius
17. 臀中肌筋膜 fascia of gluteus medius

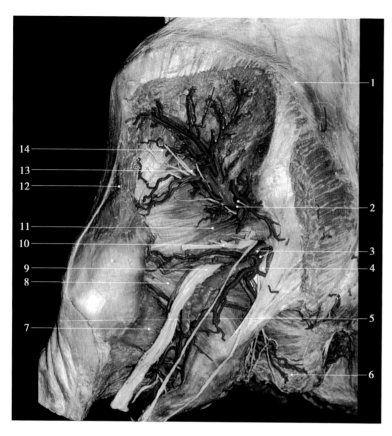

◀图 450　臀部血管、神经（3）
Blood vessels and nerves of gluteal region（3）

1. 髂嵴 iliuc crest
2. 臀上动、静脉 superior gluteal a.and v.
3. 臀下动、静脉 inferior gluteal a.and v.
4. 阴部神经 pudendal n.
5. 骶结节韧带 sacrotuberous lig.
6. 肛门外括约肌 sphincter ani externus
7. 股方肌 quadratus femoris
8. 闭孔内肌腱 tendon of obturator internus
9. 坐骨神经 sciatic n.
10. 臀下神经 inferior gluteal n.
11. 梨状肌 piriformis
12. 臀中肌 gluteus medius
13. 臀上神经 superior gluteal n.
14. 臀小肌 gluteus minimus

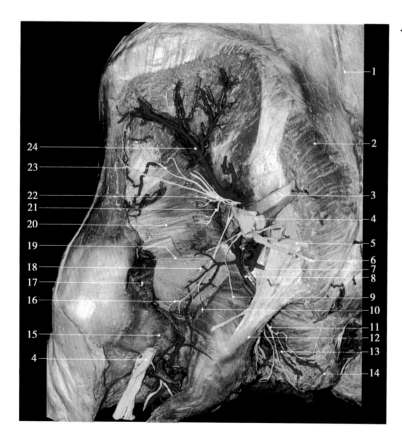

◀图 451　臀部血管、神经（4）
Blood vessels and nerves of gluteal region
（4）

1. 胸腰筋膜 thoracolumbar fascia
2. 臀大肌 gluteus maximus
3. 梨状肌（切断掀起）piriformis
4. 坐骨神经（切断掀起）sciatic n.
5. 臀下神经 inferior gluteal n.
6. 股后皮神经 posterior femoral cutaneous n.
7. 阴部神经 pudendal n.
8. 阴部内动脉 internal pudendal a.
9. 闭孔内肌神经 nerve to obturator internus
10. 下孖肌神经 nerve to gemellus inferior
11. 肛神经 anal n.
12. 骶结节韧带 sacrotuberous lig.
13. 肛动脉 anal a.
14. 肛门 anus
15. 股方肌 quadratus femoris
16. 股方肌神经 nerve to quadratus femoris
17. 下孖肌 gemellus inferior
18. 关节支 articular branch
19. 上孖肌神经 nerve to gemellus superior
20. 臀小肌 gluteus minimus
21. 臀小肌神经 nerve to gluteus minimus
22. 臀上神经 superior gluteal n.
23. 阔筋膜张肌神经 nerve to tensor fasciae latae
24. 臀上动脉 superior gluteal a.

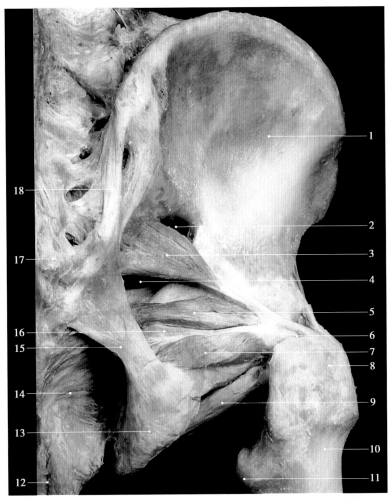

◀图 452 梨状肌上孔及梨状肌下孔
Suprapiriformis foramen and infrapiriformis foramen

1. 髂骨 ilium
2. 梨状肌上孔 suprapiriformis foramen
3. 梨状肌 piriformis
4. 梨状肌下孔 infrapiriformis foramen
5. 上孖肌 gemellus superior
6. 闭孔内肌腱 tendon of obturator internus
7. 下孖肌 gemellus inferior
8. 大转子 greater trochanter
9. 闭孔外肌 obturator externus
10. 股骨 femur
11. 小转子 lesser trochanter
12. 肛门 anus
13. 坐骨结节 ischial tuberosity
14. 肛提肌 levator ani
15. 骶结节韧带 sacrotuberous lig.
16. 闭孔内肌 obturator internus
17. 骶骨 sacrum
18. 骶髂后韧带 posterior sacroiliac lig.

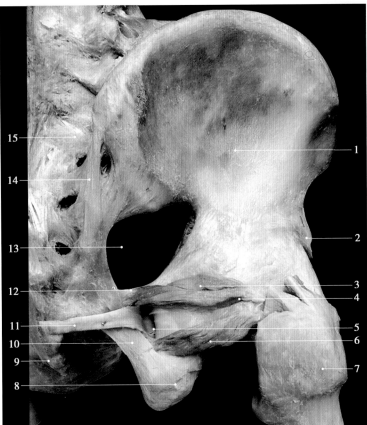

◀图 453 闭孔内肌坐骨囊
Sciatic bursa of obturator internus

1. 髂骨 ilium
2. 股直肌腱 tendon of rectus femoris
3. 上孖肌 gemellus superior
4. 闭孔内肌腱下束 subtendinous bursa of obturator internus
5. 闭孔内肌坐骨囊 sciatic bursa of obturator internus
6. 下孖肌 gemellus inferior
7. 大转子 greater trochanter
8. 坐骨结节 ischial tuberosity
9. 尾骨 coccyx
10. 骶结节韧带 sacrotuberous lig.
11. 闭孔内肌腱 tendon of obturator internus
12. 坐骨棘 ischial spine
13. 坐骨大孔 greater sciatic foramen
14. 骶髂后韧带 posterior sacroiliac lig.
15. 骶骨 sacrum

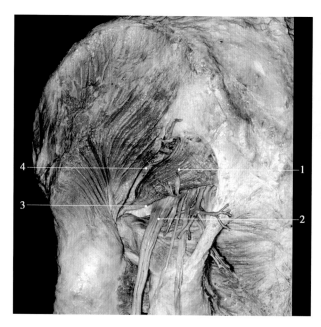

A. 常见型坐骨神经经梨状肌下孔出盆腔占 66.3%

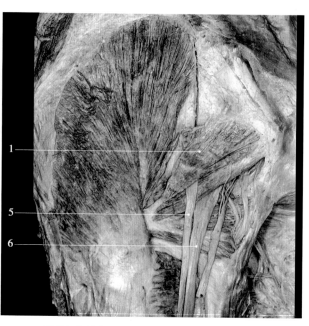

B. 胫神经穿梨状肌下孔；腓总神经穿梨状肌占 27.3%

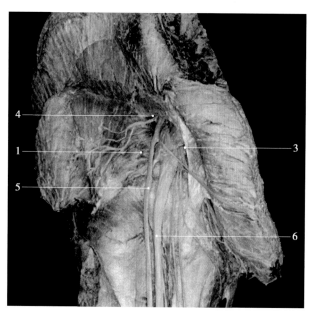

C. 胫神经穿梨状肌下孔，腓总神经穿梨状肌上孔等其他类型占 6.4%

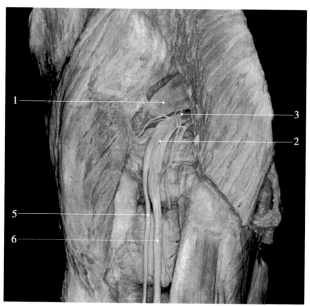

D. 坐骨神经高位分支

▲ 图 454　坐骨神经与梨状肌的关系
Relationships between sciatic nerve and piriformis

1. 梨状肌 piriformis　　　　　4. 梨状肌上孔 suprapiriformis foramen
2. 坐骨神经 sciatic n.　　　　　5. 腓总神经 common peroneal n.
3. 梨状肌下孔 infrapiriformis foramen　　6. 胫神经 tibial n.

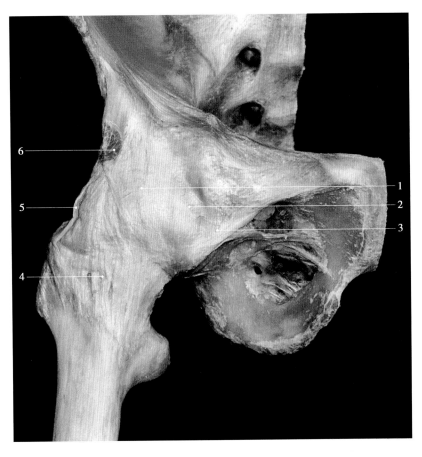

◀ 图 455　髋关节韧带（前面观）
Ligaments of hip joint.Anterior view

1. 关节囊 articular capsule
2. 髂耻囊 iliopectineal bursa
3. 耻股韧带 pubofemoral lig.
4. 髂股韧带下束 inferior bundle of iliofemoral lig.
5. 髂股韧带上束 superior bundle of iliofemoral lig.
6. 股直肌直头 straight head of rectus femoris

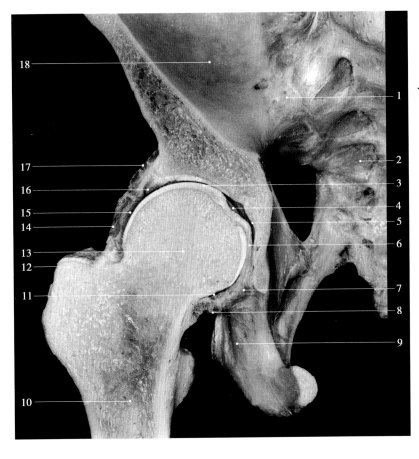

◀ 图 456　股骨头韧带
Ligament of head of femur

1. 骶髂关节 sacroiliac joint
2. 骶骨 sacrum
3. 关节软骨 articular cartilage
4. 股骨头凹 fovea of femoral head
5. 哈佛森腺 Haversian gland
6. 股骨头韧带 ligament of head of femur
7. 髋臼横韧带 transverse acetabular lig.
8. 关节囊纤维膜 fibrous membrane of articular capsule
9. 坐骨 ischium
10. 股骨 femur
11. 关节腔 articular cavity
12. 大转子 greater trochanter
13. 股骨头 femoral head
14. 轮匝带 zona orbicularis
15. 滑膜 synovium
16. 髋臼唇 acetabular labrum
17. 股直肌反折头 reflected head of rectus femoris
18. 髂骨 ilium

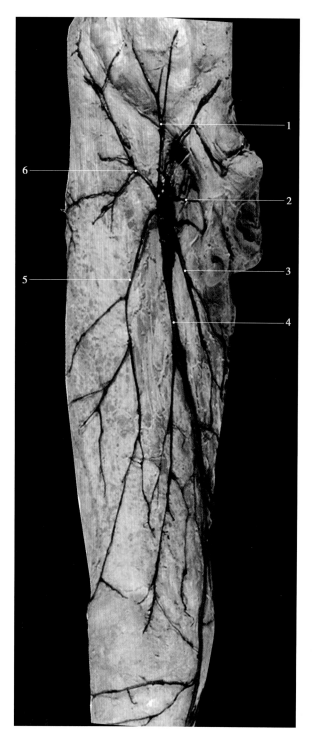

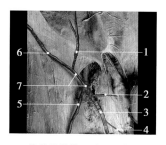

A. 旋髂浅静脉、腹壁浅静脉及
股外侧浅静脉共干，占 25.6%

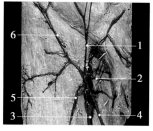

B. 5 属支单独汇入大隐静脉，
占 18.3%

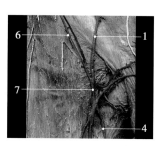

C. 旋髂浅静脉与腹壁浅静脉共
干，占 9.66%

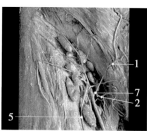

D. 腹壁浅静脉与阴部外静脉共
干，占 8.7%

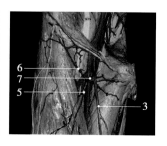

E. 旋髂浅静脉与股外浅静脉共
干，占 7.7%

▲ 图 457　大隐静脉及其属支
Great saphenous vein and its tributaries

1. 腹壁浅静脉 superficial epigastric v.
2. 阴部外静脉 external pudendal v.
3. 股内侧浅静脉 medial femoral superficial v.
4. 大隐静脉 great saphenous v.
5. 股外侧浅静脉 lateral femoral superficial v.
6. 旋髂浅静脉 superficial iliac circumflex v.

▲ 图 458　大隐静脉属支的类型
Types of tributaries of great saphenous vein

1. 腹壁浅静脉 suporficial epigastric v.
2. 阴部外静脉 external pudendal v.
3. 大隐静脉 great saphenous v.
4. 股内侧浅静脉 superficial medial femoral v.
5. 股外侧浅静脉 superficial lateral femoral v.
6. 旋髂浅静脉 superficial iliac circumflex v.
7. 共干 common trunk

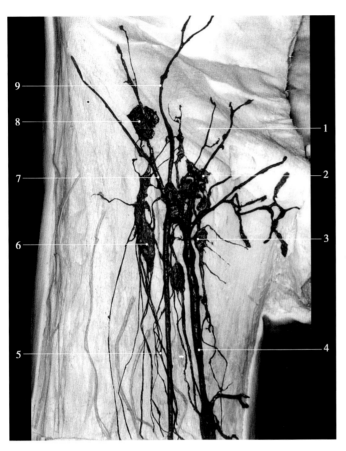

◀ 图 459　腹股沟浅淋巴结
Superficial inguinal lymph nodes

1. 腹股沟韧带 inguinal lig.
2. 腹股沟上内侧浅淋巴结 superomedial superficial inguinal lymph nodes
3. 腹股沟下内侧浅淋巴结 inferomedial superficial inguinal lymph nodes
4. 大隐静脉 great saphenous v.
5. 股淋巴管 lymph vessels of thigh
6. 腹股沟下外侧浅淋巴结 inferolateral superficial inguinal lymph nodes
7. 旋髂浅静脉 superficial iliac circumflex v.
8. 腹股沟上外侧浅淋巴结 superolateral superficial inguinal lymph nodes
9. 腹壁浅静脉 superficial epigastric v.

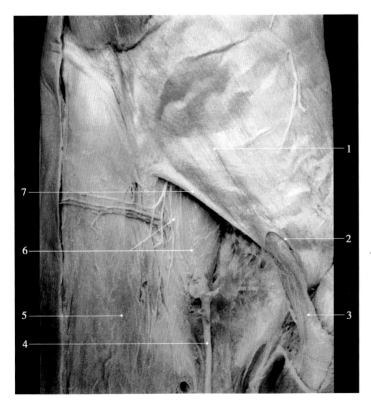

◀ 图 460　股鞘
Femoral sheath

1. 腹外斜肌腱膜 aponeurosis of obliquus externus abdominis
2. 腹股沟管浅环 superficial inguinal ring
3. 精索 spermatic cord
4. 大隐静脉 great saphenous v.
5. 阔筋膜 fascia lata
6. 股鞘 femoral sheath
7. 腹股沟韧带 inguinal lig.

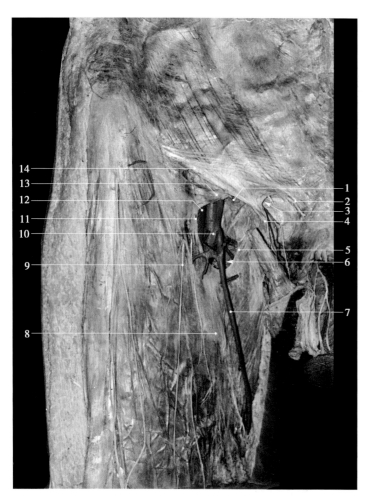

◀ 图 461　股部深筋膜
Deep fascia of thigh

1. 股管 femoral canal
2. 内侧脚 medial crus
3. 腹股沟管浅环 superficial inguinal ring
4. 外侧脚 lateral crus
5. 下角 inferior cornua
6. 隐静脉裂孔 saphenous hiatus
7. 大隐静脉 great saphenous v.
8. 阔筋膜 fascia lata
9. 前皮支 anterior cutaneous branch
10. 股静脉 femoral v.
11. 镰状缘 falciform margin
12. 股动脉 femoral a.
13. 上角 superior cornua
14. 腹股沟韧带 inguinal lig.

◀ 图 462　股管上口
Superior aperture of femoral canal

1. 髂肌 iliacus
2. 旋髂深动、静脉 deep iliac circumflex a.and n.
3. 股神经 femoral n.
4. 腹前壁 anterior abdominal wall
5. 子宫圆韧带 round ligament of uterus
6. 腹壁下动、静脉 inferior epigastric a.and v.
7. 腹股沟韧带（股环前壁）inguinal lig.（anterior wall）
8. 股环淋巴结 femoral ring lymph node
9. 股环 femoral ring
10. 腔隙韧带（股环内壁）lacunar lig.（inner wall）
11. 耻骨梳韧带（股环后壁）pectineal lig.（posterior wall）
12. 纤维隔（股环外侧壁）fibrous septum（lateral wall）
13. 闭孔动脉 obturator a.
14. 闭孔神经 obturator n.
15. 髂外静脉 exteranl iliac v.
16. 髂外动脉 exteranl iliac a.
17. 腰大肌 psoas major

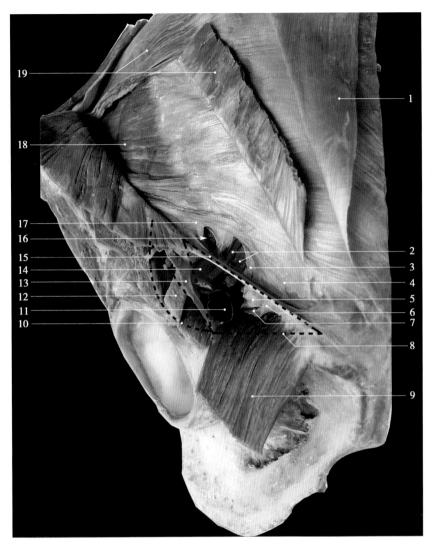

◀ 图 463　肌腔隙与血管腔隙
Lacuna musculorum and lacuna vasorum

1. 腹外斜肌腱膜 aponeurosis of obliquus externus abdominis
2. 腹壁下动、静脉 inferior epigastric a.and v.
3. 凹间韧带 interfoveolar lig.
4. 腹股沟镰 inguinal falx
5. 股环 femoral ring
6. 腔隙韧带 lacunar lig.
7. 耻骨梳韧带 pectineal lig.
8. 血管腔隙 lacuna vasorum
9. 耻骨肌 pectineus
10. 肌腔隙 lacuna musculorum
11. 股静脉 femoral v.
12. 股神经 femoral n.
13. 髂耻弓 iliopectineal arch
14. 股动脉 femoral a.
15. 腹股沟韧带 inguinal lig.
16. 腹股沟管深环 deep inguinal ring
17. 腹横筋膜 transverse fascia
18. 腹横肌 transversus abdominis
19. 腹内斜肌 obliquus internus abdominis

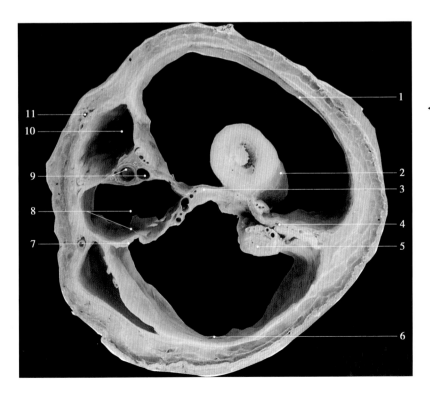

◀ 图 464　股中部骨筋膜鞘
Osseofascial sheaths of middle of thigh

1. 前骨筋膜鞘 anterior osseofascial sheath
2. 股骨 femur
3. 股内侧肌间隔 medial femoral intermuscular septum
4. 股外侧肌间隔 lateral femoral intermuscular septum
5. 坐骨神经 sciatic n.
6. 后骨筋膜鞘 posterior osseofascial sheath
7. 股后肌间隔 posterior femoral intermuscular septum
8. 内侧骨筋膜鞘 medial osseofascia sheath
9. 股动、静脉 femoral a.and v.
10. 缝匠肌鞘 sheath of sartorius
11. 大隐静脉 great saphenous v.

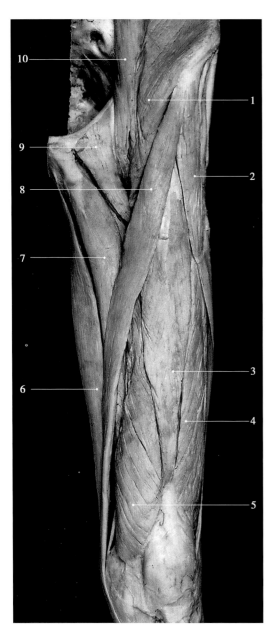

◀图 465　股部肌（前面观 1）
Muscles of thigh.Anterior view（1）

1. 髂肌 iliacus
2. 阔筋膜张肌 tensor fasciae latae
3. 股直肌 rectus femoris
4. 股外侧肌 vastus lateralis
5. 股内侧肌 vastus medialis
6. 股薄肌 gracilis
7. 长收肌 adductor longus
8. 缝匠肌 sartorius
9. 耻骨肌 pectineus
10. 腰大肌 psoas major

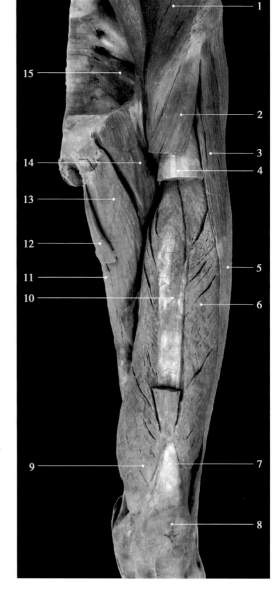

图 466　股部肌（前面观 2）▶
Muscles of thigh.Anterior view（2）

1. 髂肌 iliacus
2. 缝匠肌 sartorius
3. 阔筋膜张肌 tensor fasciae latae
4. 股直肌 rectus femoris
5. 髂胫束 iliotibial tract
6. 股外侧肌 vastus lateralis
7. 股四头肌腱 tendon of quadriceps femoris
8. 髌骨 patella
9. 股内侧肌 vastus medialis
10. 股中间肌 vastus intermedius
11. 大收肌 adductor magnus
12. 股薄肌 gracilis
13. 长收肌 adductor longus
14. 耻骨肌 pectineus
15. 梨状肌 piriformis

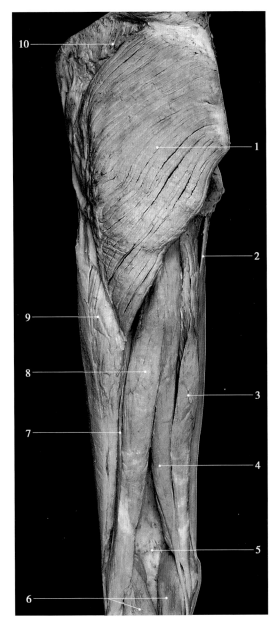

▲ 图 467 股部肌（后面观 1）
Muscles of thigh.Posterior view（1）

1. 臀大肌 gluteus maximus
2. 股薄肌 gracilis
3. 半膜肌 semimembranosus
4. 半腱肌 semitendinosus
5. 腘窝 popliteal fossa
6. 腓肠肌 gastrocnemius
7. 股二头肌短头 short head of biceps femoris
8. 股二头肌长头 long head of biceps femoris
9. 股外侧肌 vastus lateralis
10. 臀中肌 gluteus medius

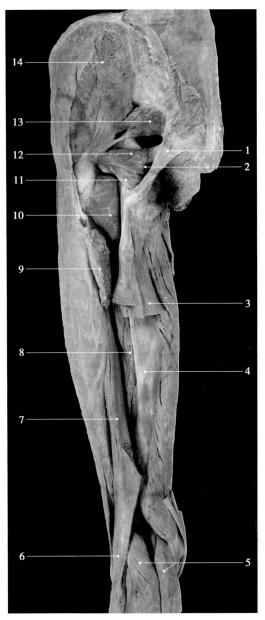

▲ 图 468 股部肌（后面观 2）
Muscles of thigh.Posterior view（2）

1. 骶结节韧带 sacrotuberous lig.
2. 闭孔内肌 obturator internus
3. 半腱肌 semitendinosus
4. 半膜肌 semimembranosus
5. 腓肠肌 gastrocnemius
6. 股二头肌腱 tendon of biceps femoris
7. 股二头肌短头 short head of biceps femoris
8. 大收肌 adductor magnus
9. 臀大肌 gluteus maximus
10. 股方肌 quadratus femoris
11. 下孖肌 gemellus inferior
12. 上孖肌 gemellus superior
13. 梨状肌 piriformis
14. 臀中肌 luteus medius

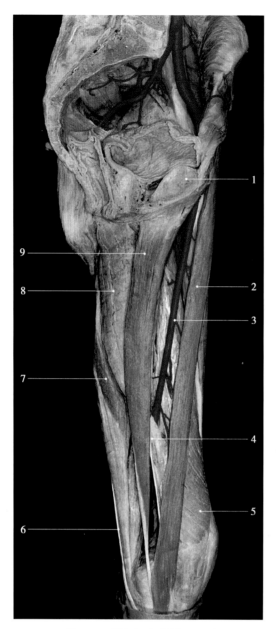

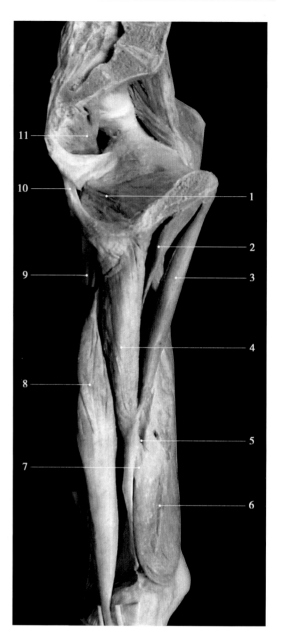

▲ 图 469　股部肌（内侧面观 1）
Muscles of thigh.Medial view（1）

1. 耻骨联合 pubic symphysis
2. 缝匠肌 sartorius
3. 股动脉 femoral a.
4. 收肌腱板 vastoadductor aponeurotic plate
5. 股内侧肌 vastus medialis
6. 半腱肌 semitendinosus
7. 半膜肌 semimembranosus
8. 大收肌 adductor magnus
9. 股薄肌 gracilis

▲ 图 470　股部肌（内侧面观 2）
Muscles of thigh.Medial veiw（2）

1. 闭孔内肌 obturator internus
2. 短收肌 adductor brevis
3. 长收肌 adductor longus
4. 大收肌 adductor magnus
5. 收肌管 adductor canal
6. 股内侧肌 vastus medialis
7. 收肌腱板 vastoadductor aponeurotic plate
8. 半膜肌 semimembranosus
9. 半腱肌 semitendinosus
10. 骶结节韧带 sacrotuberous lig.
11. 梨状肌 piriformis

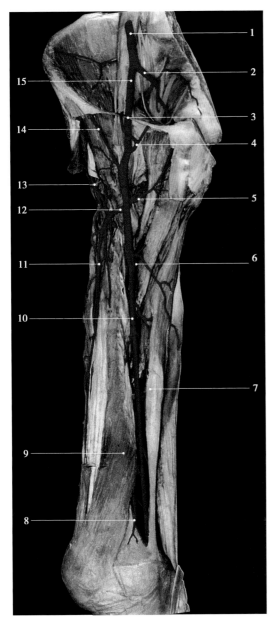

▲ 图 471 股前区的动脉
Arteries of anterior region of thigh

1. 髂总动脉 common iliac a.
2. 髂内动脉 internal iliac a.
3. 腹股沟韧带 inguinal lig.
4. 腹壁浅动脉 superficial epigastric a.
5. 旋股内侧动脉 medial femoral circumflex a.
6. 股深动脉 deep femoral a.
7. 大收肌 adductor magnus
8. 膝降动脉 descending genicular a.
9. 股内侧肌 vastus medialis
10. 股动脉 femoral a.
11. 旋股外侧动脉降支 descending branch of lateral femoral circumflex a.
12. 旋股外侧动脉 lateral femoral circumflex a.
13. 旋股外侧动脉升支 ascending branch of lateral femoral circumflex a.
14. 旋髂浅动脉 superficial iliac circumflex a.
15. 髂外动脉 external iliac a.

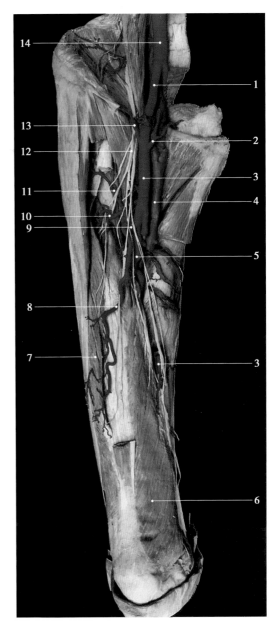

▲ 图 472 股前区的血管、神经
Blood vessels and nerves of anterior region of thigh

1. 髂外动脉 external iliac a.
2. 腹壁下动脉 inferior epigastric a.
3. 股动脉 femoral a.
4. 股静脉 femoral v.
5. 股深动脉 deep femoral a.
6. 股内侧肌 vastus medialis
7. 股外侧肌 vastus lateralis
8. 旋股外侧动脉降支 descending branch of lateral femoral circumflex a.
9. 旋股外侧动脉 lateral femoral circumflex a.
10. 旋股外侧动脉横支 transverse branch of lateral femoral circumflex a.
11. 旋股外侧动脉升支 ascending branch of lateral femoral circumflex a.
12. 股神经 femoral n.
13. 旋髂深动脉 deep iliac circumflex a.
14. 髂总动脉 common iliac a.

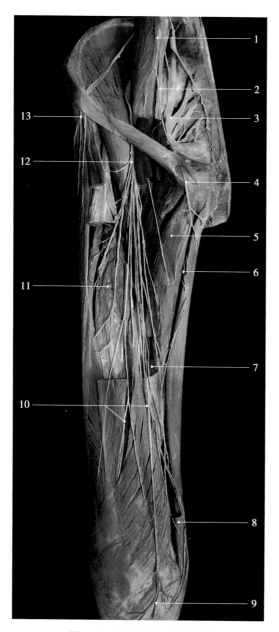

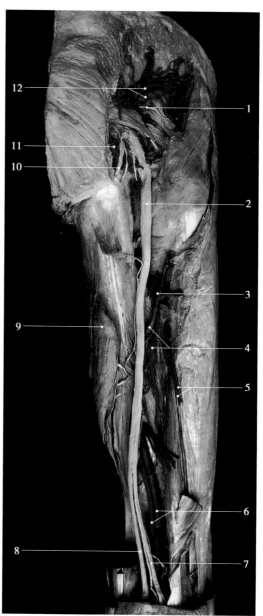

▲ 图 473　股部神经（前面观）
Nerves of thigh.Anterior view

1. 生殖股神经 genitofemoral n.
2. 股支 femoral branch
3. 骶丛 sacral plexus
4. 生殖支 genital branch
5. 长收肌 adductor longus
6. 闭孔神经皮支 cutaneous branch of obturator n.
7. 股动脉 femoral a.
8. 缝匠肌 sartorius
9. 髌下支 infrapatellar branch
10. 股神经前皮支 anterior cutaneous branches of femoral n.
11. 股中间肌 vastus intermedius
12. 股神经 femoral n.
13. 股外侧皮神经 lateral femoral cutaneous n.

▲ 图 474　臀部与股后区的血管、神经
Blood vessels and nerves of gluteal region and
posterior region of thigh

1. 臀上神经 superior gluteal n.
2. 坐骨神经 sciatic n.
3. 第 1 穿支动、静脉 the 1st perforating a. and v.
4. 第 1 穿支动、静脉降支 descending branch of the 1st
　perforating a.and v.
5. 第 2 穿支动、静脉 the 2nd perforating a. and v.
6. 腘动、静脉 popliteal a. and v.
7. 腓总神经 common peroneal n.
8. 胫神经 tibial n.
9. 大收肌 adductor magnus
10. 股后皮神经 posterior femoral cutaneous n.
11. 臀下动脉 inferior gluteal a.
12. 臀上动、静脉 superior gluteal a. and v.

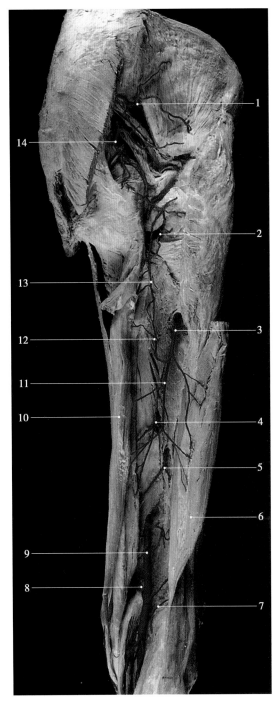

▲ 图 475　臀部与股后区的动脉
Arteries of gluteal region and posterior region of thigh

1. 臀上动脉 superior gluteal a.
2. 旋股内侧动脉 medial femoral circumflex a.
3. 第 1 穿动脉 the 1st perforating a.
4. 第 2 穿动脉 the 2nd perforating a.
5. 第 3 穿动脉 the 3rd perforating a.
6. 股二头肌 biceps femoris
7. 膝上外侧动脉 lateral superior genicular a.
8. 膝上内侧动脉 medial superior genicular a.
9. 腘动脉 popliteal a.
10. 半腱肌 semitendinosus
11. 第 1 穿动脉降支 descending branch of the 1st perforaing a.
12. 第 1 穿动脉升支 ascending bronch of the 1st perforating a.
13. 吻合支 anastomotic branch
14. 臀下动脉 inferior gluteal a.

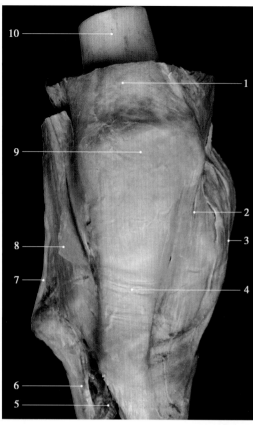

◀ 图 476　膝关节（前面观 1）
Knee joint.Anterior view（1）

1. 股四头肌腱 tendon of quadriceps femoris
2. 髌内侧支持带 medial patellar retinaculum
3. 胫侧副韧带 tibial collateral lig.
4. 髌韧带 patellar lig.
5. 骨间膜 interosseous membrane
6. 腓骨 fibula
7. 腓侧副韧带 fibular collateral lig.
8. 髌外侧支持带 lateral patellar retinaculum
9. 髌骨 patella
10. 股骨 femur

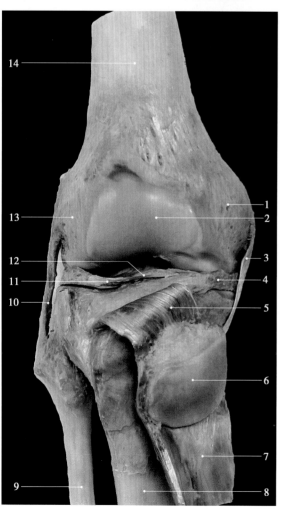

◀ 图 477　膝关节（前面观 2）
Knee joint.Anterior view（2）

1. 内上髁 medial epicondyle
2. 髌面 patellar surface
3. 胫侧副韧带 tibial collateral lig.
4. 内侧半月板 medial meniscus
5. 髌韧带 patellar lig.
6. 髌关节面 patellar articular surface
7. 股四头肌腱 tendon of quadriceps femoris
8. 胫骨 tibia
9. 腓骨 fibula
10. 腓侧副韧带 fibular collateral lig.
11. 外侧半月板 lateral meniscus
12. 膝横韧带 transverse ligament of knee
13. 外上髁 lateral epicondyle
14. 股骨 femur

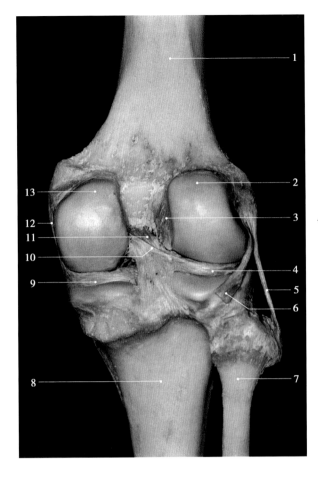

◀ 图 478 膝关节（后面观）
Knee joint.Posterior view

1. 股骨 femur
2. 股骨外侧髁 lateral condyle of femur
3. 前交叉韧带 anterior cruciate lig.
4. 外侧半月板 lateral meniscus
5. 腓侧副韧带 fibular collateral lig.
6. 腘肌腱 tendon of popliteus
7. 腓骨 fibula
8. 胫骨 tibia
9. 内侧半月板 medial meniscus
10. 板股后韧带 posterior meniscofemoral lig.
11. 后交叉韧带 posterior cruciate lig.
12. 胫侧副韧带 tibial collateral lig.
13. 股骨内侧髁 medial condyle of femur

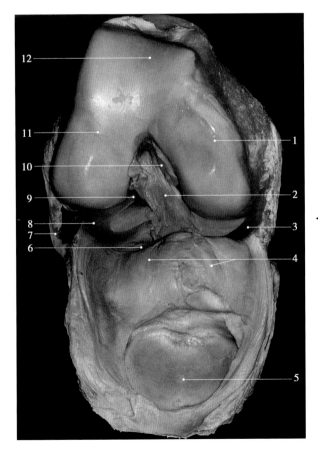

◀ 图 479 膝关节内景（前面敞开）
Interior view of knee joint.Open anteriorly

1. 股骨内侧髁 medial condyle of femur
2. 前交叉韧带 anterior cruciate lig.
3. 内侧半月板 medial meniscus
4. 翼状襞 alar folds
5. 髌关节面 patellar articular surface
6. 膝横韧带 transverse ligament of knee
7. 腓侧副韧带 fibular collateral lig.
8. 外侧半月板 lateral meniscus
9. 外侧半月板后角 posterior angle of lateral meniscus
10. 后交叉韧带 posterior cruciate lig.
11. 股骨外侧髁 lateral condyle of femur
12. 髌面 patellar surface

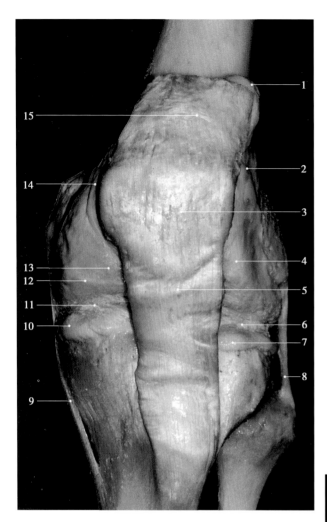

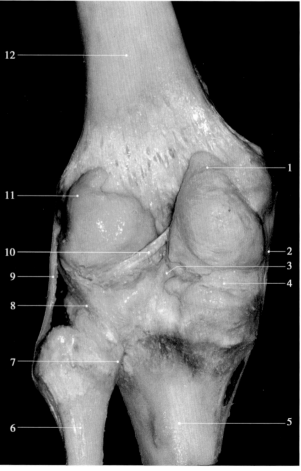

◀ 图 480 膝关节腔（前面观）
Cavity of knee joint.Anterior view

1. 髌上囊 suprapatellar bursa
2. 前上外侧隐窝 superolateral anterior recess
3. 髌骨 patella
4. 前下外侧隐窝 inferolateral anterior recess
5. 髌韧带 patellar lig.
6. 外侧半月板 lateral meniscus
7. 下部（外髁部）lower part（portion of lateral condyle）
8. 腓侧副韧带 fibular collateral lig.
9. 胫侧副韧带 tibial collateral lig.
10. 下部（内髁部）lower part（portion of medial condyle）
11. 内侧半月板 medial meniscus
12. 上部（内髁部）upper part（portion of medial condyle）
13. 前下内侧隐窝 inferomedial anterior recess
14. 前上内侧隐窝 superomedial anterior recess
15. 股四头肌腱 tendon of quadriceps femoris

图 481 膝关节腔（后面观）▶
Cavity of knee joint.Posterior view

1. 后上内侧隐窝 superomedial posterior recess
2. 胫侧副韧带 tibial collateral lig.
3. 后交叉韧带 posterior cruciate lig.
4. 内侧半月板 medial meniscus
5. 胫骨 tibia
6. 腓骨 fibula
7. 胫腓关节 tibiofibular joint
8. 腘肌腱 tendon of popliteus
9. 腓侧副韧带 fibular collateral lig.
10. 板股后韧带 posterior meniscofemoral lig.
11. 后上外侧隐窝 superolateral posterior recess
12. 股骨 femur

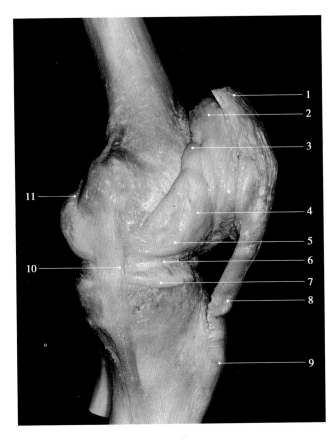

◀图 482　膝关节腔（内侧面观）
Cavity of knee joint.Medial view

1. 股四头肌腱 tendon of quadriceps femoris
2. 髌上囊 suprapatellar bursa
3. 前上内侧隐窝 superomedial anterior recess
4. 前下内侧隐窝 inferomedial anterior recess
5. 上部（内髁部）upper part（portion of medial condyle）
6. 内侧半月板 medial meniscus
7. 下部（内髁部）lower part（portion of medial condyle）
8. 髌韧带 patellar lig.
9. 胫骨粗隆 tibial tuberosity
10. 胫侧副韧带 tibial collateral lig.
11. 后上内侧隐窝 superomedial posterior recess

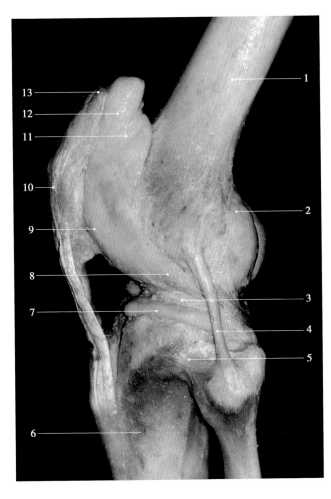

◀图 483　膝关节腔（外侧面观）
Cavity of knee joint.Lateral view

1. 股骨 femur
2. 后上外侧隐窝 superolateral posterior recess
3. 外侧半月板 lateral meniscus
4. 腓侧副韧带 fibular collateral lig.
5. 腓骨头前韧带 anterior ligament of fibular head
6. 胫骨 tibia
7. 下部（外髁部）lower part（portion of lateral condyle）
8. 上部（外髁部）upper part（portion of lateral condyle）
9. 前下外侧隐窝 inferolateral anterior recess
10. 髌骨 patella
11. 前上外侧隐窝 superolateral anterior recess
12. 髌上囊 suprapatellar bursa
13. 股四头肌腱 tendon of quadriceps femoris

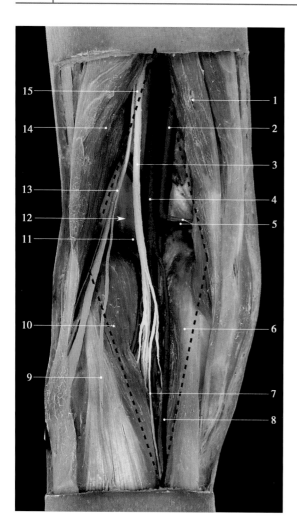

◀ 图 484　腘窝及其内容
Popliteal fossa and its contents

1. 半腱肌 semitendinosus
2. 腘动脉 popliteal a.
3. 胫神经 tibial n.
4. 腘静脉 popliteal v.
5. 膝上内侧动、静脉 medial superior genicular a.and v.
6. 腓肠肌内侧头 medial head of gastrocnemius
7. 腓肠内侧皮神经 medial sural cutaneous n.
8. 小隐静脉 small saphenous v.
9. 腓肠外侧皮神经 lateral sural cutaneous n.
10. 腓肠肌外侧头 lateral head of gastrocnemius
11. 膝上外侧动、静脉 lateral superior genicular a.and v.
12. 腘窝 popliteal fossa
13. 腓总神经 common peroneal n.
14. 股二头肌 biceps femoris
15. 坐骨神经 sciatic n.

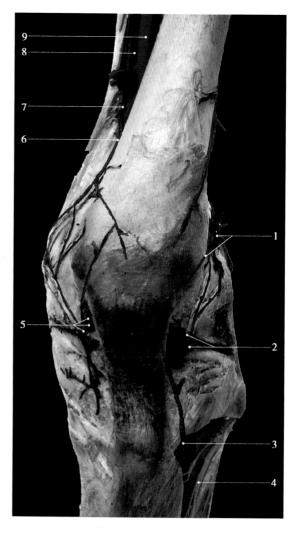

图 485　膝关节动脉网（前面观）▶
Arterial rete of knee joint.Anterior view

1. 膝上外侧动、静脉 lateral superior genicular a.and v.
2. 膝下外侧动、静脉 lateral inferior genicular a.and v.
3. 胫前返动脉 anterior tibial recurrent a.
4. 腓深神经 deep peroneal n.
5. 膝下内侧动、静脉 medial inferior genicular a.and v.
6. 膝降动脉 descending genicular a.
7. 膝降静脉 descending genicular v.
8. 股静脉 femoral v.
9. 股动脉 femoral a.

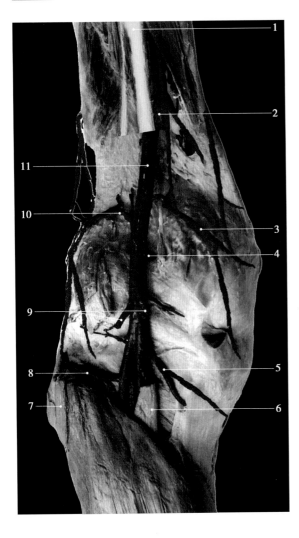

◀图 486　膝关节动脉网（后面观）
Arterial rete of knee joint.Posterior view

1. 坐骨神经 sciatic n.
2. 腘静脉 popliteal v.
3. 膝上内侧动脉 medial superior genicular a.
4. 膝中动脉 middle genicular a.
5. 膝下内侧动脉 medial inferior genicular a.
6. 胫神经 tibial n.
7. 腓总神经 common peroneal n.
8. 膝下外侧动脉 lateral inferior genicular a.
9. 腓肠动脉 sural a.
10. 膝上外侧动脉 lateral superior genicular a.
11. 腘动脉 popliteal a.

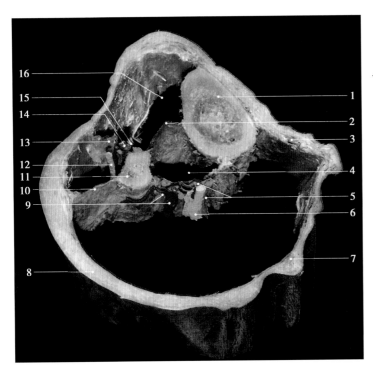

◀图 487　小腿的骨筋膜鞘
Osseofascial sheaths of leg

1. 胫骨 tibia
2. 骨间膜 interosseous membrane
3. 大隐静脉 great saphenous v.
4. 小腿后骨筋膜鞘 posterior osseofascial sheath of leg
5. 胫后动、静脉 posterior tibial a.and v.
6. 胫神经 tibial n.
7. 深筋膜 deep fascia
8. 浅筋膜 superficial fascia
9. 腓动、静脉 fibular a.and v.
10. 小腿后肌间隔 posterior intermuscular septum of leg
11. 腓骨 fibula
12. 腓浅神经 superficial peroneal n.
13. 小腿前肌间隔 anterior intermuscular septum of leg
14. 胫前动、静脉 anterior tibial a.and v.
15. 腓深神经 deep peroneal n.
16. 小腿前骨筋膜鞘 anterior osseofascial sheath of leg

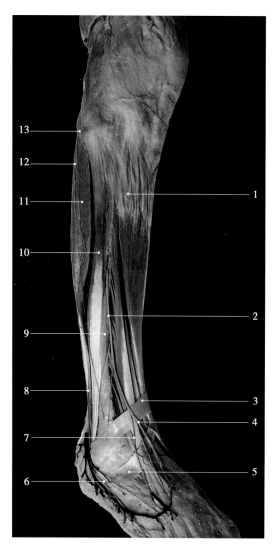

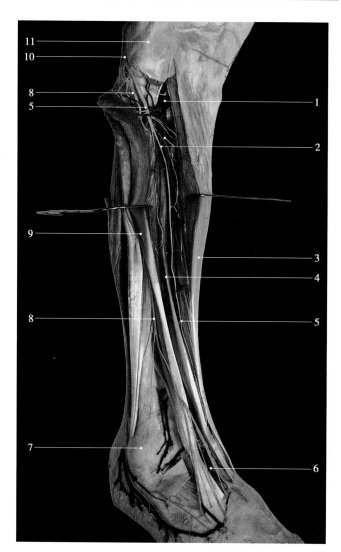

▲ 图 488　小腿的血管、神经（前外侧面 1 ）
Blood vessels and nerves of leg.Anterolateral view（1）

1. 胫骨前肌 tibialis anterior
2. 腓浅神经 superficial peroneal n.
3. 伸肌上支持带 superior extensor retinaculum
4. 足背内侧皮神经 medial dorsal cutaneous nerve of foot.
5. 伸肌下支持带 inferior extensor retinaculum
6. 足背外侧皮神经 lateral dorsal cutaneous nerve of foot
7. 足背中间皮神经 intermediate dorsal cutaneous nerve of foot.
8. 腓肠神经 sural n.
9. 腓骨短肌 peroneus brevis
10. 腓骨长肌 peroneus longus
11. 腓肠肌 gastrocnemius
12. 腓肠外侧皮神经 lateral sural cutaneous n.
13. 腓总神经 common peroneal n.

▲ 图 489　小腿的血管、神经（前外侧面 2 ）
Blood vessels and nerves of leg.Anterolateral view（2）

1. 胫前返动、静脉 anterior tibial recurrent a.and v.
2. 胫前动、静脉 anterior tibial a.and v.
3. 胫骨前肌 tibialis anterior
4. 蹋长伸肌 extensor hallucis longus
5. 腓深神经 deep peroneal n.
6. 足背动脉 dorsal artery of foot
7. 外踝 lateral malleolus
8. 腓浅神经 superficial peroneal n.
9. 趾长伸肌 extensor digitorum longus
10. 腓总神经 common peroneal n.
11. 腓骨头 fibular head

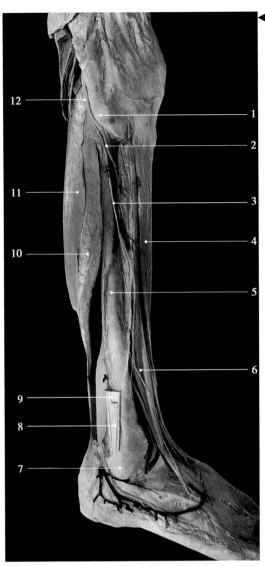

◀ 图 490　小腿的血管、神经（前外侧面 3）
Blood vessels and nerves of leg.Anterolateral view（3）

1. 腓骨头 fibular head
2. 腓深神经 deep peroneal n.
3. 腓浅神经 superficial peroneal n.
4. 胫骨前肌 tibialis anterior
5. 腓骨 fibula
6. 趾长伸肌 extensor digitorum longus
7. 外踝 lateral malleolus
8. 腓骨长肌腱 tendon of peroneus longus
9. 腓骨短肌腱 tendon of peroneus brevis
10. 比目鱼肌 soleus
11. 腓肠肌 gastrocnemius
12. 腓总神经 common peroneal n.

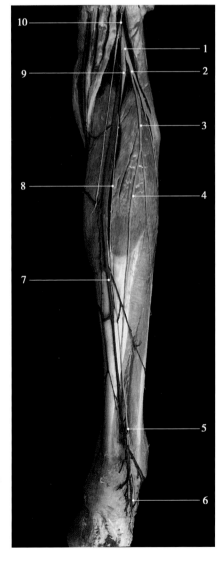

图 491　小腿的血管、神经（后面观 1）▶
Blood vessels and nerves of leg.Posterior view（1）

1. 坐骨神经 sciatic n.
2. 腓总神经 common peroneal n.
3. 腓肠外侧皮神经 lateral sural cutaneous n.
4. 腓神经交通支 communicating branch of peroneal n.
5. 腓肠神经 sural n.
6. 足背外侧皮神经 lateral dorsal cutaneous nerve of foot
7. 小隐静脉 small saphenous v.
8. 腓肠内侧皮神经 medial sural cutaneous n.
9. 胫神经 tibial n.
10. 股后皮神经 posterior femoral cutaneous n.

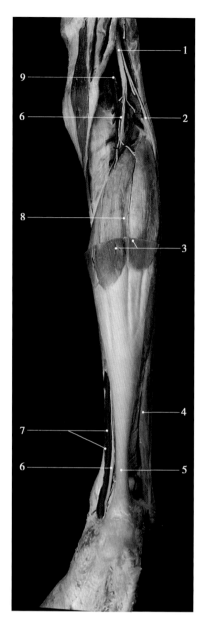

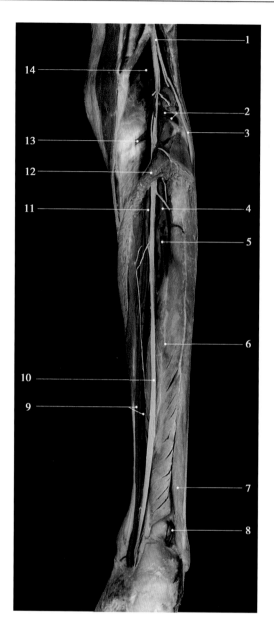

▲ 图 492　小腿的血管、神经（后面观 2 ）
Blood vessels and nerves of leg.Posterior
view（2）

1. 坐骨神经 sciatic n.
2. 腓总神经 common peroneal n.
3. 腓肠肌 gastrocnemius
4. 腓骨短肌 peroneus brevis
5. 跟腱 tendo calcaneus
6. 胫神经 tibial n.
7. 胫后动、静脉 posterior tibial a.and v.
8. 比目鱼肌 soleus
9. 腘静脉 popliteal v.

▲ 图 493　小腿的血管、神经（后面观 3 ）
Blood vessels and nerves of leg.Posterior
view（3）

1. 坐骨神经 sciatic n.
2. 膝下外侧动、静脉 lateral inferior genicular a.and v.
3. 腓总神经 common peroneal n.
4. 腓静脉 fibular v.
5. 腓动脉 fibular a.
6. 踇长屈肌 flexor hallucis longus
7. 腓骨短肌 peroneus brevis
8. 穿支 perforating branch
9. 胫后动、静脉 posterior tibial a.and v.
10. 胫神经 tibial n.
11. 胫后静脉 posterior tibial v.
12. 比目鱼肌腱弓 tendinous arch of soleus
13. 膝下内侧动、静脉 medial inferior genicular a.and v.
14. 腘静脉 popliteal v.

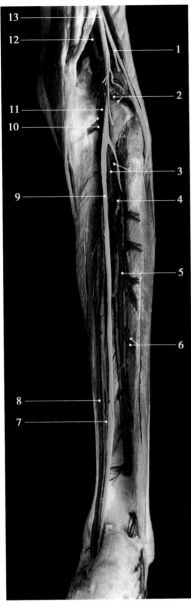

▲ 图 494　小腿的血管、神经（后面观 4）
Blood vessels and nerves of leg.Posterior view（4）

1. 腓总神经 common peroneal n.
2. 膝下外侧动、静脉 lateral inferior genicular a.and v.
3. 胫前动、静脉 anterior tibial a.and v.
4. 腓静脉 fibular v.
5. 腓动脉 fibular a.
6. 弓形动、静脉 arcuate a.and v.
7. 胫后静脉 posterior tibial v.
8. 胫后动脉 posterior tibial a.
9. 胫神经 tibial n.
10. 膝下内侧动、静脉 medial inferior genicular a.and v.
11. 腘动脉 popliteal a.
12. 腘静脉 popliteal v.
13. 坐骨神经 sciatic n.

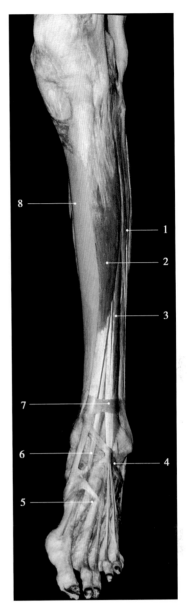

▲ 图 495　小腿肌（前面观）
Muscles of leg.Anterior view

1. 腓骨长肌 peroneus longus
2. 胫骨前肌 tibialis anterior
3. 趾长伸肌 extensor digitorum longus
4. 伸肌下支持带 inferior extensor retinaculum
5. 踇短伸肌腱 tendon of extensor hallucis brevis
6. 踇长伸肌腱 tendon of extensor hallucis longus
7. 伸肌上支持带 superior extensor retinaculum
8. 胫骨 tibia

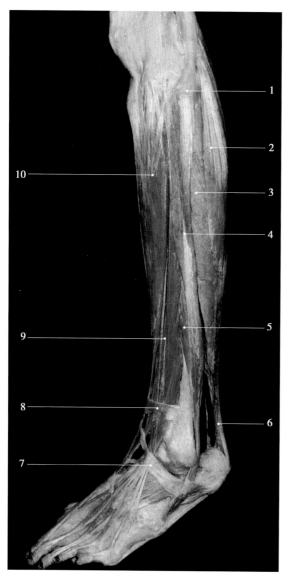

▲ 图 496　小腿肌（外侧面观）
Muscles of leg.Lateral view

1. 腓骨头 fibular head
2. 腓肠肌外侧头 lateral head of gastrocnemius
3. 比目鱼肌 soleus
4. 腓骨长肌 peroneus longus
5. 腓骨短肌 peroneus brevis
6. 跟腱 tendo calcaneus
7. 伸肌下支持带 inferior extensor retinaculum
8. 伸肌上支持带 superior extensor retinaculum
9. 趾长伸肌 extensor digitorum longus
10. 胫骨前肌 tibialis anterior

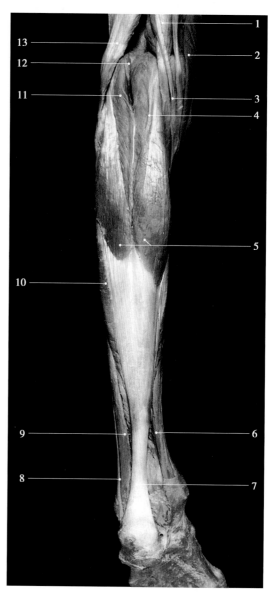

▲ 图 497　小腿肌（后面观 1）
Muscles of leg.Posterior view（1）

1. 半膜肌 semimembranosus
2. 缝匠肌 sartorius
3. 半腱肌腱 tendon of semitendinosus
4. 腓肠肌内侧头 medial head of gastrocnemius
5. 腓肠肌 gastrocnemius
6. 趾长屈肌 flexor digitorum longus
7. 跟腱 tendo calcaneus
8. 腓骨长肌腱 tendon of peroneus longus
9. 腓骨短肌 peroneus brevis
10. 比目鱼肌 soleus
11. 腓肠肌外侧头 lateral head of gastrocnemius
12. 跖肌 plantaris
13. 股二头肌 biceps femoris

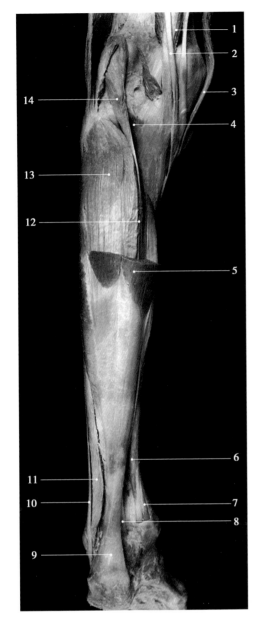

▲ 图 498　小腿肌（后面观 2）
Muscles of leg.Posterior view（2）

1. 半膜肌 semimembranosus
2. 半腱肌 semitendinosus
3. 缝匠肌 sartorius
4. 腘肌 popliteus
5. 腓肠肌 gastrocnemius
6. 趾长屈肌 flexor digitorum longus
7. 胫骨后肌腱 tendon of tibialis posterior
8. 蹞长屈肌腱 tendon of flexor hallucis longus
9. 跟腱 tendo calcaneus
10. 腓骨长肌腱 tendon of peroneus longus
11. 腓骨短肌 peroneus brevis
12. 跖肌腱 tendon of plantaris
13. 比目鱼肌 soleus
14. 跖肌 plantaris

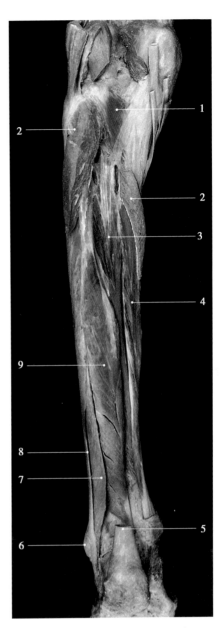

▲ 图 499　小腿肌（后面观 3）
Muscles of leg.Posterior view（3）

1. 腘肌 popliteus
2. 比目鱼肌 soleus
3. 胫骨后肌 tibialis posterior
4. 趾长屈肌 flexor digitorum longus
5. 跟腱 tendo calcaneus
6. 外踝 lateral malleolus
7. 腓骨短肌 peroneus brevis
8. 腓骨长肌腱 tendon of peroneus longus
9. 蹞长屈肌 flexor hallucis longus

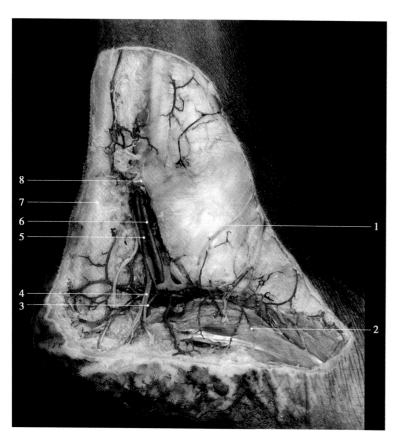

◀ 图 500　内踝区的血管、神经
Blood vessels and nerves of medial
malleolar region

1. 内踝 medial malleolus
2. 姆展肌 abductor hallucis
3. 跟支 calcanean branches
4. 跟内侧支 medial calcanean branches
5. 胫后静脉 posterior tibial v.
6. 胫后动脉 posterior tibial a.
7. 跟腱 tendo calcaneus
8. 屈肌支持带 flexor retinaculum

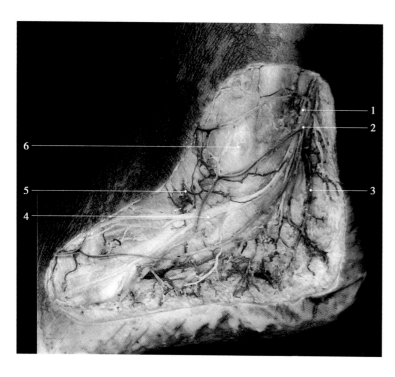

◀ 图 501　外踝区的血管、神经
Blood vessels and nerves of lateral
malleolar region

1. 腓肠神经 sural n.
2. 小隐静脉 small saphenous v.
3. 跟外侧支 lateral calcaneal branch
4. 足背外侧皮神经 lateral dorsal cutaneous nerve of foot
5. 跗外侧动脉 lateral tarsal a.
6. 外踝 lateral malleolus

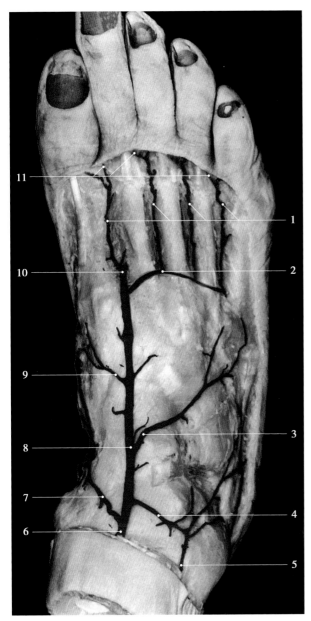

▲ 图 502 足背的动脉
Arteries of dorsum of foot

1. 跖背动脉 dorsal metatarsal a.
2. 弓状动脉 arcuate a.
3. 跗外侧动脉 lateral tarsal a.
4. 外踝前动脉 lateral anterior malleolar a.
5. 腓动脉穿支 perforating branch of peroneal a.
6. 胫前动脉 anterior tibial a.
7. 内踝前动脉 medial anterior malleolar a.
8. 足背动脉 dorsal artery of foot
9. 跗内侧动脉 medial tarsal a.
10. 足底深支 deep plantar branch
11. 趾背动脉 dorsal digital a.

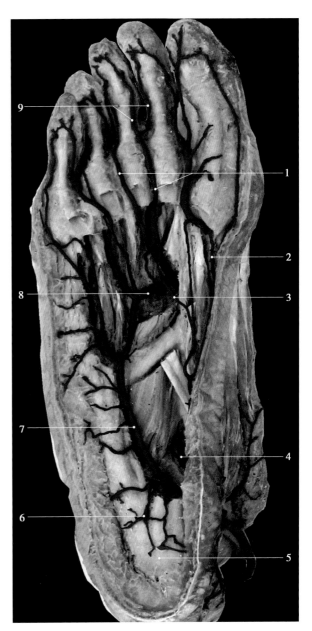

▲ 图 503 足底的动脉
Plantar arteries

1. 趾足底总动脉 common plantar digital a.
2. 足底内侧动脉浅支 superficial branch of medial plantar a.
3. 足底内侧动脉深支 deep branch of medial plantar a.
4. 足底内侧动脉 medial plantar a.
5. 跟骨 calcaneus
6. 跟网 calcaneal rete
7. 足底外侧动脉 lateral plantar a.
8. 足底深弓 deep plantar arch
9. 趾足底固有动脉 proper plantar digital a.

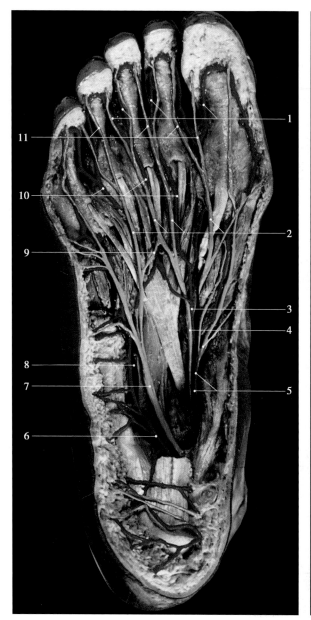

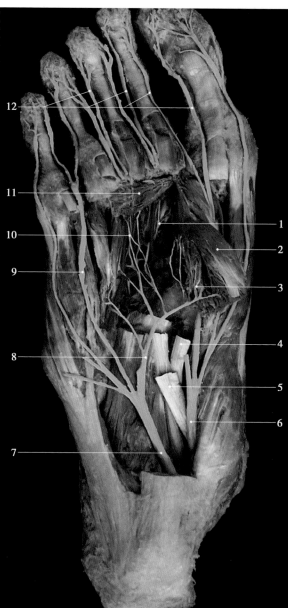

▲ 图 504　足底的血管、神经（1）
Plantar blood vessels and nerves（1）

1. 趾足底固有动脉 proper plantar digital a.
2. 趾足底总神经 common plantar digital n.
3. 足底内侧动脉 medial plantar a.
4. 足底内侧神经 medial plantar n.
5. 足底内侧动、静脉 medial plantar a .and v.
6. 足底外侧动脉 lateral plantar a.
7. 足底外侧神经 lateral plantar n.
8. 足底外侧静脉 lateral plantar v.
9. 交通支 communicating branch
10. 趾足底总动脉 common plantar digital a.
11. 趾足底固有神经 proper plantar digital n.

▲ 图 505　足底的血管、神经（2）
Plantar blood vessels and nerves（2）

1. 骨间肌神经 nerve of interossei
2. 踇收肌斜头 oblique head of adductor hallucis
3. 踇收肌斜头神经 nerve of oblique head of adductor hallucis
4. 踇长屈肌腱 tendon of flexor hallucis longus
5. 趾长屈肌腱 tendon of flexor digitorum longus
6. 足底内侧神经 medial plantar n.
7. 足底外侧神经 lateral plantar n.
8. 足底外侧神经深支 deep branch of lateral plantar n.
9. 趾足底总神经 common plantar digital n.
10. 踇收肌横头神经 nerve of transverse head of adductor hallucis
11. 踇收肌横头 transverse head of adductor hallucis
12. 趾足底固有神经 proper plantar digital n.`

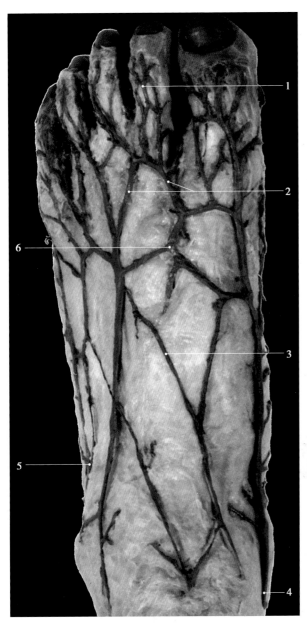

▲ 图 506 足背静脉
Veins of dorsum of foot

1. 趾背静脉 dorsal digital v.
2. 跖背静脉 dorsal metatarsal v.
3. 足背静脉网 dorsal venous rete of foot
4. 大隐静脉 great saphenous v.
5. 小隐静脉 small saphenous v.
6. 足背静脉弓 dorsal venous arch of foot

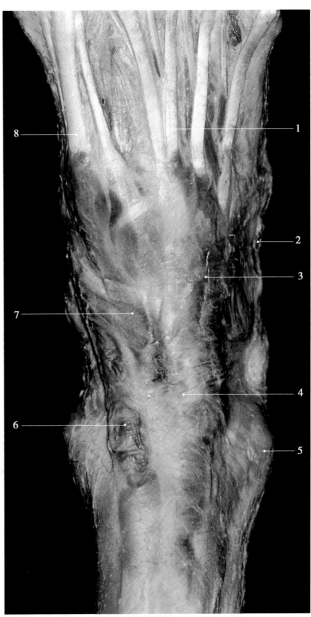

▲ 图 507 下肢肌支持带及腱鞘（前面观）
Retinaculum and tendinous sheaths of muscles of lower limb.Anterior view

1. 趾长伸肌腱 tendon of extensor digitorum longus
2. 腓骨短肌腱鞘 tendinous sheath of peroneus brevis
3. 趾长伸肌腱鞘 tendinous sheath of extensor digitorum longus
4. 伸肌支持带 extensor retinaculum
5. 外踝 lateral malleolus
6. 胫骨前肌腱鞘 tendinous sheath of tibialis anterior
7. 拇长伸肌腱鞘 tendinous sheath of extensor hallucis longus
8. 拇长伸肌腱 tendon of extensor hallucis longus

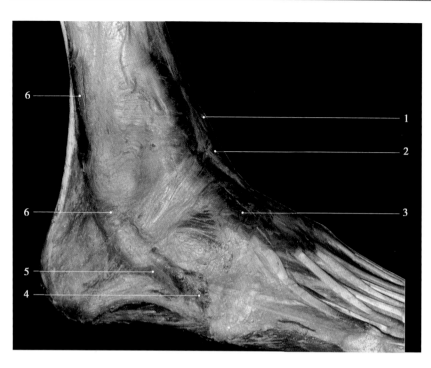

◀图 508　下肢肌支持带及腱鞘（外侧面观）
Retinaculum and tendinous sheaths of muscles of lower limb. Lateral view

1. 胫骨前肌腱鞘 tendinous sheath of tibialis anterior
2. 踇长伸肌腱鞘 tendinous sheath of extensor hallucis longus
3. 趾长伸肌腱鞘 tendinous sheath of extensor digitorum longus
4. 腓骨短肌腱鞘 tendinous sheath of peroneus brevis
5. 腓骨长肌腱鞘 tendinous sheath of peroneus longus
6. 腓骨肌总腱鞘 common sheath of peronei

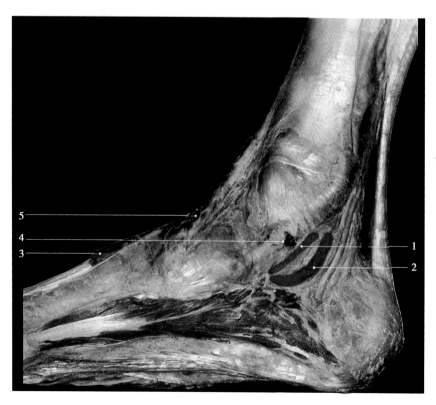

◀图 509　下肢肌支持带及腱鞘（内侧面观）
Retinaculum and tendinous sheaths of muscles of lower limb. Medial view

1. 趾长屈肌腱鞘 tendinous sheath of flexor digitorum longus
2. 踇长屈肌腱鞘 tendinous sheath of flexor hallucis longus
3. 踇长伸肌腱鞘 tendinous sheath of extensor hallucis longus
4. 胫骨后肌腱鞘 tendinous sheath of tibialis posterior
5. 胫骨前肌腱鞘 tendinous sheath of tibialis anterior

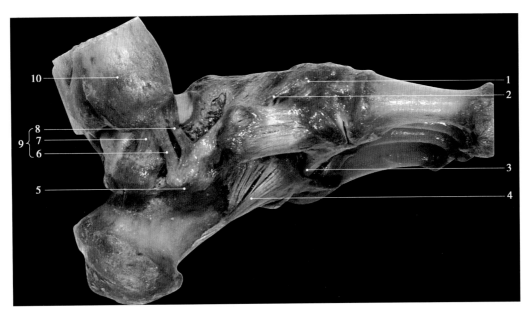

▲ 图 510 足的关节和韧带（内侧面观）
Joints and ligaments of foot.Medial view

1. 楔骨 cuneifor bone
2. 楔舟背侧韧带 dorsal cuboideonavicular lig.
3. 腓骨长肌腱 tendon of peroneus longus
4. 足底长韧带 long plantar lig.
5. 载距突 sustentaculum tali
6. 胫跟部 tibiocalcaneal part
7. 胫距后部 posterior tibiotalar part
8. 胫舟部 tibionavicular part
9. 内侧韧带 medial lig.
10. 胫骨 tabia

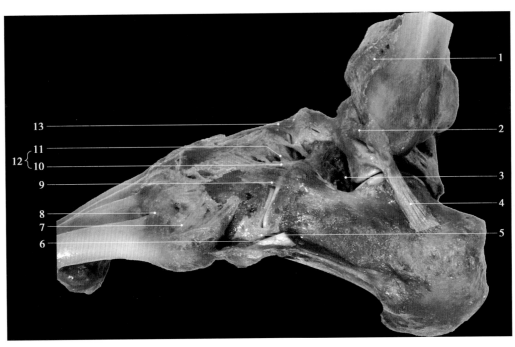

▲ 图 511 足的关节和韧带（外侧面观）
Joints and ligaments of foot.Lateral view

1. 胫腓前韧带 anterior tibiofibular lig.
2. 距腓前韧带 anterior talofibular lig.
3. 距跟骨间韧带 interosseous talocalcaneal lig.
4. 跟腓韧带 calcaneofibular lig.
5. 跟骰足底韧带 plantar calcaneocuboid lig.
6. 腓骨长肌腱 tendon of peroneus longus
7. 跗跖背侧韧带 dorsal tarsometatarsal lig.
8. 跖骨背侧韧带 dorsal metatarsal lig.
9. 跟骰背侧韧带 dorsal calcaneocuboid lig.
10. 跟骰韧带 calcaneocuboid lig.
11. 跟舟韧带 calcaneonavicular lig.
12. 分歧韧带 bifurcate lig.
13. 距舟背侧韧带 dorsal talonavicular lig.

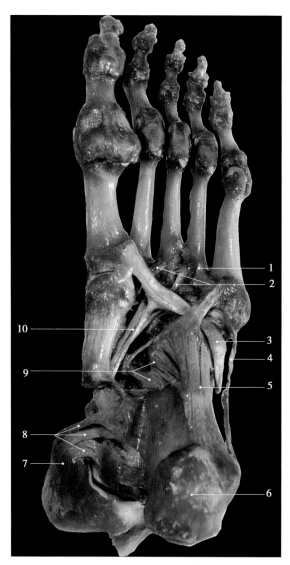

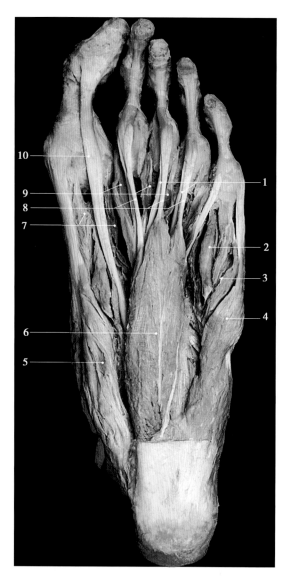

▲ 图 512　足的关节和韧带（足底面观）
Joints and ligaments of foot.Plantar view

1. 跖骨足底韧带 plantar metatarsal lig.
2. 跗跖足底韧带 plantar tarsometatarsal lig.
3. 腓骨长肌腱 tendon of peroneus longus
4. 腓骨短肌腱 tendon of peroneus brevis
5. 足底长韧带 long plantar lig.
6. 跟骨结节 calcaneal tuberosity
7. 内踝 medial malleolus
8. 内侧韧带 medial lig.
9. 跟舟足底韧带 plantar calcaneonavicular lig.
10. 胫骨后肌腱 tendon of tibialis posterior

▲ 图 513　足底肌（1）
Plantar muscles（1）

1. 趾长屈肌腱 tendon of flexor digitorum longus
2. 骨间足底肌 plantar interossei
3. 小趾短屈肌 flexor digiti minimi brevis
4. 小趾展肌 abductor digiti minimi
5. 踇展肌 abductor hallucis
6. 趾短屈肌 flexor digiti brevis
7. 踇短屈肌 flexor hallucis brevis
8. 趾短屈肌腱 tendon of flexor digiti brevis
9. 蚓状肌 lumbricales
10. 踇长屈肌腱 tendon of flexor hallucis longus

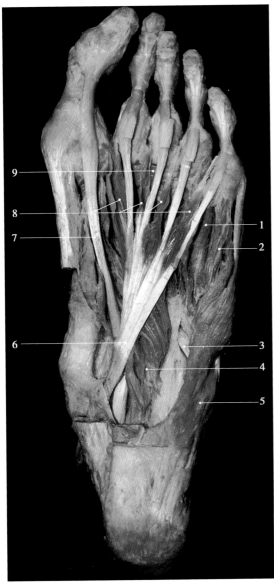

▲ 图 514 足底肌（2）
Plantar muscles（2）

1. 骨间足底肌 plantar interossei
2. 小趾短屈肌 flexor digiti minimi brevis
3. 腓骨长肌腱 tendon of peroneus longus
4. 足底方肌 quadratus plantae
5. 小趾展肌 abductor digiti minimi
6. 趾长屈肌腱 tendon of flexor digitorum longus
7. 蹈长屈肌腱 tendon of flexor hallucis longus
8. 蚓状肌 lumbricales
9. 蹈收肌横头 transversehead of adductor hallucis

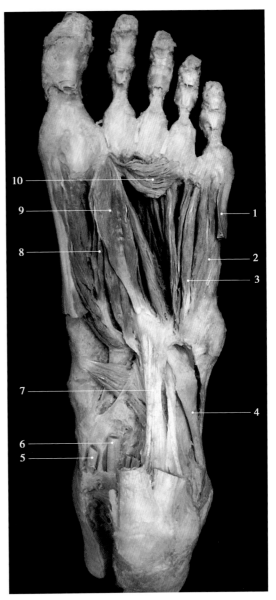

▲ 图 515 足底肌（3）
Plantar muscles（3）

1. 小趾展肌 abductor digiti minimi
2. 小趾短屈肌 flexor digiti minimi brevis
3. 骨间足底肌 plantar interossei
4. 腓骨长肌腱 tendon of peroneus longus
5. 趾长屈肌腱 tendon of flexor digitorum longus
6. 蹈长屈肌腱 tendon of flexor hallucis longus
7. 足底长韧带 long plantar lig.
8. 蹈短屈肌 flexor hallucis brevis
9. 蹈收肌斜头 oblique head of adductor hallucis
10. 蹈收肌横头 transverse head of adductor hallucis

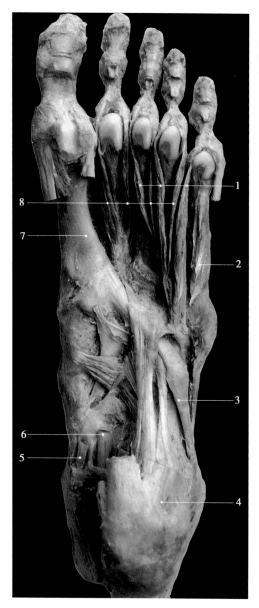

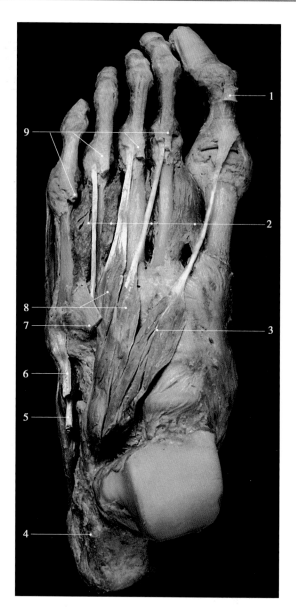

▲ 图 516　足底肌（4）
Plantar muscles（4）

1. 骨间足底肌 plantar interossei
2. 小趾短屈肌 flexor digiti minimi brevis
3. 腓骨长肌腱 tendon of peroneus longus
4. 跟骨 calcaneus
5. 趾长屈肌腱 tendon of flexor digitorum longus
6. 姆长屈肌腱 tendon of flexor hallucis longus
7. 第 1 跖骨 the 1st metatarsal bone
8. 骨间背侧肌 dorsal interossei

▲ 图 517　足背肌
Muscles of dorsum of foot

1. 姆长伸肌腱 tendon of extensor hallucis longus
2. 骨间背侧肌 dorsal interossei
3. 姆短伸肌 extensor hallucis brevis
4. 跟骨 calcaneus
5. 腓骨长肌腱 tendon of peroneus longus
6. 腓骨短肌腱 tendon of peroneus brevis
7. 第 3 腓骨肌腱 tendon of peroneus tertius
8. 趾短伸肌 extensor digitorum brevis
9. 趾长伸肌腱 tendon of extensor digitorum longus

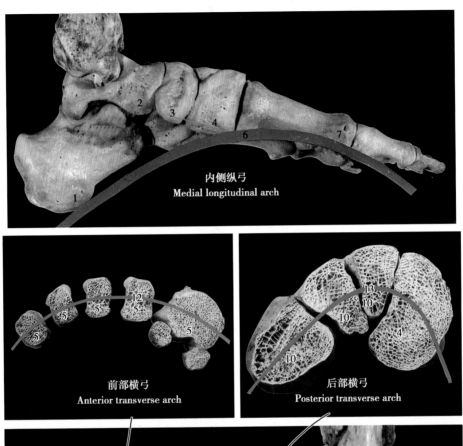

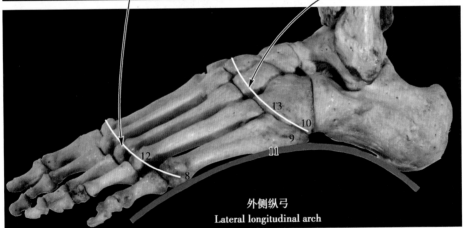

▲ 图 518　足弓 Arch of foot

1. 跟骨 calcaneus
2. 距骨 talus
3. 足舟骨 navicular bone
4. 骰骨 cuboid bone
5. 跖骨 metatarsal bone
6. 内侧纵弓 medial longitudinal arth of foot
7. 第 1 跖骨头 the 1st head of metatarsal bone

8. 第 5 跖骨头 the 5th metatarsal bone
9. 第 5 跖骨底 the 5th base of metatarsal bone
10. 楔骨 cuneiform bone
11. 外侧纵弓 lateral longitudinal arch of foot
12. 前部横弓 anterior transverse arch of foot
13. 后部横弓 posterior transverse arch of foot